Confocal Microscopy

Editors

JANE M. GRANT-KELS
GIOVANNI PELLACANI
CATERINA LONGO

DERMATOLOGIC CLINICS

www.derm.theclinics.com

Consulting Editor
BRUCE H. THIERS

October 2016 • Volume 34 • Number 4

ELSEVIER

1600 John F. Kennedy Boulevard • Suite 1800 • Philadelphia, Pennsylvania, 19103-2899

http://www.theclinics.com

DERMATOLOGIC CLINICS Volume 34, Number 4
October 2016 ISSN 0733-8635, ISBN-13: 978-0-323-46308-9

Editor: Jessica McCool
Developmental Editor: Alison Swety

Dermatologic Clinics (ISSN 0733-8635) is published quarterly by Elsevier Inc., 360 Park Avenue South, New York, NY 10010-1710. Months of publication are January, April, July, and October. Business and editorial offices: 1600 John F. Kennedy Blvd., Suite 1800, Philadelphia, PA 19103-2899. Customer service office: 11830 Westline Drive, St. Louis, MO 63146. Periodicals postage paid at New York, NY, and additional mailing offices. Subscription prices are USD 370.00 per year for US individuals, USD 618.00 per year for US institutions, USD 425.00 per year for Canadian individuals, USD 754.00 per year for Canadian institutions, USD 495.00 per year for international individuals, USD 754.00 per year for international institutions, USD 100.00 per year for US students/residents, and USD 240.00 per year for Canadian and international students/residents. International air speed delivery is included in all *Clinics* subscription prices. All prices are subject to change without notice. **POSTMASTER:** Send address changes to *Dermatologic Clinics*, Elsevier Health Sciences Division, Subscription Customer Service, 3251 Riverport Lane, Maryland Heights, MO 63043. **Customer Service: 1-800-654-2452 (U.S. and Canada); 314-447-8871 (outside U.S. and Canada). Fax: 314-447-8029. E-mail: journalscustomerservice-usa@elsevier.com (for print support); journalsonlinesupport-usa@elsevier.com (for online support).**

Reprints. For copies of 100 or more, of articles in this publication, please contact the Commercial Reprints Department, Elsevier Inc., 360 Park Avenue South, New York, New York 10010-1710. Tel.: 212-633-3874; Fax: 212-633-3820; Email: reprints@elsevier.com.

The *Dermatologic Clinics* is covered in *MEDLINE/PubMed (Index Medicus)*, *Current Contents/Clinical Medicine*, *Excerpta Medica*, *Chemical Abstracts*, and *ISI/BIOMED*.

Contributors

CONSULTING EDITOR

BRUCE H. THIERS, MD
Professor and Chairman, Department of
Dermatology and Dermatologic Surgery,
Medical University of South Carolina,
Charleston, South Carolina

EDITORS

JANE M. GRANT-KELS, MD
Professor of Dermatology, Pathology, and
Pediatrics; Director of the Cutaneous Oncology
Center and Melanoma Program; Vice Chair,
Department of Dermatology, University of
Connecticut Health Center, Farmington,
Connecticut

GIOVANNI PELLACANI, MD
Professor of Dermatology, Dermatology Unit,
Dean of the Faculty of Medicine and Surgery,
Chairman, Department of Dermatology,
University of Modena and Reggio Emilia,
Modena, Italy

CATERINA LONGO, MD, PhD
Skin Cancer Unit, Professor of Dermatology,
Arcispedale Santa Maria Nuova-Istituto di
Ricovero e Cura a Carattere Scientifico, Reggio
Emilia, Italy

AUTHORS

MARINA AGOZZINO, MD
Clinical Dermatology Department, San
Gallicano Dermatological Institute, Rome, Italy

MARCO ARDIGO, MD, PhD
Clinical Dermatology Department, San
Gallicano Dermatological Institute,
Rome, Italy

**JULIANA ARÊAS DE SOUZA LIMA
BELTRAME FERREIRA, MD**
Cutaneous Oncology Department, AC
Camargo Cancer Center, Sao Paulo, Brazil

ALICIA BARREIRO CAPURRO, MD
Melanoma Unit, Department of Dermatology,
Hospital Clínic de Barcelona, IDIBAPS,
Barcelona University; Centre of Biomedical
Research on Rare Diseases (CIBERER), ISCIII,
Barcelona, Spain

ANTONI BENNASSAR, MD
Melanoma Unit, Dermatology Department,
Hospital Clìnic of Barcelona, Institut
d'Investigacions Biomediques August Pi I
Sunyer, Barcelona, Spain

FRÉDÉRIC CAMBAZARD, PhD
Professor, Head of the Department,
Dermatology Department, University
Hospital of Saint-Etienne, Saint-Etienne,
France

CRISTINA CARRERA ALVÁREZ, MD, PhD
Melanoma Unit, Department of Dermatology,
Hospital Clínic de Barcelona, IDIBAPS,
Barcelona University; Centre of Biomedical
Research on Rare Diseases (CIBERER), ISCIII,
Barcelona, Spain

ELISA CINOTTI, MD, PhD
Senior Staff Specialists; Dermatology
Department, University Hospital of
Saint-Etienne, Saint-Etienne, France

RAQUEL DE PAULA RAMOS CASTRO, MD
Cutaneous Oncology Department, AC
Camargo Cancer Center, Sao Paulo,
Brazil

CHIARA FRANCESCHINI, MD
Department of Dermatology, University of
Rome Tor Vergata, Rome, Italy

MELISSA GILL, MD
SkinMedical Research and Diagnostics, PLLC,
Dobbs Ferry, New York

DAVID R. GOLDMANN, MD
Department of Medicine, Perelman School of
Medicine, University of Pennsylvania,
Philadelphia, Pennsylvania

SALVADOR GONZÁLEZ, MD, PhD
Professor, Medicine and Medical Specialities
Department, Medicine and Health Sciences
Faculty, Alcalá University, Madrid, Spain;
Consultant, Dermatology Service, Memorial
Sloan-Kettering Cancer Center, New York,
New York

JANE M. GRANT-KELS, MD
Professor of Dermatology, Pathology, and
Pediatrics; Director of the Cutaneous Oncology
Center and Melanoma Program; Vice Chair,
Department of Dermatology, University of
Connecticut Health Center, Farmington,
Connecticut

PASCALE GUITERA, MD, PhD, FACD
Associate Professor, Dermatology, Sydney
Melanoma Diagnostic Centre (SMDC), Royal
Prince Alfred Hospital, Melanoma Institute
Australia, Central Clinical School, Sydney
University, Camperdown, New South Wales,
Australia

RAPHAELA KÄSTLE
Department of Dermatology and Allergology,
General Hospital Augsburg, Augsburg,
Germany

BRUNO LABEILLE, MD
Senior Staff Specialists; Dermatology
Department, University Hospital of
Saint-Etienne, Saint-Etienne, France

FRANCESCO LACARRUBBA, MD, PhD
Dermatology Clinic, University of Catania,
Catania, Italy

CATERINA LONGO, MD, PhD
Skin Cancer Unit, Professor of Dermatology,
Arcispedale Santa Maria Nuova-Istituto di
Ricovero e Cura a Carattere Scientifico, Reggio
Emilia, Italy

JOANNA ŁUDZIK, MD
Department of Bioinformatics and
Telemedicine, Jagiellonian University Medical
College, Krakow, Poland

JOSEP MALVEHY GUILERA, MD, PhD
Melanoma Unit, Department of Dermatology,
Hospital Clínic de Barcelona, IDIBAPS,
Barcelona University; Centre of Biomedical
Research on Rare Diseases (CIBERER), ISCIII,
Barcelona, Spain

ASHFAQ A. MARGHOOB, MD
Dermatology Service, Department of Medicine,
Memorial Sloan Kettering Cancer Center,
Hauppauge, New York

**TATIANA CRISTINA MORAES PINTO
BLUMETTI, MD**
Cutaneous Oncology Department, AC
Camargo Cancer Center, Sao Paulo,
Brazil

KISHWER NEHAL, MD
Dermatology Service, Memorial Sloan
Kettering Cancer Center, New York,
New York

MARGARET OLIVIERO, FNP-C
Department of Dermatology, University of
Miami School of Medicine, Miami, Florida

GIOVANNI PELLACANI, MD
Professor of Dermatology, Dermatology Unit,
Dean of the Faculty of Medicine and Surgery,
Chairman, Department of Dermatology,
University of Modena and Reggio Emilia,
Modena, Italy

JEAN-LUC PERROT, MD
Senior Staff Specialists; Dermatology
Department, University Hospital of
Saint-Etienne, Saint-Etienne, France

SYRIL KEENA T. QUE, MD
Department of Dermatology, University of Connecticut Health Center, Farmington, Connecticut

HAROLD S. RABINOVITZ, MD
Department of Dermatology, University of Miami School of Medicine, Miami, Florida

MOIRA RAGAZZI, MD
Pathology Unit, Arcispedale Santa Maria Nuova-Istituto di Ricovero e Cura a Carattere Scientifico, Reggio Emilia, Italy

MILIND RAJADHYAKSHA, PhD
Dermatology Service, Memorial Sloan Kettering Cancer Center, New York, New York

GISELE GARGANTINI REZZE, MD, PhD
DermaImage Associates, Avenida General Furtado do Nascimento, Sao Paulo, Brazil

FERNANDA BERTI ROCHA MENDES, MD
Cutaneous Oncology Department, AC Camargo Cancer Center, Sao Paulo, Brazil

MEGAN SANDS-LINCOLN, PhD, MPH
Elsevier Clinical Solutions, Evidence-Based Medicine Center, Philadelphia, Pennsylvania

SUSANA PUIG SARDÁ, MD, PhD
Melanoma Unit, Department of Dermatology, Hospital Clínic de Barcelona, IDIBAPS, Barcelona University; Centre of Biomedical Research on Rare Diseases (CIBERER), ISCIII, Barcelona, Spain

ELKE C. SATTLER, MD
Department of Dermatology and Allergology, Ludwig-Maximilian University of Munich, Munich, Germany

ALON SCOPE, MD
Department of Dermatology, Sheba Medical Center Affiliated with the Sackler School of Medicine of Tel Aviv University, Ramat Gan, Israel

H. PETER SOYER, MD, FACD
Dermatology Research Centre, Translational Research Institute, School of Medicine, The University of Queensland, Brisbane, Australia

PHOEBE STAR, MBBS, BSc, BA
Dermatology Research Fellow, Department of Dermatology, Melanoma Institute Australia, North Sydney, New South Wales, Australia

RODOLFO SUÁREZ, MD
Melanoma Unit, Dermatology Department, Hospital Clìnic of Barcelona, Institut d'Investigacions Biomediques August Pi I Sunyer, University of Barcelona, Barcelona, Spain

JULIANA CASAGRANDE TAVOLONI BRAGA, MD, PhD
Cutaneous Oncology Department, AC Camargo Cancer Center, Sao Paulo, Brazil

MARTIN ULRICH, MD
Private Dermatology Office/CMB Collegium Medicum Berlin, Berlin, Germany

J. WELZEL, MD
Department of Dermatology and Allergology, General Hospital Augsburg, Augsburg, Germany

ALEXANDER WITKOWSKI, MD, PhD
Department of Dermatology, University of Modena and Reggio Emilia, Modena, Italy

IRIS ZALAUDEK, MD
Non-Melanoma Skin Cancer Unit, Department of Dermatology and Venereology, Medical University of Graz, Graz, Austria

Contents

The use of reflectance confocal microscopy (RCM) and other noninvasive imaging devices can potentially streamline clinical care, leading to more precise and efficient management of skin cancer. This article explores the potential role of RCM in cutaneous oncology, as an adjunct to more established techniques of detecting and monitoring for skin cancer, such as dermoscopy and total body photography. Discussed are current barriers to the adoption of RCM, diagnostic workflows and standards of care in the United States and Europe, and medicolegal issues. The potential role of RCM and other similar technological innovations in the enhancement of dermatologic care is evaluated.

The knowledge of histopathology and in vivo reflectance confocal microscopy correlation has several potential applications. Reflectance confocal microscopy can be performed in all skin tumors, and in this article, the most common histopathologic features of confocal microscopic findings in melanocytic skin tumors and nonmelanocytic skin tumors are described.

Reflectance confocal microscopy (RCM) together with dermoscopy enables improved differentiation of melanomas from most nevi. The resulting high sensitivity for detecting melanoma with RCM is complemented by a concomitant increased specificity, which results in the reduction of unnecessary biopsies of nevi. Although RCM can achieve high diagnostic accuracy for early melanoma detection, false-negative and false-positive cases of melanoma are occasionally encountered. This article reviews the essential clues and pitfalls for the diagnosis of melanoma via RCM and highlights the importance of evaluating RCM findings in light of the clinical scenario and dermoscopic features.

Melanomas are a wide range of tumors that differ in their epidemiology, morphology, genetic profile, and biological behavior. They can be grouped as superficial spreading melanoma, lentigo maligna, and nodular melanoma. Reflectance confocal microscopy is useful for the evaluation of skin lesions that are dermoscopically doubtful by increasing diagnostic accuracy and specificity. This article provides a comprehensive overview of the different confocal main morphologies of distinct melanoma types as a function of the anatomic location of the tumor.

Distinguishing lentigo maligna (LM) and lentigo maligna melanoma (LMM) from background pigmented non-melanoma lesions is challenging. The field of solar damage can obscure clinical assessment, and diagnostic ambiguities are created due to the overlap of the clinical features of LM with other benign lesions. Moreover, margin assessment on histology is limited by the resemblance between melanocytic hyperplasia of actinically damaged skin and scattered atypical melanocytes of LM/LMM. Dermoscopy has made a significant contribution but is often not sufficient for diagnosis and margin assessment. Confocal microscopy has become an important complementary tool in enhancing the management of these complex lesions.

Reflectance confocal microscopy patterns and structures of clinically dark lesions are described. Because many of the dark lesions have melanin in superficial skin layers these lesions show great semiology by confocal. Limitations and pitfalls of reflectance confocal microscopy in clinically dark lesions are also detailed.

Solitary pink lesions can pose a particular challenge to dermatologists because they may be almost or completely featureless clinically and dermoscopically, previously requiring biopsy to exclude malignancy. However, these lesions usually are not particularly challenging histopathologically. Thus, the incorporation of in vivo reflectance confocal microscopy into the clinical practice, which allows for noninvasive examination of the skin at the cellular level revealing features previously seen only on histopathology, is particularly useful for this subset of clinically difficult lesions.

Actinic keratosis, Bowen disease, and invasive squamous cell carcinoma represent different steps within the disease continuum of squamous neoplasia. Although these stages of squamous neoplasia share common findings, reflectance confocal microscopy may be applied for their differentiation and distinction from other benign or malignant lesions. Hyperkeratosis represents the most important limitation in the evaluation of squamous neoplasia as it may impair the analysis of deeper epidermal and dermal structures significantly.

The clinical diagnosis of tumors on the curved surfaces of the face, around the eyes, and on the mucosal surfaces can be difficult, while biopsies and excisions can have functional and aesthetic consequences. To avoid unnecessary surgery, clinicians have been aiming to attain accurate noninvasive diagnosis of lesions at these sites. However, acquisition of high-quality images with dermoscopy and with traditional wide-probe reflectance confocal microscopy (WP-RCM) have been hampered with technical difficulties. This article discusses the technical parameters of the handheld reflectance confocal microscope and discusses its advantages and limitations compared with the WP-RCM.

 Video content accompanies this article at http://www.derm.theclinics.com.

This article describes the use of confocal microscopy devices dedicated to the skin for special sites and unconventional applications. These new applications have been made possible thanks to the introduction on the market of a hand-held camera and an ex vivo device. Special sites discussed include oral, genital and ocular mucosa, nails, and palms and soles. Special uses discussed include infections and infestations; tumor mapping; understanding clinical, dermoscopic, and histology features; and videos.

Reflectance confocal microscopy (RCM) allows real-time, noninvasive microscopic view of the skin at nearly histologic resolution serially over time. RCM increases the sensibility and sensitivity of the diagnosis of skin tumours. RCM evaluates descriptive features of psoriasis, lupus erythematosus, contact dermatitis, and others. Three groups of optical histology have been described: psoriasiform, spongiotic, and interface dermatitis. In a multicenter study, RCM patterns of spongiotic, hyperkeratotic, and interface dermatitis have been analyzed and an algorithmic method of analysis for fast application in the clinical setting based on a multivariate analysis has been proposed. A tree decision diagram has been also established.

Confocal microscopy is a modern imaging device that has been extensively applied in skin oncology. More specifically, for tumor margin assessment, it has been used in two modalities: reflectance mode (in vivo on skin patient) and fluorescence mode (on freshly excised specimen). Although in vivo reflectance confocal microscopy is an add-on tool for lentigo maligna mapping, fluorescence confocal microscopy is far superior for basal cell carcinoma and squamous cell carcinoma margin assessment in the Mohs setting. This article provides a comprehensive overview of the use of confocal microscopy for skin cancer margin evaluation.

Reflectance confocal microscopy (RCM) is becoming more popular among dermatologists aiming to improve their bedside diagnostic accuracy and reduce unnecessary removal of benign cutaneous lesions. With increased interest in the field, limitation of experts and dedicated training programs, telemedicine application to RCM (teleconfocal) helps to connect patients with experts at a distance. Diagnostic accuracy of store-and-forward telemedicine review of RCM images, patient safety, and cost-effectiveness are important considerations for proper acceptance and usage of the technology in the medical community.

The aim of the current review is to provide an overview of the use of reflectance confocal microscopy to detect early skin aging signs. This new imaging tool holds the promise to morphologically explore the epidermis and upper dermis at nearly histologic resolution and over time. The main confocal findings of aged skin include the presence of irregular honeycombed pattern, linear skin furrows, mottled pigmentation, and distinct collagen types (coarse and huddled).

Reflectance confocal microscopy (RCM) allows the evaluation with superb accuracy of some skin tumors before, during, and after treatment. In clinical trials RCM has been shown to provide useful information for evaluation of efficacy of topical or systemic medication. With the recent introduction of handheld RCM a fast examination of the tumor can be done in minutes. In patients treated with surgery RCM plays a unique role to precisely map margins of the tumor in the skin surface and for the detection of subclinical recurrences. This article reviews the use of RCM in the research of different skin cancer tumor treatments.

In addition to reflectance confocal microscopy, multiwave confocal microscopes with different laser wavelengths in combination with exogenous fluorophores allow fluorescence confocal microscopy in vivo and ex vivo. Fluorescence confocal microscopy improves the contrast between the epithelium and the surrounding soft tissue and allows the depiction of certain structures, like epithelial tumors, nerves, and glands.

Special Articles

DERMATOLOGIC CLINICS

THE CLINICS ARE AVAILABLE ONLINE!
Access your subscription at:
www.theclinics.com

Preface

Reflectance Confocal Microscopy Clinical Applications: The Skin from Inside

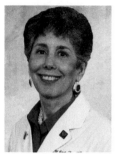
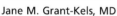

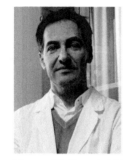

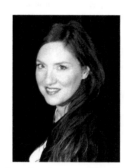

Jane M. Grant-Kels, MD   Giovanni Pellacani, MD   Caterina Longo, MD, PhD

Editors

We are constantly seeking ways to improve our clinical acumen and reduce unnecessary biopsies. Reflectance confocal microscopy (RCM) is an approved technology that is now available to add to our armamentarium. This high-resolution, noninvasive, and safe diode laser (830-nm)–based device allows us to visualize on a cellular level at the bedside the epidermis, dermal-epidermal junction, and papillary dermis of the skin of our patients. The resulting images are dependent on inherent differences in refractivity of the various structures of the skin. The pixels that are converted to an image result in horizontal sections of the skin with a field as large as 8×8 mm^2.

In the hands of experienced confocalists, RCM has demonstrated a sensitivity of 68% to 99% and a specificity of 60% to 99%. In different skin cancer centers where RCM is routinely applied for supporting the diagnostic and decisional process, the number of unnecessary biopsies has been reduced up to 60%! At present, there are only 350 RCM devices worldwide being used for research and clinical endeavors. The use of RCM in clinical practice is today largely diffused in Europe, with more than 200 sites (university clinics, hospitals, and private dermatologists), but seeds of interest and practical applications are present and growing also in United States thanks to pioneers and passionate colleagues throughout the

country, like New York, Miami, Los Angeles, Connecticut, and many others. The hope of all the authors included herein is that the numbers of clinicians taking advantage of this technology will increase dramatically now that valued CPT codes have been assigned by the American Medical Association in the United States.

RCM has been studied extensively, and there are more than 600 peer-reviewed articles on confocal microscopy, with approximately 500 of those reviewing in vivo skin imaging applications. However, in this issue of *Dermatology Clinics*, we have dedicated the entire issue to RCM. Herein, we have gathered the world's experts on RCM to review this topic in-depth, including all the new advances that have been accomplished in the last few years. We start the issue by covering the basics of the technology and how it is used in clinical practice at the bedside. We have also reviewed the fact that in many cases local expertise is still not available on how best to interpret the images; therefore, one of the articles reviews how this technology lends itself to tele-confocal with the images transmitted via the cloud to an expert for their interpretation. Various articles are dedicated to the features we have come to recognize with RCM that help us differentiate various neoplasms, both benign and malignant. Many of these articles delve deeply into the distinguishing

Dermatol Clin 34 (2016) xiii–xiv
http://dx.doi.org/10.1016/j.det.2016.08.003
0733-8635/16/© 2016 Published by Elsevier Inc.

derm.theclinics.com

features of melanocytic lesions, nonpigmented lesions, epithelial neoplasms, RCM features in various inflammatory diseases, and the exciting new ways Mohs surgeons can take advantage of this technology, including the use of fluorescence confocal microscopy.

All of the guest editors are grateful to our distinguished group of authors who have contributed to this issue dedicated to RCM. We hope that the articles will inspire more dermatologists and clinicians to become confocalists like us!

Jane M. Grant-Kels, MD
Department of Dermatology
University of Connecticut Health Center
21 South Road
Farmington, CT 06032, USA

Giovanni Pellacani, MD
Department of Dermatology
University of Modena and Reggio Emilia
Via del Pozzo 71
41100 Modena, Italy

Caterina Longo, MD, PhD
Skin Cancer Unit
Arcispedale Santa Maria Nuova-Istituto di
Ricovero e Cura a
Carattere Scientifico
Reggio Emilia, Italy

E-mail addresses:
grant@uchc.edu (J.M. Grant-Kels)
pellacani.giovanni@gmail.com (G. Pellacani)
longo.caterina@gmail.com (C. Longo)

Basics of Confocal Microscopy and the Complexity of Diagnosing Skin Tumors

New Imaging Tools in Clinical Practice, Diagnostic Workflows, Cost-Estimate, and New Trends

 CrossMark

Syril Keena T. Que, MD[a],*, Jane M. Grant-Kels, MD[a],
Caterina Longo, MD, PhD[b], Giovanni Pellacani, MD[c]

KEYWORDS

- Confocal microscopy • Melanoma • Nonmelanoma skin cancer • Cost-estimates
- Standard of care • Medicolegal issues

KEY POINTS

- A review of the literature shows that the overall sensitivity of RCM for melanoma detection is 91% to 100%, with a specificity ranging from 68% to 98%. The overall RCM sensitivity for BCC is 85% to 97%, with a specificity ranging from 89% to 99%.
- A cost-benefit analysis performed in Europe showed that RCM reduced the number of unnecessary biopsies and led to an overall cost savings in the management of melanoma and nonmelanoma skin cancer.
- Barriers to the adoption of RCM include the image processing time, limited depth of imaging, need for extensive training to master image interpretation, and potential medicolegal risks.
- Proposed methods for overcoming barriers include the continued development of RCM devices to improve speed, diagnostic accuracy, and ease of use; incorporation of RCM training into dermatology residencies and dermatopathology fellowships; and further research studies to justify the use of RCM in dermatology.

INTRODUCTION

The incidence rate of melanoma and nonmelanoma skin cancer is increasing in the United States and in most parts of Europe.[1,2] With this increased burden on the health care system, strides have been made to reduce costs while maintaining a high quality of care. This article examines the complexity of diagnosing skin cancers, discusses

Conflicts of Interest: None.
[a] Department of Dermatology, University of Connecticut Health Center, 263 Farmington Avenue, MC 6231, Farmington, CT 06030-6231, USA; [b] Skin Cancer Unit, Arcispedale S. Maria Nuova-IRCCS, viale risorgimento, 80, 42100 Reggio Emilia, Italy; [c] Department of Dermatology, University of Modena and Reggio Emilia, via del Pozzo 71, Modena 41124, Italy
* Corresponding author.
E-mail address: keenaq@gmail.com

Dermatol Clin 34 (2016) 367–375
http://dx.doi.org/10.1016/j.det.2016.05.001

the diagnostic workflows and current standards of care in the United States and Europe, and assesses the role of reflectance confocal microscopy (RCM) and other similar technological innovations in the enhancement of dermatologic care.

COMPLEXITY OF DIAGNOSING SKIN TUMORS

Skin cancers can sometimes be difficult, even for experienced dermatologists, to recognize and diagnose. Basal cell carcinomas (BCCs) often resemble scars, intradermal nevi, benign lichenoid keratoses, and benign adnexal neoplasms. Squamous cell carcinomas (SCCs) may be difficult to differentiate from hyperplastic actinic keratoses or irritated seborrheic keratoses.

Although some melanomas are diagnosed by gestalt, the diagnosis of many melanocytic lesions is indeterminate without a multidimensional analytical approach that entails assessment of patient history, pattern analysis, comparison with neighboring lesions on the patient, and evaluation of subtle changes over time.[3] Diagnostic algorithms and technological innovations can aid the clinician in developing a clinical impression.

The clinician's ultimate goal is to diagnose skin cancers at an early stage while maintaining a high enough specificity to differentiate between malignant and benign lesions. The number needed to excise (NNE), also known as the number needed to treat (NNT), is a useful measure of diagnostic accuracy. The NNE expresses the ratio between the number of benign lesions biopsied to rule out skin cancer and the number of actual skin cancers biopsied during the same timeframe. Technological innovations, such as RCM, have made it possible to increase diagnostic accuracy and reduce the NNE, thereby decreasing the number of unnecessary procedures.

UNITED STATES STANDARD APPROACH TO SKIN CANCER
Skin Cancer Screening

Several studies have shown that physician detection of melanoma is associated with thinner tumors at the time of diagnosis.[4–6] Nevertheless, there is no consensus in the United States about who should be screened or the frequency with which these patients should be screened.[7] In 2009, the US Preventive Services Task Force concluded there is not enough evidence to recommend for or against routine skin cancer screening in the adult general population.[8] Patient populations that should regularly be screened for skin cancer have the following risk factors: fairer skin types,

older age, the presence of atypical moles or more than 50 moles, family history of melanoma, personal history, and sunburns. A sentinel study performed in Germany, however, demonstrated that in general skin cancer screening decreased melanoma mortality by 47% to 49% compared with adjacent communities not undergoing screenings.[9]

Dermoscopy and total body photography (TBP) allow the clinician to diagnose skin cancers more effectively than unaided visual inspection, making them relatively mainstream methods for skin cancer screening.[10] One meta-analysis established that dermoscopy could raise the sensitivity of melanoma diagnosis from 74% to 90%, while maintaining the specificity associated with unaided visual inspection.[11] Dermoscopy can also decrease the number of benign lesions biopsied by dermatologists.[12] The use of dermoscopy in the United States is increasing, with a recent survey in 2014 showing that 80.7% of surveyed US dermatologists used dermoscopy, a rate higher than previously reported.[13]

TBP is also used by 67% of US dermatologists,[14] especially in patients with several risk factors for melanoma. TBP involves taking a series of photographs covering the full body surface area and monitoring for the development of new melanocytic nevi or any change in existing nevi. When used as an adjunct to dermoscopy in high-risk patients, TBP can help detect de novo melanomas[15] and leads to the diagnosis of thinner melanomas.[16]

Melanoma

The American Academy of Dermatology has published a set of guidelines for the management of primary cutaneous melanoma.[17] For a lesion clinically suspicious for melanoma, the ideal biopsy is a narrow excisional biopsy with 1- to 3-mm margins. For very large lesions and for lesions on the face or acral sites, an incisional biopsy of the most atypical portion is acceptable. If this initial biopsy is inadequate to make a diagnosis or to stage the lesion, a repeat biopsy is indicated.

Surgical excision is the standard of care for the treatment of melanoma, with recommended margins based on prospective randomized controlled trials or consensus opinion[16]; follow-up and diagnosis of eventual regional or distant metastases are outlined by the National Comprehensive Cancer Network.[18]

Nonmelanoma Skin Cancer

In 2015, the American Society for Dermatologic Surgery published its consensus statement on the treatment of BCC[19] and SCC.[20] Although the American Society for Dermatologic Surgery guidelines do not specify the follow-up interval for BCCs, patients with a history of BCC are typically followed every 6 months for the first few years, with the interval extended to 9 to 12 months, and then yearly.

EUROPEAN APPROACH TO SKIN CANCER AND GUIDELINES

Guidelines for the management of melanoma in Europe have been set forth by the European Association of Dermato-Oncology.[21] Briefly, the European Association of Dermato-Oncology recommends the excision of cutaneous melanoma with 1- to 2-cm margins and advocates for sentinel lymph node dissection for patients with tumors more than 1 mm in thickness.

There have been numerous skin cancer prevention campaigns and screenings organized throughout Europe, such as the Euromelanoma initiative, all with the intent of promoting primary and secondary skin cancer screening. European dermatologists are more likely to report the use of dermoscopy[22,23] than US dermatologists and were pioneers in the adoption and implementation of dermoscopy as a diagnostic tool.

WHY REFLECTANCE CONFOCAL MICROSCOPY REPRESENTS AN INNOVATION AND HOW IT CAN CHANGE THE STANDARDS

Recently there has been a surge of RCM research in the dermatologic literature. Researchers have investigated the application of RCM in dermatooncology for the following purposes: improving diagnosis of skin tumors,[24,25] monitoring of melanocytic nevi over time, monitoring after treatment with nonsurgical approaches, selection of biopsy sites, and surgical margin delineation.

RCM can be used as an adjunct to dermoscopy to determine whether a biopsy is indicated. It can potentially reduce the number of unnecessary biopsies. A study by Alarcon and colleagues[26] showed that use of RCM could lower the hypothetical NNT. The authors included a set of lesions showing dermoscopic patterns suggestive of melanoma. Analysis of lesions with dermoscopy alone resulted in an NNT of 3.73, the combination of dermoscopy and RCM resulted in a lower NNT of 2.87, and RCM alone reduced NNT even more to 1.12. There was no significant difference between the specificities of dermoscopy and RCM versus RCM alone.

However, a prospective interventional study on a cohort of approximately 1000 patients referred to a skin cancer unit showed that the number of unnecessary excisions of benign nevi could be reduced by more than 50% using RCM. This reduces the NNE from a potential 14.6 without RCM to an actual NNE of 6.8 with the systematic use of RCM on equivocal lesions.[27]

In cases where an incisional or partial biopsy of a large melanoma is warranted, RCM can help to indicate which site is best to biopsy to establish the diagnosis. In the setting of dermatologic surgery, RCM can potentially be used to indicate surgical margins before Mohs micrographic surgery.[28] For lesions that are treated with nonsurgical approaches, RCM can be used to monitor the clearance of tumor with topical chemotherapy agents.[29,30]

HOW THE CONFOCAL MICROSCOPE WORKS

The confocal microscope uses near-infrared light at 830 nm and focuses the light through a gating pinhole before it enters the detector. The gating pinhole effectively filters out the extraneous light, thus improving the resolution. Images obtained are horizontal and parallel to the surface of the skin. Images can be viewed in stack mode, which enables the viewing of each consecutive level from the epidermis to the dermoepidermal junction down to the papillary dermis (up to a depth of 200 μm). They can also be viewed in mosaic mode, where optical sections are stitched together into a larger image.[31]

Several confocal microscopy models are currently in use. The wide-probe RCM (VivaScope 1500; CaliberID, Rochester, NY) can piece together optical sections into an 8 × 8 mm mosaic image. The handheld RCM (VivaScope 3000; Caliber ID), a newer device, is more ideal for imaging lesions on concave surfaces but has a limited field of view of 1 × 1 mm. Other confocal microscopes use fluorescence, which has been especially useful in ex vivo examination of specimens during Mohs micrographic surgery.[32,33]

SHORT LITERATURE OVERVIEW AND THE ACCURACY OF REFLECTANCE CONFOCAL MICROSCOPY

A review of the literature reveals high sensitivity and specificity for the diagnosis of melanoma and BCC using RCM (Table 1). The overall sensitivity of RCM for melanoma detection is 87% to 100%, with a specificity ranging from 68% to 98%. The overall RCM sensitivity for BCC is 85% to 97%, with a specificity ranging from 89% to 99%.

Table 1
Studies demonstrating diagnostic accuracy of reflectance confocal microscopy

First Author, Year	Country of Study	Study Type	Number of Lesions	Number of Tumors (MM-NMSC)	Accuracy	Tumor Type
Witkowski et al,[34] 2016	Italy	Retrospective	260	114 BCC; 12 MM; 13 SCC; 1 other	Sn: 85.1% Sp: 93.8%	BCC
Kadouch et al,[35] 2015	Netherlands	Meta-analysis of 6 studies	6 studies	—	Sn: 97% Sp: 93%	BCC
Farnetani et al,[36] 2015	Italy, United States, Australia, Spain, Switzerland	Retrospective World Wide Web–based study	100	55 melanocytic nevi; 20 MM; 15 BCC; 7 solar lentigines or SK; 3 AK	Sn: 88.9% Sp: 79.3%	Melanoma, BCC
Lovatto et al,[26] 2015	Spain	Retrospective	64	8 MM; 5 invasive MM; 51 melanocytic nevi	Sn: 100% Sp: 69%	Melanoma
Cinotti et al,[37] 2014	France	Prospective, noninterventional	47	5 MM; 9 melanocytic nevi; 14 BCC; 3 SCC	Sn: 100% Sp: 69.20%	Melanoma, SCC, BCC (eyelid margin tumors)
Bennassar et al,[32] 2014	Spain	Prospective, noninterventional, detection of residual tumor in Mohs sections	80	80 BCC	Sn: 88% Sp: 99%	BCC
Larson et al,[38] 2013	United States	Retrospective	17	17 BCC	Sn: 94% Sp: 94%	BCC
Longo et al,[39] 2013	Italy	Retrospective	140	23 nodular MM; 9 MM mets; 28 BCC; 6 SCC; 32 nevi; 14 SK; 17 dermatofibromas; 5 vascular lesions; 6 other	MM accuracy Sn: 96.5% Sp: 94.1%	Melanoma data (overall study about nodular lesions)
Gareau et al,[33] 2009	United States	Retrospective, Mohs excisions	45 confocal mosaics	BCC	Sn: 96.6% Sp: 89.2%	BCC
Guitera et al,[40] 2009	Australia	Prospective, noninterventional	326	203 melanocytic nevi; 123 MM	Sn: 91% Sp: 68%	Melanoma, nevi
Horn et al,[41] 2007	Austria	Retrospective	120	—	Sn: 95% Sp: 96.25%	SCC

Study	Country	Study type	No.	Lesions	Sn/Sp	Diagnosis
Langley et al,[42] 2007	Canada	Prospective, noninterventional	125	88 melanocytic nevi; 37 MM	Sn: 97.3% Sp: 83%	Melanoma, nevi
Gerger et al,[43] 2005	Austria	Retrospective	117	90 melanocytic nevi; 27 MM	Sn: 98.15% Sp: 98.89%	Melanoma, nevi
Guitera et al,[44] 2010	Australia	Retrospective	284	81 MM; 203 benign macules	Sn: 93% Sp: 82%	Lentigo maligna
Witkowski et al,[34] 2016	Italy, United States, Poland	Retrospective, combined dermoscopy-RCM evaluation	260	144 BCC; 12 MM; 13 SCC; 1 other	Sn: 77.2% Sp: 96.6%	Pink cutaneous lesions, melanoma, SCC, BCC
Guitera et al,[45] 2012	Australia	Prospective noninterventional	710	216 MM; 266 melanocytic nevi; 119 BCC; 67 pigmented facial macules; 42 other	MM accuracy Sn: 87.6% Sp: 70.8% BCC accuracy Sn: 100% Sp: 88.5%	Melanoma/BCC
Pellacani et al,[25] 2005	Italy	Retrospective	102	37 MM; 49 acquired nevi; 16 Spitz/Reed nevi	Sn: 97% Sp: 72%	Melanoma/nevi
Pellacani et al,[24] 2007	Italy	Retrospective	351	136 MM; 215 melanocytic nevi	Sn: 92% Sp: 69%	Melanoma/nevi
Segura et al,[46] 2009	Spain	Retrospective	154	36 MM; 64 melanocytic nevi; 27 BCC; 8 SK; 5 solar lentigines; 4 BLK; 4 vascular lesions; 3 AKs; 2 dermatofibromas; 1 sebaceous hyperplasia	MM accuracy Sn: 100% Sp: 57%	Melanocytic and BCC
Ferrari et al,[47] 2015	Italy	Retrospective	322	70 MM; 252 melanocytic nevi	Sn: 96% Sp: 70%	Melanoma/nevi

Abbreviations: AK, actinic keratosis; BLK, benign lichenoid keratosis; MM, malignant melanoma; NMSC, nonmelanoma skin cancer; SK, seborrheic keratosis; Sn, sensitivity; Sp, specificity.

On a cautious note, most studies involve expert readers, with prior experience in RCM interpretation. More data are needed regarding the sensitivity and specificity of RCM among novice readers. There is also a lack of trials involving the use of RCM for the diagnosis of SCC.

DIAGNOSTIC WORKFLOWS COMPARISON AND ROLE/POSITION OF REFLECTANCE CONFOCAL MICROSCOPY

Although the data reveal a high level of diagnostic accuracy with RCM use, the actual implementation of this technology will have to take into account the workflow of a busy dermatology office. In the ideal scenario, the device would be used for same-day diagnostic confirmation of skin cancers or as a perioperative tool to aid in cutaneous surgeries.

Yet multiple barriers exist. The image processing time is approximately 7 to 10 minutes. To streamline the process in a high-risk or pigmented lesion clinic, trained staff would be hired solely to operate the machine and obtain the images.

In the setting of Mohs micrographic surgery, RCM would have to be incorporated in a way that enhances surgical flow. Using RCM to examine ex vivo Mohs surgical specimens, for example, could decrease the time currently used for slide preparation by frozen sections.[32,33]

The implementation of RCM into clinical practice involves a balance between diagnostic accuracy and time expenditure. As handheld machines with faster image processing time and a live video stream capture mode become available, it becomes more feasible to use RCM in dermatology.

COST-BENEFIT ANALYSIS

The diagnosis of melanoma is often suboptimal, leading to a large number of unnecessary procedures and unwarranted costs associated with the biopsies and excision of benign nevi. Cost-analysis estimates by Pellacani and colleagues[48] show a cost reduction when RCM is incorporated into the diagnostic workflow. The use of RCM led to a decrease in NNE from 19.41 (dermoscopy only) to 6.25 (dermoscopy + RCM). RCM reduced more than 70% of benign lesions biopsied. By reducing the number of unnecessary excisions, RCM could potentially add 280,000 Euros in yearly savings to the European health care system. Patient satisfaction secondary to reduced unnecessary biopsies is immeasurable.

COMMENTARY AND TRANSLATION OF COST-EFFECTIVE STUDY TO THE UNITED STATES SYSTEM

To date, no cost-effective study has been performed in the United States. There is currently no assigned reimbursement for the use of confocal microscopy, although CPT codes have been assigned suggesting that reimbursement will be in place in 2017. Presently, patients are paying out of pocket for this service. At this time, it is unknown whether RCM would lead to cost savings in the context of the US health care system but cost savings are anticipated based on the European literature.

STRATEGIES TO OVERCOME BARRIERS TO THE ADOPTION OF REFLECTANCE CONFOCAL MICROSCOPY

The following lists the proposed ways to overcome current barriers in the adoption of RCM:

1. Assignment of reimbursement value for RCM use in the United States
2. Conduction of further research studies to justify RCM use in various dermatologic settings
3. Development of specialized skin cancer clinics incorporating RCM
4. Incorporation of RCM into teledermatology
5. Development of more training courses for dermatologists; incorporation of RCM training into residency curriculum and dermatopathology and Mohs fellowship training
6. Continued improvement in speed, accuracy of imaging, and ease of use for RCM devices; use of stains and computer-reconstructed images that mimic histopathology

MEDICOLEGAL ISSUES AND THE BARRIERS TO CHANGE THE STANDARDS

By introducing an alternative means of skin cancer diagnosis, RCM can potentially supplement and even replace histopathology, which carries with it some unique medicolegal implications. To reduce the risk of misdiagnosis and malpractice risk, the clinician would biopsy any lesions that demonstrate atypical features on RCM and follow lesions that appear benign.

Another issue with RCM is the need for extensive training and the present dearth of experienced RCM readers. On a positive note, studies have shown high diagnostic accuracy with RCM in teleconsultation use.[49]

OTHER EMERGING TECHNOLOGIES

Aside from RCM, other new and emerging technologies may increase the sensitivity of clinical evaluation for melanoma. The SIAscope (Biocompatibles, Farnham, Surrey, UK) is a multispectral device that measures melanin, blood, and collagen in the epidermis and papillary dermis. It has a similar sensitivity and specificity to dermoscopy by experienced dermatologists[50]; however, the possibility of replacing the standard of care in skin cancer diagnosis (which includes clinical and dermoscopic examination) remains controversial.[51]

The MelaFind (MELA Sciences, Inc, Irvington, NY) is another multispectral device that analyzes images using automated software and provides a score indicating whether or not a lesion should be biopsied. Although this device is targeted to achieve a very high sensitivity, its low specificity will likely limit its use.[52,53] Electrical impedence spectroscopy, another technology, measures impedance to current flow to predict the likelihood that a lesion is skin cancer. Although sensitivity is high, specificity ranges from 24% to 49%.[54]

SUMMARY

There is a significant potential role of RCM in cutaneous oncology, as an adjunct to more established techniques of detecting and monitoring for skin cancer, such as dermoscopy and TBP. RCM has demonstrated high rates of diagnostic accuracy and can potentially simplify the decision-making process with regard to skin cancer recognition and confirmation. For the technology to enter real-world clinical practice, clinicians must assess how it can fit in with the standards of care in the United States and Europe and evaluate its role in cost savings and quality improvement.

REFERENCES

1. Lomas A, Leonardi-Bee J, Bath-Hextall F. A systematic review of worldwide incidence of non-melanoma skin cancer. Br J Dermatol 2012;166(5): 1069–80.
2. National Program of Cancer Registries (NPCR) and Surveillance, Epidemiology, and End Results (SEER) Program. Atlanta, GA: Centers for Disease Control and Prevention and Bethesda, MD: National Cancer Institute. Data from 2002–2011. Available at: http://seer.cancer.gov/
3. Gachon J, Beaulieu P, Sei JF, et al. First prospective study of the recognition process of melanoma in dermatological practice. Arch Dermatol 2005; 141(4):434–8.
4. Schneider JS, Moore DH 2nd, Mendelsohn ML. Screening program reduced melanoma mortality at the Lawrence Livermore National Laboratory, 1984 to 1996. J Am Acad Dermatol 2008;58(5):741–9.
5. Aitken JF, Elwood M, Baade PD, et al. Clinical whole-body skin examination reduces the incidence of thick melanomas. Int J Cancer 2010;126(2):450–8.
6. Swetter SM, Pollitt RA, Johnson TM, et al. Behavioral determinants of successful early melanoma detection: role of self and physician skin examination. Cancer 2012;118(15):3725–34.
7. American Academy of Dermatology. Skin cancer: tips for preventing and finding. Available at: www.aad.org/dermatology-a-to-z/diseases-and-treatments/q–t/skin cancer/tips. Accessed December 5, 2015.
8. U.S. Preventive Services Task Force. Screening for skin cancer: U.S. Preventive Services Task Force recommendation statement. Ann Intern Med 2009; 150(3):188–93.
9. Katalinic A, Waldmann A, Weinstock MA, et al. Does skin cancer screening save lives?: an observational study comparing trends in melanoma mortality in regions with and without screening. Cancer 2012; 118(21):5395–402.
10. Psaty EL, Halpern AC. Current and emerging technologies in melanoma diagnosis: the state of the art. Clin Dermatol 2009;27(1):35–45.
11. Vestergaard ME, Macaskill P, Holt PE, et al. Dermoscopy compared with naked eye examination for the diagnosis of primary melanoma: a meta-analysis of studies performed in a clinical setting. Br J Dermatol 2008;159:669–76.
12. Carli P, de Giorgi V, Chiarugi A, et al. Addition of dermoscopy to conventional naked-eye examination in melanoma screening: a randomized study. J Am Acad Dermatol 2004;50:683–9.
13. Murzaku EC, Hayan S, Rao BK. Methods and rates of dermoscopy usage: a cross-sectional survey of US dermatologists stratified by years in practice. J Am Acad Dermatol 2014;71(2):393–5.
14. Rice ZP, Weiss FJ, DeLong LK, et al. Utilization and rationale for the implementation of total body (digital) photography as an adjunct screening measure for melanoma. Melanoma Res 2010;20(5):417–21.
15. Goodson AG, Florell SR, Hyde M, et al. Comparative analysis of total body and dermatoscopic photographic monitoring of nevi in similar patient populations at risk for cutaneous melanoma. Dermatol Surg 2010;36:1087–98.
16. Rademaker M, Oakley A. Digital monitoring by whole body photography and sequential digital dermoscopy detects thinner melanomas. J Prim Health Care 2010;2:268–72.
17. Bichakjian CK, Halpern AC, Johnson TM, et al. Guidelines of care for the management of primary cutaneous melanoma. American Academy of Dermatology. J Am Acad Dermatol 2011;65(5): 1032–47.

18. Colt DG, Andtbacka R, Bichakjian CK, et al. Melanoma. J Natl Compr Canc Netw 2009;7:250–75.

19. Kauvar AN, Cronin T, Roenigk R, et al. Consensus for nonmelanoma skin cancer treatment: basal cell carcinoma, including a cost analysis of treatment methods. Dermatol Surg 2015;41(5):550–71.

20. Kauvar AN, Arpey CJ, Hruza G, et al. Consensus for nonmelanoma skin cancer treatment. Part II: squamous cell carcinoma, including a cost analysis of treatment methods. Dermatol Surg 2015;41(11): 1214–40.

21. Garbe C, Peris K, Hauschild A, et al, European Dermatology Forum, European Association of Dermato-Oncology, European Organization of Research and Treatment of Cancer. Diagnosis and treatment of melanoma. European consensus-based interdisciplinary guideline–Update 2012. Eur J Cancer 2012;48(15):2375–90.

22. Moulin C, Poulalhon N, Duru G, et al. Dermoscopy use by French private practice dermatologists: a nationwide survey. Br J Dermatol 2013;168(1):74–9.

23. Butler TD, Matin RN, Affleck AG, et al. Trends in dermoscopy use in the UK: results from surveys in 2003 and 2012. Dermatol Pract Concept 2015; 5(2):29–38.

24. Pellacani G, Guitera P, Longo C, et al. The impact of in vivo reflectance confocal microscopy for the diagnostic accuracy of melanoma and equivocal melanocytic lesions. J Invest Dermatol 2007;127(12): 2759–65.

25. Pellacani G, Cesinaro AM, Seidenari S. Reflectance-mode confocal microscopy of pigmented skin lesions: improvement in melanoma diagnostic specificity. J Am Acad Dermatol 2005;53(6):979–85.

26. Lovatto L, Carrera C, Salerni G, et al. In vivo reflectance confocal microscopy of equivocal melanocytic lesions detected by digital dermoscopy follow-up. J Eur Acad Dermatol Venereol. 2015;29(10):1918–25.

27. Pellacani G, Pepe P, Casari A, et al. Reflectance confocal microscopy as a second-level examination in skin oncology improves diagnostic accuracy and saves unnecessary excisions: a longitudinal prospective study. Br J Dermatol 2014;171(5):1044–51.

28. Venturini M, Gualdi G, Zanca A, et al. A new approach for pre-surgical margin assessment of basal cell carcinoma by reflectance confocal microscopy. Br J Dermatol 2016;174(2):380–5.

29. Curiel-Lewandrowski C, Williams CM, Swindells KJ, et al. Use of in vivo confocal microscopy in malignant melanoma: an aid in diagnosis and assessment of surgical and nonsurgical therapeutic approaches. Arch Dermatol 2004;140(9):1127–32.

30. Torres A, Niemeyer A, Berkes B, et al. 5% imiquimod cream and reflectance-mode confocal microscopy as adjunct modalities to Mohs micrographic surgery for treatment of basal cell carcinoma. Dermatol Surg 2004;30(12 Pt 1):1462–9.

31. Que SK, Fraga-Braghiroli N, Grant-Kels JM, et al. Through the looking glass: basics and principles of reflectance confocal microscopy. J Am Acad Dermatol 2015;73(2):276–84.

32. Bennàssar A, Vilata A, Puig S, et al. Ex vivo fluorescence confocal microscopy for fast evaluation of tumour margins during Mohs surgery. Br J Dermatol 2014;170(2):360–5.

33. Gareau DS, Karen JK, Dusza SW, et al. Sensitivity and specificity for detecting basal cell carcinomas in Mohs excisions with confocal fluorescence mosaicing microscopy. J Biomed Opt 2009;14(3): 034012.

34. Witkowski AM, Łudzik J, DeCarvalho N, et al. Non-invasive diagnosis of pink basal cell carcinoma: how much can we rely on dermoscopy and reflectance confocal microscopy? Skin Res Technol 2016;22(2):230–7.

35. Kadouch DJ, Wolkerstorfer A, Elshot Y, et al. Treatment of basal cell carcinoma using a one-stop-shop with reflectance confocal microscopy: study design and protocol of a randomized controlled multicenter trial. JMIR Res Protoc 2015;4(3):e109.

36. Farnetani F, Scope A, Braun RP, et al. Skin cancer diagnosis with reflectance confocal microscopy: reproducibility of feature recognition and accuracy of diagnosis. JAMA Dermatol 2015;151(10): 1075–80.

37. Cinotti E, Perrot JL, Campolmi N, et al. The role of in vivo confocal microscopy in the diagnosis of eyelid margin tumors: 47 cases. J Am Acad Dermatol 2014;71(5):912–8.e2.

38. Larson B, Abeytunge S, Seltzer E, et al. Detection of skin cancer margins in Mohs excisions with high-speed strip mosaicing confocal microscopy: a feasibility study. Br J Dermatol 2013;169(4):922–6.

39. Longo C, Farnetani F, Ciardo S, et al. Is confocal microscopy a valuable tool in diagnosing nodular lesions? A study of 140 cases. Br J Dermatol 2013; 169(1):58–67.

40. Guitera P, Pellacani G, Longo C, et al. In vivo reflectance confocal microscopy enhances secondary evaluation of melanocytic lesions. J Invest Dermatol 2009;129(1):131–8.

41. Horn M, Gerger A, Koller S, et al. The use of confocal laser-scanning microscopy in microsurgery for invasive squamous cell carcinoma. Br J Dermatol 2007;156(1):81–4.

42. Langley RG, Walsh N, Sutherland AE, et al. The diagnostic accuracy of in vivo confocal scanning laser microscopy compared to dermoscopy of benign and malignant melanocytic lesions: a prospective study. Dermatology 2007;215(4):365–72.

43. Gerger A, Koller S, Kern T, et al. Diagnostic applicability of in vivo confocal laser scanning microscopy in melanocytic skin tumors. J Invest Dermatol 2005;124(3):493–8.

44. Guitera P, Pellacani G, Crotty KA, et al. The impact of in vivo reflectance confocal microscopy on the diagnostic accuracy of lentigo maligna and equivocal pigmented and nonpigmented macules of the face. J Invest Dermatol 2010;130(8):2080–91.

45. Guitera P, Menzies SW, Longo C, et al. In vivo confocal microscopy for diagnosis of melanoma and basal cell carcinoma using a two-step method: analysis of 710 consecutive clinically equivocal cases. J Invest Dermatol 2012;132(10):2386–94.

46. Segura S, Puig S, Carrera C, et al. Development of a two-step method for the diagnosis of melanoma by reflectance confocal microscopy. J Am Acad Dermatol 2009;61(2):216–29.

47. Ferrari B, Pupelli G, Farnetani F, et al. Dermoscopic difficult lesions: an objective evaluation of reflectance confocal microscopy impact for accurate diagnosis. J Eur Acad Dermatol Venereol 2015; 29(6):1135–40.

48. Pellacani G, Witkowski A, Cesinaro AM, et al. Cost-benefit of reflectance confocal microscopy in the diagnostic performance of melanoma. J Eur Acad Dermatol Venereol 2015;30(3):413–9.

49. Rao BK, Mateus R, Wassef C, et al. In vivo confocal microscopy in clinical practice: comparison of bedside diagnostic accuracy of a trained physician and distant diagnosis of an expert reader. J Am Acad Dermatol 2013;69(6):e295–300.

50. Haniffa MA, Lloyd JJ, Lawrence CM. The use of a spectrophotometric intracutaneous analysis device in the real-time diagnosis of melanoma in the setting of a melanoma screening clinic. Br J Dermatol 2007; 156:1350–2.

51. Sgouros D, Lallas A, Julian Y, et al. Assessment of SIAscopy in the triage of suspicious skin tumours. Skin Res Technol 2014;20(4):440–4.

52. Monheit G, Cognetta AB, Ferris L, et al. The performance of MelaFind: a prospective multicenter study. Arch Dermatol 2011;147:188–94.

53. Wells R, Gutkowicz-Krusin D, Veledar E, et al. Comparison of diagnostic and management sensitivity to melanoma between dermatologists and MelaFind: a pilot study. Arch Dermatol 2012;148:1083–4.

54. Mayer JE, Swetter SM, Fu T, et al. Screening, early detection, education, and trends for melanoma: current status (2007-2013) and future directions. Part I: epidemiology, high-risk groups, clinical strategies, and diagnostic technology. J Am Acad Dermatol 2014;71(4):599.e1-12.

Opening a Window into Living Tissue
Histopathologic Features of Confocal Microscopic Findings in Skin Tumors

Juliana Casagrande Tavoloni Braga, MD, PhD[a],
Raquel de Paula Ramos Castro, MD[a],
Tatiana Cristina Moraes Pinto Blumetti, MD[a],
Fernanda Berti Rocha Mendes, MD[a],
Juliana Arêas de Souza Lima Beltrame Ferreira, MD[a],
Gisele Gargantini Rezze, MD, PhD[b],*

KEYWORDS

- Reflectance confocal microscopy • Histopathology • Skin tumors • Melanoma • Melanocytic nevi
- Actinic keratosis • Squamous cell carcinoma • Basal cell carcinoma

KEY POINTS

- Several histopathologic features of skin tumors can be characterized individually through reflectance confocal microscopy (RCM) examination.
- As a result, RCM has significant correlation with histopathologic final diagnosis.
- RCM can improve noninvasive in vivo diagnosis of skin tumors and prevent biopsy of benign lesions.

INTRODUCTION

The knowledge of histopathology and in vivo reflectance confocal microscopy (RCM) correlation has several potential applications.[1,2] First, it enables the skin tissue evaluation of specific sites for a punch biopsy, improving its diagnostic accuracy and reducing the need of repetitive investigation in heterogeneous lesions. Second, it may differentiate skin tumors and reassure confidence in clinical diagnosis of doubtful lesions.[3,4]

Notably, RCM evaluation of a given lesion is made in sections parallel to skin (en face), where each section is at a different skin depth.[1]

Oppositely, conventional histopathology sections are made perpendicular to the skin, and each section shows different depths of a given lesion.[1] This technical difference makes the histopathology-RCM correlation challenging for the general pathologist/dermatologist, who is used to studying the skin according to perpendicular sections.[1] Braga and colleagues[5] described the value of transverse histologic sections as a tool to better understand the structures observed in dermoscopy and RCM.

In this article, the most common skin tumors observed in clinical practice as seen on RCM are described.

Disclosure Statement: All authors have seen and agree with the contents of the article and there is no financial interest to report.
[a] Cutaneous Oncology Department, AC Camargo Cancer Center, Rua Prof. Antônio Prudente, 211-Liberdade, Sao Paulo, Sao Paulo 01509-010, Brazil; [b] Dermalmage associates, Avenida General Furtado do Nascimento, 740, cj. 24. São Paulo, SP 05465-070, Brazil
* Corresponding author.
E-mail address: ggrezze@hotmail.com

derm.theclinics.com

Table 1
Reflectance confocal microscopy features for nevi and correlation with histopathology

RCM	Histopathology
Ring pattern	Junctional nevus: individual melanocytes at the DEJ, elongated papillae, and lentiginous pattern
Meshwork and junctional thickening (enlargement of the junctional space)	Junctional nevus: junctional nests located at the tips of epidermal ridges
Meshwork and junctional thickening with junctional and dermal nests	Compound nevus: nests at the DEJ and papillary dermis (more superficial)
Meshwork with junctional and dermal nests, predominantly with clod pattern	Compound nevus: nests at the DEJ, papillary dermis, and reticular dermis (deeper)
Dense or dense and sparse nests	Dermal nevus: nevus cells nests at the dermis

CONFOCAL MICROSCOPY CORRELATION IN MELANOCYTIC SKIN TUMORS

Melanocytic nevi are seen in histopathology as a benign proliferation of nevus cells with monomorphic pattern.[6–8] When the proliferation occurs initially at the epidermis, more precisely at the dermal-epidermal junction (DEJ), it is known as junctional nevi.[6–8] On the other hand, when the nevus cells are located at the dermis, the lesion is classified as dermal nevus.[6–8] Finally, when it is located in both compartments (epidermis and dermis), it is named compound nevus.[6–8]

Junctional Nevi

Junctional nevi can be seen in RCM with 2 patterns: ringed and/or meshwork[8–11] (**Table 1**).

The ringed pattern is the most commonly observed. It presents as edged papillae with intense bright basal keratinocytes surrounding a dark center. In histopathology, it corresponds to a lentiginous proliferation of single melanocytes at the DEJ[8–11] (see **Table 1**; **Fig. 1**).

In the meshwork pattern, a proliferation of nevus cells organized in nests is seen at the interpapillary space by histopathology and, consequently, by RCM as well[8–11] (see **Table 1**; **Fig. 2**).

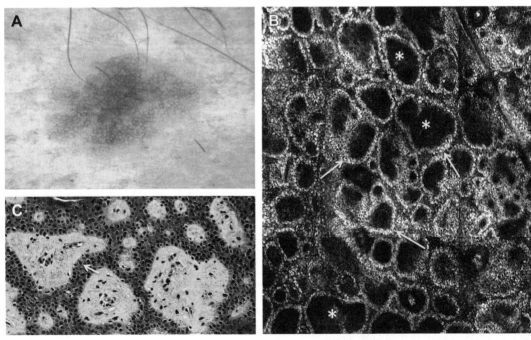

Fig. 1. Junctional nevus. (*A*) Dermatoscopy shows typical network. (*B*) RCM mosaic image (1 × 1.25 mm) at the level of the DEJ shows ringed pattern: rings of bright polygonal cells (*arrows*) surrounding roundish to oval dark areas corresponding to dermal papillae at DEJ (*asterisks*). (*C*) Histopathologic transverse section shows isolated melanocytes arranged around the dermal papillae (*arrow*) (H&E, original magnification × 100).

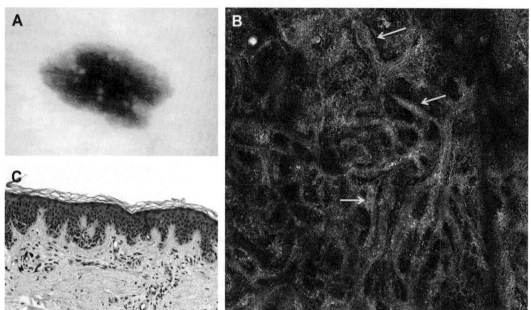

Fig. 2. Junctional nevus. (*A*) Dermatoscopy of a junctional reticular nevus. (*B*) RCM mosaic image (1 × 1 mm) at the level of the DEJ shows meshwork pattern with regular junctional nests enlarging the interpapillary space (*arrows*). (*C*) Histopathology showing single cell and nested proliferation at the DEJ (H&E, original magnification × 100).

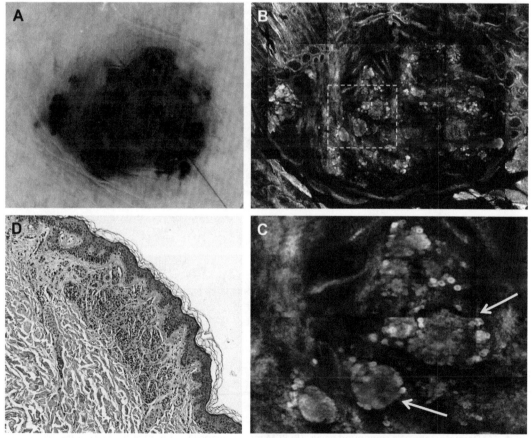

Fig. 3. (*A*) Dermoscopy of a dermal nevus with a cobblestone pattern. (*B*) RCM mosaic image (2.5 × 2 mm) at the level of the dermis showing clod pattern. (*C*) RCM mosaic image (0.75 × 0.5 mm) at the level of the dermis showing dense and sparse nests (*arrows*). (*D*) Histopathology of the intradermal nevus showing predominant dermal nests (H&E, original magnification × 100).

Dermal Nevi

The main RCM characteristic of this lesion is the clod pattern that shows intradermal nests (clods) occupying at least 50% of the lesion. This pattern corresponds to the cobblestone pattern in dermoscopy, and in histopathology, this feature represents nests of melanocytes at the dermal level[8–13] (see **Table 1**; **Fig. 3**).

Compound Nevi

Compound nevi can present both junctional nevus patterns and intradermal nests (clods) in the papillary dermis.[13,14] The nests can be dense, observed like compact dense aggregates, or dense and sparse, observed like compact dense aggregates with large cells detectable within[13,14] (see **Table 1**; **Fig. 4**).

Dysplastic Nevi

Dysplastic nevi or atypical nevi are benign lesions that might show few features of melanoma in dermoscopy, RCM, or histopathology and can be extremely challenging at all levels.[15] Some RCM features have been described[8,15] (**Fig. 5**, **Table 2**), as follows:

- Slightly irregular epidermal architecture with few sporadic pagetoid cells mainly in the center of the lesion;
- Papillae contours are mostly edged and, when nonedged papillae are observable, they rarely extend more than 10% of the lesion surface;
- Presence of some large nucleated atypical cells at the DEJ, usually found in the center of the lesion;
- Junctional and/or intradermal nests, usually observed like compact dense aggregates with large cells detectable within (dense and sparse nests);
- Junctional nests can present an elongated shape or short interconnections, which correspond to nest fusion and bridging at histopathology;

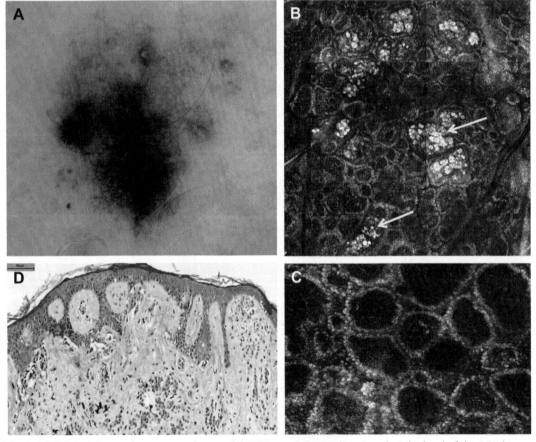

Fig. 4. (*A*) Dermatoscopy of a compound nevus. (*B*) RCM mosaic image (1 × 1 mm) at the level of the DEJ shows a pattern of ringed and clod with nests in the dermal papillae (*arrows*). (*C*) RCM individual image at the level of the DEJ showing a ringed pattern. (*D*) Histopathology of the compound nevus with dermal nests (correlated with the clod pattern) and single cell and nested proliferation at the DEJ (correlated with the ringed pattern) (H&E, original magnification × 100).

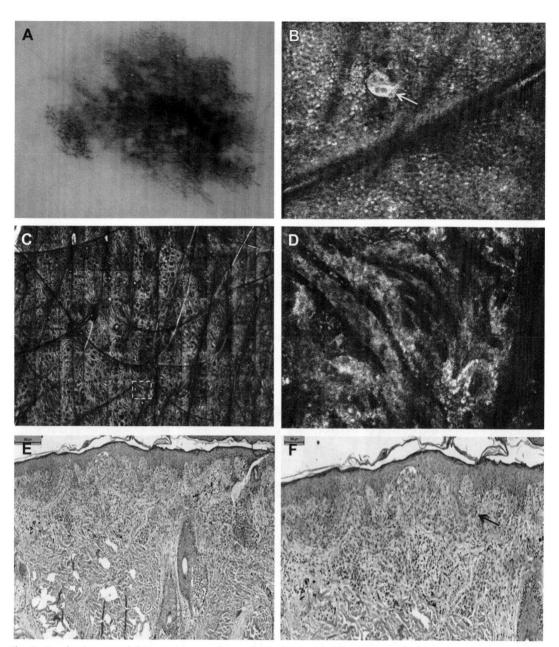

Fig. 5. Dysplastic nevus. (*A*) Dermatoscopy shows atypical network. (*B*) RCM individual image at the spinous layer showing few dendritic pagetoid cells (*yellow arrow*). (*C*) RCM mosaic image (5 × 3.75 mm) at the level of the DEJ showing meshwork pattern (*the area inside the dashed square* is represented in *D*). (*D*) RCM individual image at the DEJ shows junctional nests with elongated shape or short interconnection, which correspond to nest fusion and bridging at histopathology. (*E*) Histopathology of the compound dysplastic nevus (H&E, original magnification × 100). (*F*) Histopathology showing nest fusion and bridging (*black arrow*) (H&E, original magnification × 100).

- Bright particles (corresponding to inflammatory infiltrate), plump bright round and stellate cells (corresponding to melanophages), and coarse collagen fibers. These fibers assume a bandlike disposition that corresponds in histopathology to lamellar and concentric fibrosis around epidermal ridges.

Spitz/Reed Nevus

RCM features found in Spitz/Reed nevi are in most cases indistinguishable from melanoma, and good correlation has been found between some RCM features and histopathologic examination.[8] Although there are several types of dermoscopy

Table 2
Reflectance confocal microscopy features for dysplasic nevi (atypical nevi) and correlation with histopathology

RCM	Histopathology
Edged papillae are prevalent at the lesion (<10% nonedged papillae)	Focal disorganization at DEJ
Low presence of atypical cells at epidermis	Few atypical melanocytic cells at epidermis (focal atypia)
Atypical cells at DEJ	Few atypical melanocytic cells at DEJ (focal atypia)
Nests usually with dense and sparse pattern	Nests at DEJ and/or dermis
Short interconnections	Nest fusion and bridging at DEJ
Bright particles, plump bright round and stellate cells at dermis	Inflammatory infiltrate and melanophages at dermis
Collagen in bandlike disposition at dermis	Lamellar and concentric fibrosis around epidermal ridges at dermis

patterns for Spitz nevus, the most prevalent is the starburst pattern, and the RCM features found for this pattern are[8] (Fig. 6) as follows:

- Typical regular epidermis (honeycombed or cobblestone), sometimes with pagetoid infiltration;
- Nonedged papillae with atypical cells and junctional thickenings at DEJ;
- Spindled cells and dendritic cells at epidermis and DEJ;
- Dense regular nests at DEJ and papillary dermis;

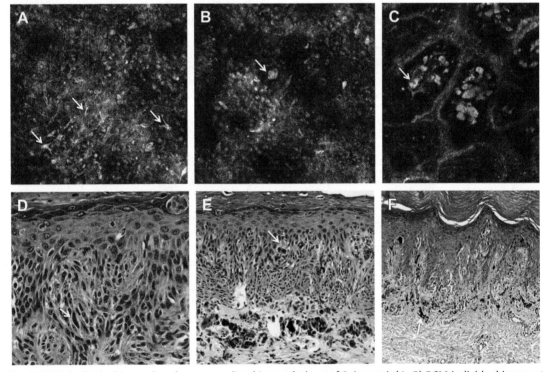

Fig. 6. RCM (individual images) and corresponding histopathology of Spitz nevi. (*A, D*) RCM individual image at the suprabasal/basal layer showing a few elongated (*spindled*) cells regularly distributed (*arrow*). The histopathology shows dense nest of elongated cells at the level of the DEJ (*arrow*) (H&E, original magnification × 100). (*B, E*) RCM individual image at the basal/DEJ showing bright round cells (*arrow*) corresponding to an agglomerate of pigment on histopathology (*arrow*) (H&E, original magnification × 100). (*C, F*) RCM individual image at the DEJ/papillary dermis showing plump cells (*arrow*) corresponding to melanophages in the dermis on histopathology (*arrow*) (H&E, original magnification × 100).

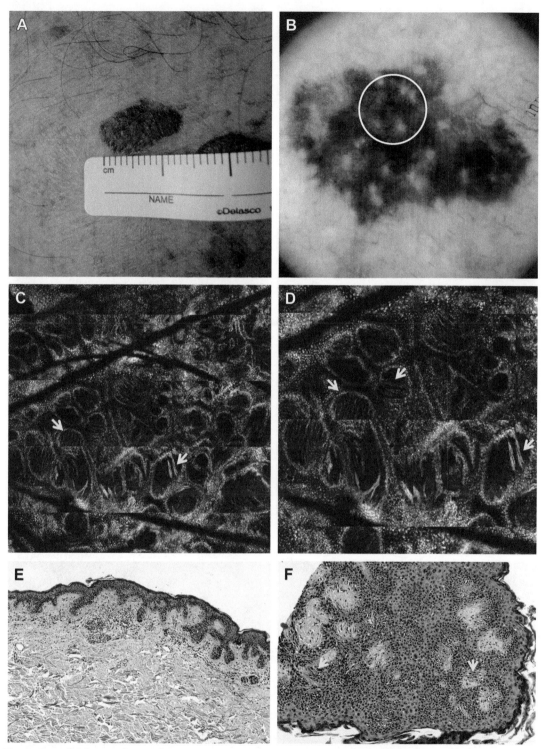

Fig. 7. Superficial spreading melanoma in situ. (*A*) Clinical image. (*B*) Dermoscopy shows atypical pigmented network (*area inside the white circle*). (*C*) RCM mosaic image (2 × 2 mm) at the DEJ showing irregular dermal papillae with dendritic cells (*arrows*). (*D*) RCM mosaic image (1.5 × 1.5 mm) at the level of the DEJ shows dendritic cells forming "bridges" called mitochondria-like structures (*arrows*). (*E*) Histopathologic perpendicular section shows disarrangement of the rete ridge and the increased number of atypical melanocytes (H&E, original magnification × 100). (*F*) Histopathologic transverse section shows atypical melanocytes protruding into the dermal papillae forming bridges (*arrows*) (H&E, original magnification × 100).

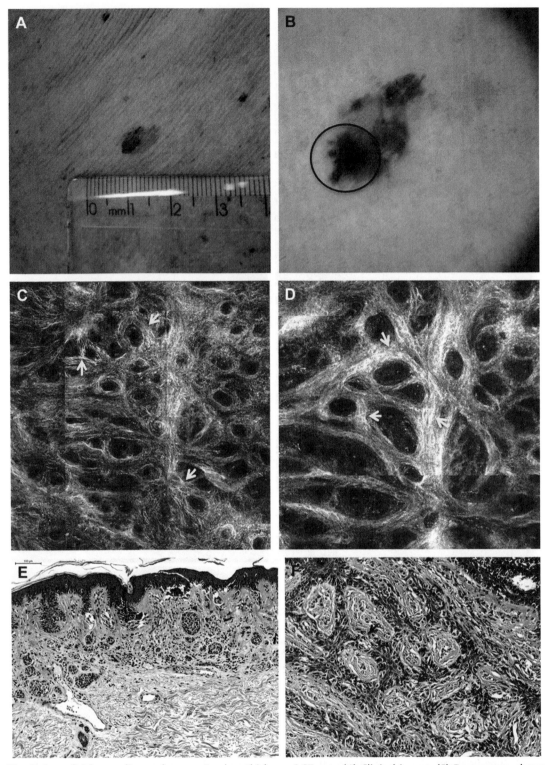

Fig. 8. Superficial spreading melanoma, Breslow thickness 0.27 mm. (*A*) Clinical image. (*B*) Dermoscopy shows atypical pigmented network (*area inside the black circle*). (*C*) RCM mosaic image (1.5 × 1.5 mm) at the level of the DEJ shows non-demarcated rings separated by loosely thick interpapillary spaces (*yellow arrows*). (*D*) RCM mosaic image (0.75 × 0.75 mm) at the level of the DEJ showing dendritic cells enlarging the interpapillary spaces (*yellow arrows*). (*E*) Histopathologic perpendicular section shows disarrangement of the rete ridge and the increased number of atypical melanocytes in the epidermis (H&E, original magnification × 100). (*F*) Histopathologic transverse section shows predominance of atypical melanocytes, isolated or in nests, enlarging the interpapillary spaces (*black arrows*) (H&E, original magnification × 100).

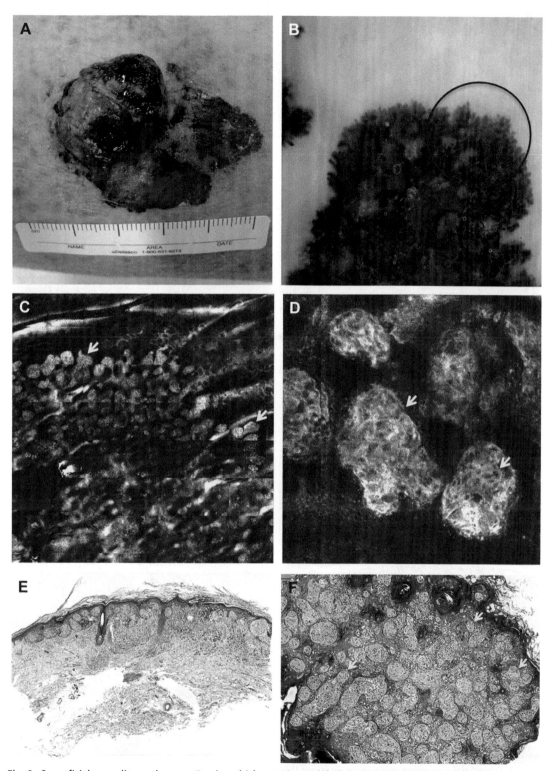

Fig. 9. Superficial spreading melanoma, Breslow thickness 10 mm. (*A*) Clinical image. (*B*) Dermoscopy shows pseudopods (*area inside the black circle*). (*C*) RCM mosaic image (3.5 × 3.5 mm) at the level of the DEJ showing compact aggregates of atypical cells distributed in a linear arrangement toward the periphery with a dense nest at the extremity (*arrows*). (*D*) RCM individual image at the level of the DEJ shows the pseudopods in detail, characterized by elongated, dense, and bright peripheral aggregate (*arrows*). (*E*) Histopathologic perpendicular section shows nests of atypical melanocytes distributed contiguously toward the periphery along the DEJ (H&E, original magnification × 40). (*F*) Histopathologic transverse section shows nests of atypical cells arranged in a linear manner throughout the periphery of the lesion (*arrows*) (H&E, original magnification × 100).

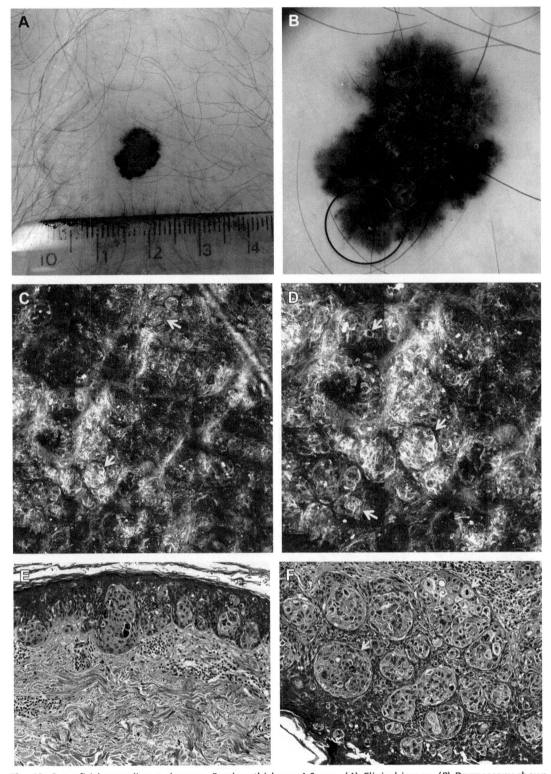

Fig. 10. Superficial spreading melanoma, Breslow thickness 1.0 mm. (*A*) Clinical image. (*B*) Dermoscopy shows irregular globules (*area inside the black circle*). (*C*) RCM mosaic image (2 × 2 mm) at the level of the DEJ showing irregularly shaped clusters (*arrows*). (*D*) RCM mosaic image (1 × 1 mm) at the level of the DEJ shows clusters with cells that are nonhomogeneous in morphologic features and reflectivity (*arrows*). (*E*) Histopathologic perpendicular section shows compact aggregates of atypical melanocytes with a slight intercellular discohesion (H&E, original magnification × 100). (*F*) Histopathologic transverse section shows large amount of atypical melanocytes predominantly in nests with variable size and shape (*arrows*) (H&E, original magnification × 200).

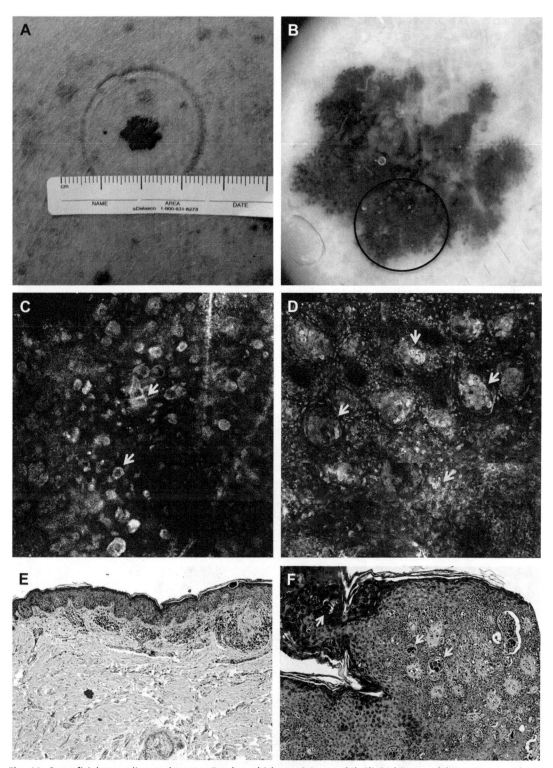

Fig. 11. Superficial spreading melanoma, Breslow thickness 0.5 mm. (*A*) Clinical image. (*B*) Dermoscopy shows blotch (*area inside the black circle*). (*C*) RCM individual image at the level of the epidermis showing round pagetoid cells (*arrows*). (*D*) RCM mosaic image (0.75 × 0.75 mm) at the level of the basal layer/DEJ shows bright clusters with atypical cells (*arrows*). (*E*) Histopathologic perpendicular section shows important pigmentation in the epidermis and dermis (H&E, original magnification × 40). (*F*) Histopathologic transverse section shows large amount of pigmented nests in the epidermis and orthokeratosis (*arrows*) (H&E, original magnification × 100).

- Sharp borders constituted by a peripheral rim of dense nests;
- Bright particles (corresponding to inflammatory infiltrate);
- Plump bright round and stellate cells (corresponding to melanophages).

Melanoma

There are several subtypes of melanoma, and the most prevalent is the superficial spreading melanoma.[16] There are well-described RCM features for diagnosis of superficial spreading melanoma that has close relationship with histopathology[5,8,16–18] (**Figs. 7–12, Table 3**), as follows:

- Loss of typical arrangement of the epidermis;
- Atypical cobblestone pattern, which is defined by atypical keratinocytes at the top of papillae;
- Pagetoid cells that could have roundish shape and hyporeflective nucleus or dendritic shape, scattered within the epidermis;
- Nonedged papillae in more than 10% of the lesion;

- Sheet of atypical melanocytes presenting a lot of bright cytoplasm and short and thick dendrites (atypical melanocytes) at epidermis and DEJ;
- Dendritic cells forming "bridges," called mitochondria-like structures, at the DEJ;
- Atypical meshwork, represented by junctional clusters with dendritic bright cells;
- Junctional and/or intradermal nests, which are usually dense and sparse with irregular shape and size (corresponding to irregular globules and/or pseudopods on dermoscopy);
- Coarse and huddle collagen, corresponding to solar elastosis in histopathology, and bright cells (inflammatory cells) and plump bright cells (melanophages) can be seen at the upper dermis.[18]

CONFOCAL MICROSCOPY CORRELATION IN NONMELANOCYTIC SKIN TUMORS
Basal Cell Carcinoma

The RCM features of basal cell carcinoma (BCC) lesions have already been described by previous studies and shown to have a good correlation

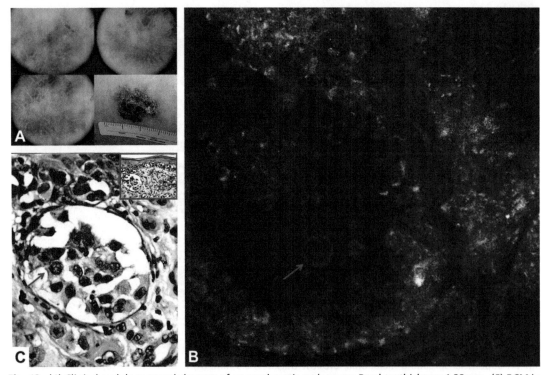

Fig. 12. (*A*) Clinical and dermoscopic images of an amelanotic melanoma, Breslow thickness 1.32 mm. (*B*) RCM individual image showing sparse nest with atypical melanocytes that are nonhomogeneous in morphologic features and reflectivity. Red arrow indicates an isolated atypical melanocyte in "B" and "C". (*C*) Histopathology shows aggregates of atypical melanocytes with an intercellular discohesion (H&E, original magnification × 200; inset × 100). Red arrow indicates single detached atypical tumoral cell inside nest in histopathology and confocal microscopy.

Table 3
Reflectance confocal microscopy features for melanoma and correlation with histopathology

RCM	Histopathology
Dendritic cells forming "bridges," called mitochondria-like structures, at the DEJ	Disarrangement of the rete ridges and increased number of atypical melanocytes (it is possible to see the mitochondrial structure in transverse section)
Nonedged papillae	Disarrangement of the rete ridges and increased number of atypical melanocytes in the epidermis
Cells with roundish shape and hyporeflective nucleus (pagetoid)	Pagetoid cells spreading in the epidermis
Sheet of cells with a lot of bright cytoplasm and short and thick dendrites in the epidermis and DEJ	Atypical melanocytes in the epidermis
Atypical meshwork, represented by junctional clusters with dendritic bright cells	Junctional clusters with atypical melanocytes cells
Dense and sparse nests, compact aggregates with large cells (atypical cells) at DEJ and dermis (irregular globules in dermoscopy)	Nest with atypical melanocytes cells in the DEJ and dermis
Dense nest, compact aggregates of atypical cells at DEJ toward the periphery (pseudopods in dermoscopy)	Nest with atypical melanocytes cells distributed contiguously toward the periphery along the DEJ
Bright coarse and huddle collagen at dermis	Elastosis
Bright cells at DEJ and dermis	Inflammatory infiltrated in the dermis
Plump cells are bright, round, and stellate cells in the dermis	Melanophages in the dermis

with the histopathologic diagnostic criteria of BCC.[16] Also, the utility of RCM for identification of BCC and for differentiation of BCC from other pigmented and pink neoplasms has been reported.[19]

The RCM features for BCC diagnosis are[8,20,21] described as follows; (**Figs. 13, 14** and **Table 4**)

- The presence of basaloid islands, seen as dark silhouettes or as bright tumor islands at the level of the DEJ or upper dermis;
- Streaming polarization of nuclei in neoplastic aggregates along the same axis of orientation, which corresponds to the tumor pushing the epidermis;

Table 4
Reflectance confocal microscopy features for BCC and correlation with histopathology

RCM	Histopathology
Dark silhouettes or bright islands at DEJ or upper dermis	Neoplastic aggregates or tumor islands at DEJ or upper dermis
Streaming polarization of nuclei along the same axis of orientation	Neoplastic aggregates pushing the epidermis
Peripheral palisading of nuclei at the tumor islands periphery	Peripheral palisading of nuclei at the tumor islands periphery
Dark peritumoral clefts around the tumor islands	Peritumoral clefts around the tumor islands
Bright thickened collagen bundles	Fibrotic stroma with thickened collagen bundles around the tumor islands
Linear blood vessels and coiled blood vessels	Dilated vessels around the tumor islands
Bright dendritic structures within tumor islands	Melanocytes within the tumor islands
Bright round cells in the stroma	Inflammatory cells and free melanin

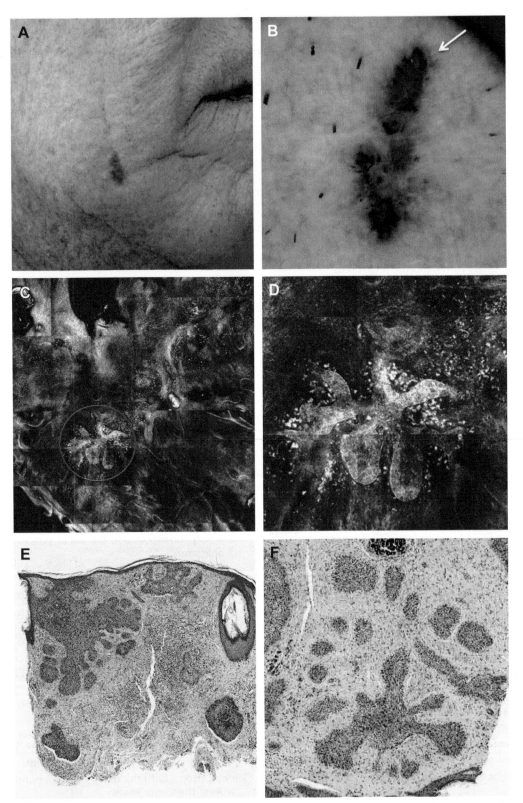

Fig. 13. Pigmented BCC. (*A*) Clinical image. (*B*) Dermoscopy shows leaflike area (*arrow*). (*C*) RCM mosaic image (3.5 × 3.5 mm) showing tumor islands (*circle*) in the dermis. (*D*) RCM mosaic image (1 × 1 mm) shows bright tumor islands in detail at the level of the upper dermis. (*E*) Histopathologic perpendicular section shows basaloid tumoral clusters enclosed by connective tissue stroma. Melanin was present inside the tumoral nests (H&E, original magnification × 40). (*F*) Histopathologic transverse section shows pigmented tumor clusters (H&E, original magnification × 100).

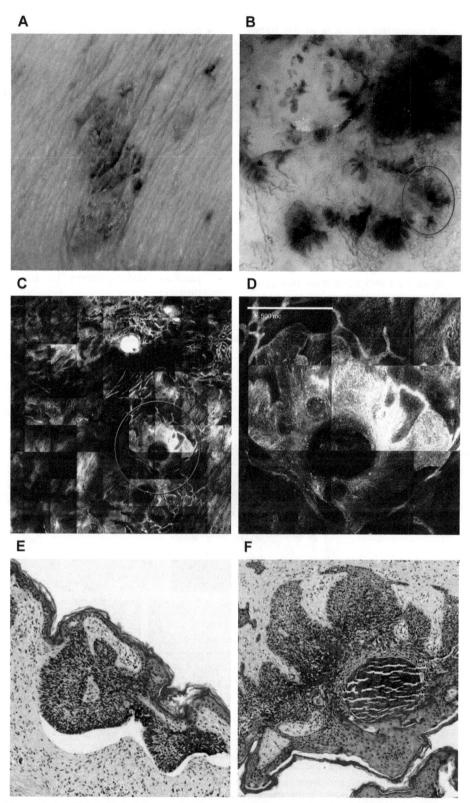

Fig. 14. Pigmented BCC. (*A*) Clinical image. (*B*) Dermoscopy shows spoke-wheel (*circle*). (*C*) RCM mosaic image (4.5 × 4.5 mm) showing bright tumor islands (*circle*) in the dermis. (*D*) RCM mosaic image (1.5 × 1.5 mm) shows bright tumor islands in detail at the level of the upper dermis. (*E*) Histopathologic perpendicular section shows basaloid tumoral clusters enclosed by connective tissue stroma (H&E, original magnification × 100). (*F*) Histopathologic transverse section shows pigmented tumor clusters (H&E, original magnification × 100).

- Peripheral palisading of nuclei at the tumor islands periphery;
- Dark peritumoral clefts around the tumor islands;
- Fibrotic stroma with thickened collagen bundles;
- Dilated and tortuous linear blood vessels and coiled blood vessels;
- Bright dendritic structures that correspond to melanocytes within tumor islands;
- Bright round cells in the stroma that correspond to inflammatory cells or free melanin found in histopathology.

Actinic Keratosis and Squamous Cell Carcinoma

Actinic keratosis (AK) and squamous cell carcinoma (SCC) have some overlapping features in RCM and histopathology, but their presence and architectural disarrangement at the epidermis are more pronounced and prevalent in SCC.[2,8,22]

The RCM features of AK lesions have also been described by previous studies and shown to have a good correlation with the histopathologic diagnostic criteria of AK. The RCM for AK diagnosis are as follows[2,8,22]:

- Superficial scale and detached corneocytes, corresponding to hyperkeratosis in histopathology;
- Nucleated cells with dark center and sharp demarcation at the level of the stratum corneum, corresponding to parakeratosis;
- Atypical honeycomb pattern, defined as variation of size and shape of keratinocytic nuclei and irregular cell borders with architectural disruption, corresponding to atypical proliferation of keratinocytes in histopathology;
- Collagen in bundles, corresponding to solar elastosis in histopathology;
- Small, highly refractive cells at the epidermal layer and/or superficial dermis, corresponding to inflammatory infiltrate;
- Round blood vessels in the center of dermal papillae, corresponding to blood vessel dilatation.

The examination of SCC by RCM reveals (Fig. 15) the following:

- Presence of scale at the stratum corneum level;
- Atypical honeycomb and/or a disarranged pattern at the spinous and granular layers, more pronounced than observed in AK;

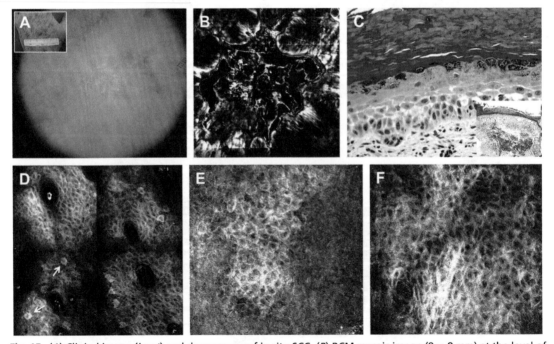

Fig. 15. (A) Clinical image (inset) and dermoscopy of in situ SCC. (B) RCM mosaic image (8 × 8 mm) at the level of the epidermis showing central scale at the stratum corneum. (C) Histopathology showing parakeratosis and atypical proliferation of keratinocytes in the entire epidermis thickness (H&E, original magnification × 200; inset × 40). (D) RCM individual image at the stratum corneum/granulosum showing polygonal nucleated cells (parakeratosis;arrow). (E, F) RCM individual images at the spinous-granular layer showing atypical honeycomb pattern, more pronounced than observed in AK.

- Polygonal nucleated cells at the stratum corneum, representing parakeratosis, and round nucleated cells at the spinous-granular layer corresponding to dyskeratotic cells;
- Large bright round and dendritic cells in spinous-granular layer, representing pigmented keratinocytes or melanocytes;
- Edged papillae with widened interpapillary spaces that are usually seen in solar lentigos, may also be seen in pigmented SCCs;
- Round or coiled (glomerular) blood vessels running perpendicular to the horizontal surface in the center of dermal papillae;
- Collagen in bundles at the dermis, corresponding to solar elastosis in histopathology;
- Small, highly refractive cells at the epidermal layer and/or superficial dermis, corresponding to inflammatory infiltrate;
- Plump, bright round and stellate cells within the dark dermal papillae, corresponding to melanophages can be present in pigmented SCC;
- The presence of nestlike structures in the dermis, which are highly suggestive of invasive SCC.

REFERENCES

1. Rajadhyaksha M, Gonzalez S, Zavislan JM, et al. In vivo confocal laser microscopy of human skin II: advances in instrumentation and comparison with histology. J Invest Dermatol 1999;113:293–303.
2. Pellacani G, Ulrich M, Casari A, et al. Grading keratinocyte atypia in actinic keratosis: a correlation of reflectance confocal microscopy and histopathology. J Eur Acad Dermatol Venereol 2015;29(11):2216–21.
3. Gill M, Longo C, Farnetani F, et al. Non-invasive in vivo dermatopathology: identification of reflectance confocal microscopic correlates to specific histological features seen in melanocytic neoplasms. J Eur Acad Dermatol Venereol 2014;28(8):1069–78.
4. Alarcon I, Carrera C, Palou J, et al. Impact of in vivo reflectance confocal microscopy on the number needed to treat melanoma in doubtful lesions. Br J Dermatol 2014;170(4):802–8.
5. Braga JC, Macedo MP, Pinto C, et al. Learning reflectance confocal microscopy of melanocytic skin lesions through histopathologic transversal sections. PLoS One 2013;8:e81205.
6. Pellacani G, Scope A, Farnetani F, et al. Towards an in vivo morphologic classification of melanocytic nevi. J Eur Acad Dermatol Venereol 2014;28(7):864–72.
7. Guitera P, Pellacani G, Longo C, et al. In vivo reflectance confocal microscopy enhances secondary evaluation of melanocytic lesions. J Invest Dermatol 2009;129:131–8.
8. Hofmann-Wellenhof R, Pellacani G, Malvehy J, et al. Reflectance confocal microscopy for skin diseases. 1st edition. Berlin (heidelberg): Springer-Verlag; 2012.
9. Pellacani G, Scope A, Ferrari B, et al. New insights into nevogenesis: in vivo characterization and follow-up of melanocytic nevi by reflectance confocal microscopy. J Am Acad Dermatol 2009; 61(6):1001–13.
10. Pellacani G, Vinceti M, Bassoli S, et al. Reflectance confocal microscopy and features of melanocytic lesions: an internet-based study of the reproducibility of terminology. Arch Dermatol 2009;145:1137–43.
11. Ahlgrimm-Siess V, Massone C, Koller S, et al. In vivo confocal scanning laser microscopy of common naevi with globular, homogeneous and reticular pattern in dermoscopy. Br J Dermatol 2008;158(5):1000–7.
12. Pellacani G, Cesinaro AM, Seidenari S. In vivo confocal reflectance microscopy for the characterization of melanocytic nests and correlation with dermoscopy and histology. Br J Dermatol 2005b;152:384–6.
13. Pellacani G, Longo C, Malvehy J, et al. In vivo confocal microscopic and histopathologic correlations of dermoscopic features in 202 melanocytic lesions. Arch Dermatol 2008;144:1597–608.
14. Scope A, Benvenuto-Andrade C, Agero AL, et al. Correlation of dermoscopic structures of melanocytic lesions to reflectance confocal microscopy. Arch Dermatol 2007;143:176–85.
15. Pellacani G, Farnetani F, Gonzalez S, et al. In vivo confocal microscopy for detection and grading of dysplastic nevi: a pilot study. J Am Acad Dermatol 2012;66:e109–21.
16. González S, Tannous Z. Real-time in vivo confocal reflectance confocal microscopy of basal cell carcinoma. J Am Acad Dermatol 2002;47:869–74.
17. Stevenson AD, Mickan S, Mallett S, et al. Systematic review of diagnostic accuracy of reflectance confocal microscopy for melanoma diagnosis in patients with clinically equivocal skin lesions. Dermatol Pract Concept 2013;3(4):19–27.
18. Longo C, Casari A, Beretti F, et al. Skin aging: in vivo microscopic assessment of epidermal and dermal changes by means of confocal microscopy. J Am Acad Dermatol 2013;68(3):e73–82.
19. Braga JC, Scope A, Klaz I, et al. The significance of reflectance confocal microscopy in the assessment of solitary pink skin lesions. J Am Acad Dermatol 2009;61:230–41.
20. Castro RP, Stephens A, Fraga-Braghiroli NA, et al. Accuracy of in vivo confocal microscopy for diagnosis of basal cell carcinoma: a comparative study between handheld and wide-probe confocal imaging. J Eur Acad Dermatol Venereol 2015;29(6):1164–9.

21. Longo C, Lallas A, Kyrgidis A, et al. Classifying distinct basal cell carcinoma subtype by means of dermatoscopy and reflectance confocal microscopy. J Am Acad Dermatol 2014;71(4): 716–24.e1.

22. Peppelman M, Nguyen KP, Hoogedoorn L, et al. Reflectance confocal microscopy: non-invasive distinction between actinic keratosis and squamous cell carcinoma. J Eur Acad Dermatol Venereol 2015; 29(7):1302–9.

Discriminating Nevi from Melanomas: Clues and Pitfalls

Cristina Carrera, MD, PhD[a], Ashfaq A. Marghoob, MD[b],*

KEYWORDS

- Atypical nevi • Confocal • Diagnostic accuracy • Differential diagnosis • Early detection • Nevus
- Melanoma

KEY POINTS

- The improved ability to differentiate nevi from melanoma via reflectance confocal microscopy (RCM) has the potential to greatly impact the management of patients with multiple atypical nevi, changing nevi, and hypomelanotic or amelanotic lesions.
- Clinically subtle melanomas usually reveal architectural disarray of the dermoepidermal junction (DEJ) with nonedged papillae and atypical nucleated cells along the basal layer; in addition, the presence of pagetoid cells consisting of large roundish and/or dendritic refractile cells is a prominent feature seen in many melanomas.
- Most nevi manifest edged papillae with a combination of benign patterns at DEJ (ie, clod pattern, ringed pattern, meshwork pattern). Mild focal architectural disarray may also be seen.
- False-positive cases of melanoma on RCM are often encountered when evaluating nevi that prove on histology to have a high degree of dysplasia, a spitzoid morphology, or are inflamed.
- False-negative cases of melanoma often reveal minimal architectural disarray on RCM. Although they tend to lack pagetoid cells, they also do not display any of the benign RCM nevus patterns.

INTRODUCTION

Challenges in Early Detection of Melanoma

Despite great advances made in the treatment of late-stage melanoma, the best chance of survival hinges on early detection.[1,2] However, detection pressure leading to a heightened sensitivity for finding thinner and smaller melanomas is usually coupled to a lowering of specificity, which results in the biopsy of many nevi. Ideally, surveillance of high-risk patients for melanoma via total-body skin examination aided by technology (eg, dermoscopy, reflectance confocal microscopy [RCM]) should aim to maintain a high sensitivity for the detection of melanoma while at the same time prevent the excision of as many nevi as possible.[3] Parameters that can be used to track surveillance efficiency is monitoring ones benign to malignant

No conflict of interests.
Funding Sources: The research at the Melanoma Unit in Barcelona is partially funded by: Spanish Fondo de Investigaciones Sanitarias grants 09/01393 and 12/00840; CIBER de Enfermedades Raras of the Instituto de Salud Carlos III, Spain; AGAUR 2009 SGR 1337 and AGAUR 2014_SGR_603 of the Catalan Government, Spain; European Commission under the 6th Framework Programme, Contract No. LSHC-CT-2006-018702 (GenoMEL) and by the European Commission under the 7th Framework Programme, Diagnoptics (CE_CIP-ICT-PSR-13-7); The National Cancer Institute (NCI) of the US National Institute of Health (NIH) (CA83115) and a grant from "Fundació La Marató de TV3, 201331-30", Catalonia, Spain.
[a] Melanoma Unit, Department of Dermatology, Hospital Clinic, Institut d'Investigacions Biomèdiques August Pi i Sunyer, CIBER de Enfermedades Raras, Instituto de Salud Carlos III, University of Barcelona, Villarroel 170, Escala 1-4, Barcelona 08036, Spain; [b] Dermatology Service, Department of Medicine, Memorial Sloan Kettering Cancer Center, 800 Veterans Memorial Highway, 2nd Floor, Hauppauge, NY 11788, USA
* Corresponding author.
E-mail address: marghooa@mskcc.org

Dermatol Clin 34 (2016) 395–409
http://dx.doi.org/10.1016/j.det.2016.05.003
0733-8635/16/$ – see front matter © 2016 Elsevier Inc. All rights reserved.

biopsy ratio (B:M ratio), ratio of thick to thin melanomas, and mean/median melanoma thickness. Total-body photography was one of the first technologies introduced aimed at improving the sensitivity and specificity for melanoma detection. It has been shown that total-body photographs lead to the detection of thinner melanomas and less biopsies of benign nevi with a B:M ratio of 17:1 compared with 45:1 when the examination is performed without photographs.[4] Dermoscopy has also been shown to lead to the diagnosis of thinner melanomas.[5] Dermoscopy and digital monitoring has further improved the B:M ratio to between 4 to 7:1[6–10] and RCM has continued to improved this ratio to about 2:1.[11–14] RCM has demonstrated an improvement in the diagnostic accuracy of physicians for melanoma detection with a mean sensitivity of 93% and specificity of 76%.[15]

Of course, although RCM can greatly impact diagnostic accuracy, it does require learning the features associated with melanoma and nevi. The first section of this article reviews the common clinical scenarios in which RCM can enhance the detection of early melanoma. The second part focuses on the main RCM features used to differentiate nevi from melanoma. Lastly, the RCM pitfalls, including the false-positive nevi and false-negative melanomas, are discussed.

ROLE OF REFLECTANCE CONFOCAL MICROSCOPY IN DETECTING MELANOMA: CLINICAL APPLICATIONS
Patients with the Atypical Mole Syndrome

Numerous studies have shown that individuals with many nevi and individuals with large acquired nevi (>5 mm in diameter) are at increased risk for developing melanoma. The presence of many nevi displaying increased variability of size, shape, and color allows easy identification of this high-risk population. Although melanoma may develop in association with any nevus, most melanomas develop de novo; thus, prophylactic excision of nevi is an inefficient strategy to prevent melanoma.[16] The methods used to find melanoma within a sea of many nevi relies on finding outlier lesions (the ugly duckling sign)[17,18] and in identifying lesions that are new or have changed over time. Although change is a highly sensitive criterion for melanoma detection, it lacks specificity. Less than 10% of changing lesions identified during digital total-body photography and digital sequential dermoscopy prove to be melanoma.[8,19] Several studies have demonstrated that focal dermoscopic structural changes are significantly associated with melanoma, however; it remains extremely difficult to differentiate changing atypical nevi from early melanoma via dermoscopy.[20]

Approximately 8% to 10% of lesions monitored with dermoscopy, total-body photography, and sequential digital dermoscopy end up getting biopsied.[8] If RCM is added as another investigative layer, approximately 70% of the excisions of changing or equivocal nevi could potentially be avoided without decreasing the sensitivity for melanoma detection.[20,21] Table 1 summarizes the RCM features used to help differentiate melanoma from nevi. The main RCM features associated with melanoma include the presence of roundish pagetoid cells, atypical cells at the basal layer, non-edged papilla, and nucleated atypical cells within the dermis. Based on the aforementioned features, 2 algorithms have been published that are designed to help diagnose melanoma via RCM with high sensitivity and specificity[11,12] (Figs. 1 and 2). In addition, another algorithm was created (Fig. 3) to assist in characterizing the degree of atypia present within melanocytic lesions.[22] The combination of dermoscopy, digital follow-up, and RCM in the evaluation of equivocal melanocytic lesions has dramatically reduced the number of excisions of benign lesions in patients with the atypical mole syndrome while at the same time improved our ability to detect subtle melanomas.[23] Figs. 4 and 5 showcase 2 lesions for which dermoscopy was unable to correctly diagnose the lesion as melanoma or dysplastic nevus; however, RCM was able to make the correct diagnosis.

Patients Receiving BRAF Inhibitors for BRAF Mutant-Metastatic Melanoma

It is well documented that nevi in patients receiving BRAF inhibitors frequently undergo changes. These patients are also at increased risk for developing new primary BRAF wild-type melanomas.[24–26] Although the natural biology of nevi changing under the influence of a BRAF inhibition remains unclear, many of these changing nevi have clinical, dermoscopic, RCM, and histopathology morphologic features that overlap with melanoma. Thus, any changing nevus that has RCM features suggestive of malignancy should be excised.[24,26]

Other Patients at High Risk for Melanoma

Carriers of mutations in high-susceptibility melanoma genes, such as CDKN2A, BAP1, POT1,[27] as well as patients with xeroderma pigmentosum,[28] albinism, red-hair MC1R polymorphisms, or immunosuppressed patients (eg, transplant recipients) may all benefit from surveillance to help find early curable melanoma using all of the aforementioned tools, including RCM.

Table 1
Confocal features used to differentiate melanoma from nevi

Evaluation Level	Melanoma	Atypical Nevus	Nevus
Epidermis	Marked or complete loss of honeycomb and/or cobblestone patterns Widespread pagetoid cells and large atypical bright cells	Variably disarranged honeycomb and/or cobblestone patterns A few focal isolated atypical cells mostly located towards the center of the lesion Pagetoid spread is absent or very limited in its extent	Well-conserved honeycombed pattern and/or Regular cobblestone pattern (when keratinocytes are pigmented)
DEJ	Poorly demarcated lesion Moderate to severe distortion of DEJ architecture Nonedged papillae (ill-defined dermal papillae) Irregular, elongated, and fused interpapillary crests resulting in junctional thickenings Moderate to severe cellular atypia at the basal layer	Well-circumscribed lesion Mild to severe distortion of DEJ architecture Focal areas of nonedged papillae and meshwork pattern Irregular, elongated, and fused interpapillary crests resulting in junctional thickenings Junctional nests with irregular shape, size, and location Variable atypia with hyper-refractile cells at basal layer	Well-circumscribed lesion Well-defined DEJ architecture Edged papillae (well-defined margins), regular in shape and distribution Bright basal cells forming cobblestone and ringed pattern Dense clusters and/or interpapillary processes forming meshwork and/or clod patterns
Dermis	Atypical nucleated cells within dermal papillae Cerebriform nests Bright non-nucleated plump cells (melanophages) Bright triangle particles (inflammation) Prominent and atypical vessels Coarse collagen bundles forming a gross networklike structure	Bright non-nucleated plump cells (melanophages) Bright triangle particles (inflammation) Coarse collagen bundles forming networklike structure	Regular dense and/or some sparse cells within the clods or clusters of cells at DEJ and superficial dermis Uniform cellularity within the clods (occasionally bright roundish nucleated uniform cells can be seen in congenital nevi) Regular vessels in the center of the papilla

Abbreviation: DEJ, dermoepidermal junction.

Dermoscopically Feature-Poor and Amelanotic Tumors

Lesions that reveal nonspecific or few to no dermoscopic structures are known as featureless or structureless lesions. These dermoscopic feature-poor lesions pose a challenge because melanomas as well as benign lesions can present in this manner. Before availability of RCM, the management of these lesions was to biopsy them or to subject them to digital monitoring and resort to biopsy if changes developed. RCM has facilitated our ability to correctly diagnose many of these dermoscopic

RISK CRITERIA Barcelona Algorithm (Melanoma ≥−1)

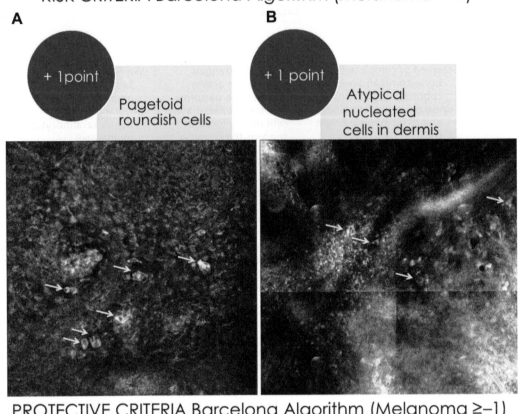

A + 1 point — Pagetoid roundish cells

B + 1 point — Atypical nucleated cells in dermis

PROTECTIVE CRITERIA Barcelona Algorithm (Melanoma ≥−1)

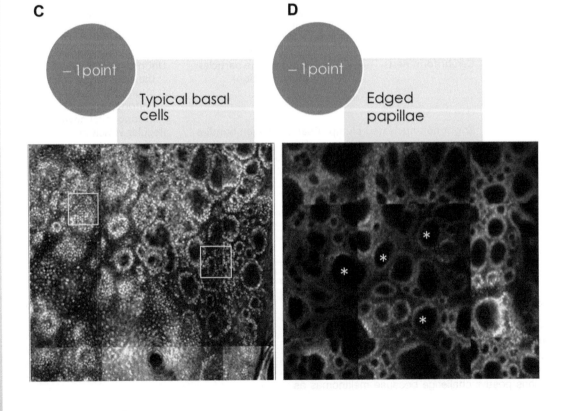

C − 1 point — Typical basal cells

D − 1 point — Edged papillae

feature poor. A recent retrospective study demonstrated that among 130 featureless lesions,[29] all the melanomas (n = 6 cases) were correctly diagnosed based on the presence of many roundish pagetoid cells (5 or more per square millimeter) and/or by marked disarrangement of the junctional architecture. In contrast, only 17.7% (n = 30) of nevi were incorrectly diagnosed as melanoma (false positive).[30] In addition, RCM was also found to be helpful in evaluating small-diameter (ie, incipient melanomas) melanomas.[31] With RCM, the combination of cytologic atypia with cellular pleomorphism and architectural disorder with irregular clods was found to be strong criteria for the identification of incipient melanomas. Each of the following 3 RCM features were found to be independently associated with small melanomas: the presence of at least 5 pagetoid cells per square millimeter, dendrites or tangled lines (meaning short fine lines with no visible nucleus interlacing the keratynocytes) within the epidermis, and atypical roundish cells at the dermoepidermal junction (DEJ) (see **Fig. 4**).

Amelanotic melanomas are by definition feature-poor lesions. However, because melanocytes, including melanocytes in amelanotic tumors, contain highly refractile melanosomes, RCM has proven to be an ideal instrument for analyzing these lesions. RCM enables the visualization of architectural and cytologic structures in melanocytic tumors, including tumors lacking pigment on dermoscopy (**Fig. 6**). It has been shown that RCM improves the ability to correctly identify both nevi and early melanomas in red-haired and fair skin–type patients, such as those with albinism.[32–34]

Collision Tumors

Collision tumors can be difficult to diagnose based on dermoscopy findings. This difficulty is especially true for collision tumors composed of a malignancy arising in association with a benign lesion. In one study, RCM was able to identify the malignant component in 19 out of 20 collision tumors.[35]

REFLECTANCE CONFOCAL MICROSCOPY FEATURES USED TO DIFFERENTIATE NEVI FROM MELANOMA

Histopathologic-proven benign nevi that are dermoscopically equivocal or atypical (ie, false positive for melanoma on dermoscopy) are usually easy to differentiate from melanoma by RCM. Melanoma can be ruled out if the lesion displays typical RCM features encountered in nevi while at the same time lacking the features associated with melanoma. The following 5 scenarios are most commonly encountered in routine practice. In all 5 cases the nevi are found to be clinically or dermoscopically equivocal, but RCM reveals a benign pattern.

a. Dermoscopy reveals an atypical or irregular pigment pattern (eg, atypical network, irregular globules, eccentric asymmetric dermoscopic islands with darker pigment; RCM shows a well-circumscribed nevus with edged papilla and a clod, ringed or meshwork pattern.[36]

b. Dermoscopy reveals a hyperpigmented structureless pattern (black lamella and/or black-blue area), and RCM shows a regular cobblestone pattern of the epidermis and/or a dense infiltration of melanophages appearing as bright plump cells in the superficial dermis. The cobblestone pattern corresponds to melanized keratinocytes situated in the basal and spinous layers of the skin.

c. Dermoscopy of a pink macule reveals a nonspecific vascular pattern; RCM demonstrates one of the aforementioned benign nevus patterns or a Spitz nevus pattern consisting of regular

---

Fig. 1. The Barcelona algorithm[12] is a 2-step process. The first step requires the clinician to differentiate melanocytic from nonmelanocytic tumors. A melanocytic lesion should be suspected if the dermal papillae are visualized and at least one of the following features is also seen: cobblestone pattern, pagetoid cells, and/or refractile nests. Lesions not displaying any of the aforementioned features are then evaluated to determine if they have any RCM features diagnostic of basal cell carcinoma, seborrheic keratosis, angioma, or dermatofibroma. If not, then by default the lesion is considered to be a melanocytic tumor. The second step of the *Barcelona algorithm helps to differentiate melanoma from nevus.* Lesions that are dermoscopically suspicious for melanoma are evaluated via RCM for the presence of 2 risk features (+1 point) and 2 protective features (−1 point) for melanoma diagnosis. The high-risk criteria include (*A*) pagetoid roundish cells in the superficial epidermal layers (*yellow arrows*) and (*B*) atypical nucleated cells in the papillary dermis (*yellow arrows*). The protective criteria include (*C*) presence of typical basal cells (*squares*) and (*D*) presence of edged papillae (*asterisks*) at the dermoepidermal junction. The points for the presence of any of the 4 features are summed together, and the final score is used to predict the probability of melanoma. Lesions with a score of −1 or greater have a sensitivity of 100% and specificity of 57.1% for melanoma. Lesions with scores of 0 or greater have a high probability of being melanoma with a sensitivity of 86.1% and specificity of 95.3%.

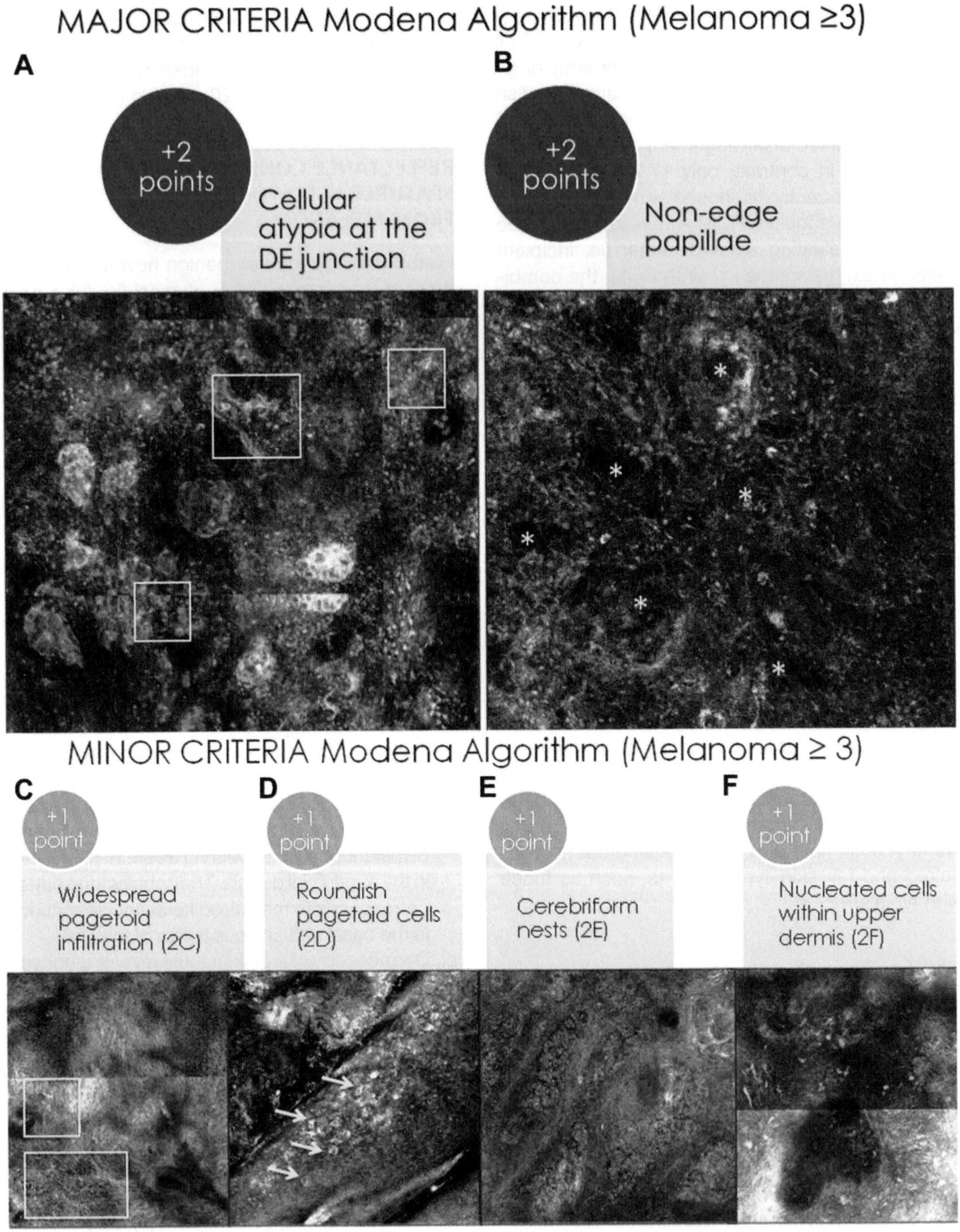

MAJOR CRITERIA Modena Algorithm (Melanoma ≥3)

A

+2 points

Cellular atypia at the DE junction

B

+2 points

Non-edge papillae

MINOR CRITERIA Modena Algorithm (Melanoma ≥ 3)

C

+1 point

Widespread pagetoid infiltration (2C)

D

+1 point

Roundish pagetoid cells (2D)

E

+1 point

Cerebriform nests (2E)

F

+1 point

Nucleated cells within upper dermis (2F)

Fig. 2. Modena algorithm[11] classifies lesions into melanoma or nevus based on the presence of 2 main risk features (+2 points for the presence of each, for a maximum of 4 points) observed at dermoepidermal (DE) junction: (1) cellular atypia at basal layer (*A, squares*); (2) nonedged papillae (*B, asterisks*). In addition, the lesion is evaluated for the presence of 4 minor risk features (+1 point for the presence of each, for a maximum of 4 points): (1) widespread pagetoid infiltration of spinous layer (*C, squares*); (2) roundish pagetoid cells (*D, arrows*); (3) cerebriform nests in dermis (*E, squares*); (4) nucleated atypical cells in upper dermis (*F, arrows*). Lesions with a total score of 3 or greater should be excised to rule out melanoma (sensitivity 91.9%, specificity 69.3%).

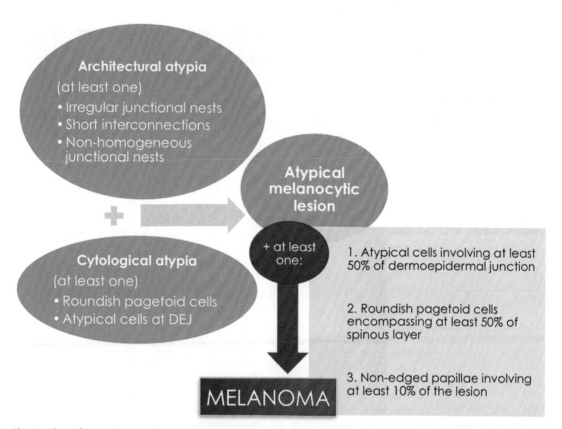

Architectural atypia
(at least one)
• Irregular junctional nests
• Short interconnections
• Non-homogeneous junctional nests

+

Cytological atypia
(at least one)
• Roundish pagetoid cells
• Atypical cells at DEJ

Atypical melanocytic lesion

+ at least one:

1. Atypical cells involving at least 50% of dermoepidermal junction

2. Roundish pagetoid cells encompassing at least 50% of spinous layer

3. Non-edged papillae involving at least 10% of the lesion

MELANOMA

Fig. 3. Algorithm to distinguish dysplastic nevi from melanoma as described by Pellacani and colleagues.[22] First step requires evaluation of the lesion for the presence or absence of cytologic and architectural atypia; junctional nests of different size or with sparse cells of differing refractility (nonhomogeneous) are considered irregular. Junctional thickenings or short interconnections are irregular refractile aggregates between papillae. Absence of atypical cells in epidermis and atypical junctional nests or aggregates is suggestive of a benign nondysplastic nevus. The second step quantifies the degree of atypia and allows differentiation of probable dysplastic nevi from melanoma. The presence of widespread pagetoid infiltration encompassing at least 50% of lesion, diffuse cytologic atypia at the dermoepidermal junction (DEJ) involving at least 50% of lesion, or nonedged papillae encompassing at least 10% of the lesion is suggestive of melanoma.

dense uniform clods occupying the entire epidermis, DEJ, and superficial dermis.[37]

d. Many melanomas found because of changes noted on sequential digital dermoscopy are dermoscopically featureless lesions and, based on primary morphology alone, are not distinguishable from nevi. It has also been shown that less than 20% of changing lesions found on sequential digital dermoscopy prove to be melanoma.[8] However, as discussed previously, these dermoscopically featureless melanomas can usually be correctly diagnosed with RCM. And according to recent publications, approximately 70% of the changing nevi reveal one of the benign RCM nevus patterns mentioned previously[20,21,34] (see **Fig. 5**).

e. Recurrent pigmentation in a scar of a previously biopsied presumed nevus can be disconcerting. In most cases the repigmentation

is due to benign reactive pigmentation or due to persistence of an incompletely excised nevus. However, on rare occasions, the recurrent pigmentation may represent melanoma. RCM can assist in evaluating these lesions. In the absence of atypical RCM features, such as pagetoid infiltration of the epidermis or atypical nucleated cells at the DEJ, the likelihood of melanoma becomes exceeding remote.[38]

CHALLENGING LESIONS ON REFLECTANCE CONFOCAL MICROSCOPY: PITFALLS OF REFLECTANCE CONFOCAL MICROSCOPY

Unfortunately, diagnostic accuracy by RCM is not 100% and therefore it is necessary to acknowledge some limitations of the technique and to interpret the findings in context with the entire clinical scenario (**Box 1**).

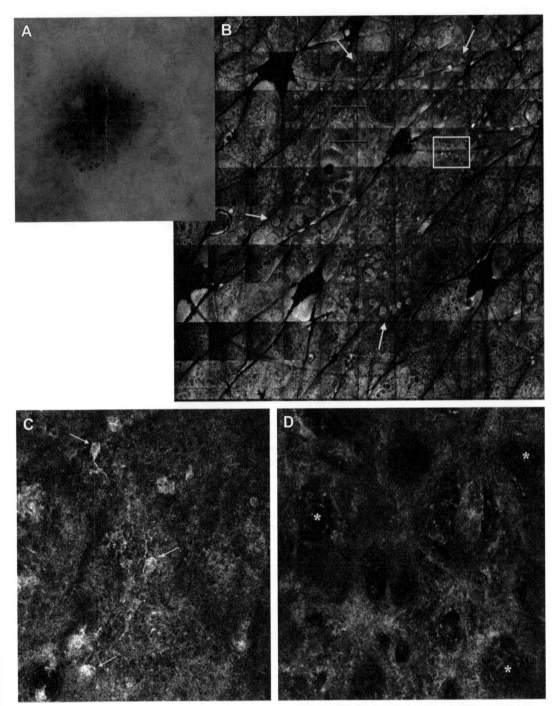

Fig. 4. (*A*) Dermoscopy of a 3.0 × 3.5-mm new pigmented lesion noted on the forearm of a patient with a history of multiple primary melanomas. The lesion has a globular pattern with an irregular arrangement of globules at the periphery. (*B*) A 5 × 5-mm RCM mosaic at the dermoepidermal junction (DEJ) layer shows a well-demarcated lesion that is predominantly composed of a clod pattern at the periphery (*arrows*). A few small irregular nonaggregated clusters are visible (*red square*) and isolated eccentric pagetoid cells can also be seen (*yellow square*). (*C*) Single RCM image shows large atypical roundish and dendritic pagetoid cells within the superficial epidermis (*yellow arrows*). (*D*) Single RCM image at DEJ displaying nonedged papillae (*asterisks*) and junctional thickenings (*red arrow*) with dendritic cells along the basal layer. DIAGNOSIS: in situ melanoma.

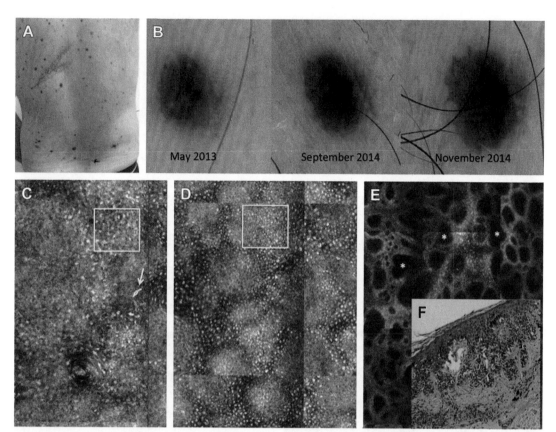

Fig. 5. (*A*) This patient has a history of multiple primary melanomas. Two changing lesions were detected on his back during digital surveillance. (*B*) Sequential digital dermoscopy of the 3-mm lesion on the central lumbar area disclosed progressive enlargement of the lesion with development of an atypical network and peripheral blotch. (*C*, *D*) RCM mosaics of epidermal layers show a well-conserved cobblestone pattern (*yellow squares*). One single isolated small dendritic cell was visible in the superficial layers (*arrow*). (*E*) Mosaic at dermoepidermal junction level shows typical architecture composed of edged papillae (*asterisks*) and meshwork pattern with typical basal cells between the dermal papillae. (*F*) A compound nevus with a lentiginous growth pattern, bridging of rete ridges, and moderate dysplasia (hematoxylin-eosin, original magnification ×20). These features correlate to the meshwork pattern and junctional thickening seen in (*E*). DIAGNOSIS: Compound melanocytic nevus with moderate atypia.

False-Negative Melanomas

False-negative melanomas are those that manifest a morphology resembling a benign lesion. Recently it was estimated that less than 4% of melanomas fail to be detected with RCM alone; however, just one case out of 201 would have failed detection if the RCM findings were seen in context with the clinical and/or dermoscopic examination. Thus, placing RCM findings in context with patient-related information and clinical history will help avoid missing most of these melanomas.[39]

Nodular/dermal/desmoplastic melanoma

Melanomas in which the diagnostic pathology features are located below the papillary dermis cannot be diagnosed with RCM because the

imaging of RCM is unable to penetrate past the depth of approximately 150 to 200 μm. Pure nodular melanomas[40] often reveal a thin and well-conserved epidermis with a normal honeycombed pattern with fewer atypical features, such as pagetoid cells in the suprabasal layer. In such cases, the RCM findings can mistakenly lead to a benign diagnosis. In some cases, RCM may only reveal inflammation and a disarranged architectural pattern that may lead to an incorrect diagnosis of an irritated nevus. However, a retrospective study by Longo and colleagues[41] evaluated 140 nodular lesions (including 23 pure nodular melanomas) and they found that approximately 86% of nodular lesions that were not ulcerated or hyperkeratotic were correctly diagnosed via RCM examination. Remarkably, RCM reached

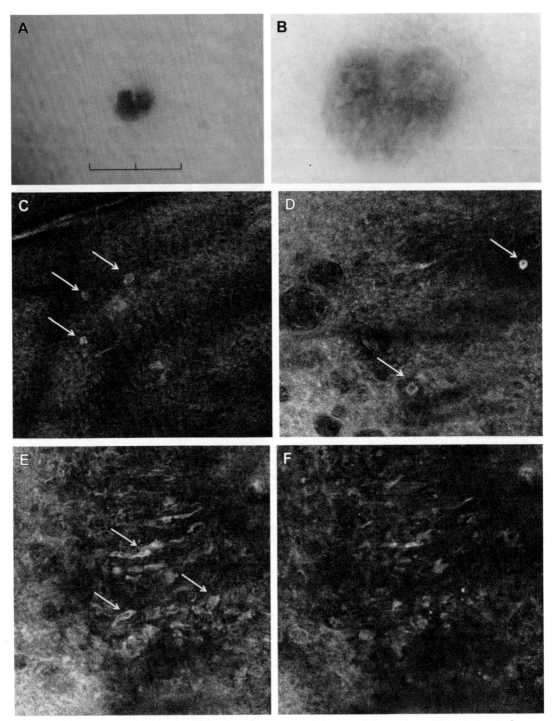

Fig. 6. (A) This 5-mm hypomelanotic lesion was noted on the abdomen of this patient. (B) Dermoscopy features were nondiagnostic revealing erythema, milky red area, dotted and linear irregular vessels. (C) RCM examination shows pagetoid roundish cells (*arrows*) both in the superficial epidermal layers (C) and at the DEJ (*D–F*). Atypical roundish and dendritic large cells are seen along the basal layer resulting in disruption of the DEJ, and nonedged papillae can also be seen (*F*). DIAGNOSIS: Superficial spreading melanoma, Breslow 0.5 mm.

Box 1
Pitfalls in reflectance confocal microscopy

Possible false-positive melanoma by RCM

1. Atypical nevi with a high degree of atypia

2. Nevi with focal pagetoid cells infiltrating the epidermis as can occur in nevi of special sites or in acral or mucosal nevi; can also be seen in inflamed nevi, such as halo nevi

3. Spitz nevi or spitzoid lesions

4. Nevi after acute UV light exposure

Possible false-negative melanomas by RCM

1. There is a nodular, dermal, or desmoplastic melanoma. Deep component of melanomas cannot be assessed via RCM because of limitations in the depth of RCM light penetration, which is about 200 μm.

2. Nevoid melanoma may only have focal pagetoid infiltration and may consist of small monomorphic melanoma cells, which can resemble the cells seen in nevi.

3. Focal melanoma arising in a nevus. The focal melanoma features may get overlooked in an otherwise benign appearing RCM background revealing features of the nevus.

4. Verrucous melanomas or seborrheic keratosis–like melanomas with heavily pigmented epidermis.

96.5% sensitivity and 94.1% specificity for the diagnosis of melanoma despite the fact that all lesions were nodular palpable lesions.[41] In nodular melanoma, one may observe a disarranged DEJ, nonedged papillae, and/or cerebriform nests in the superficial dermis. It should be noted that the presence of cerebriform nests on RCM is highly specific for nodular areas of invasive melanoma.

Nevoid melanoma

Melanomas composed cytologically of mostly small-melanocytes forming nests are diagnostically challenging not only by RCM but also by histopathology.

Verrucous melanoma

RCM of lesions, including melanomas, that are heavily pigmented and associated with hyperkeratosis or ulceration are challenging. This challenge stems from the fact that, in hyperkeratotic lesions, the RCM light penetration often does not reach to a sufficient depth to allow clear visualization of DEJ. However, a few cases have been reported whereby RCM allowed for the observation of melanocytic proliferation at the DEJ.[42]

Early melanomas arising in melanocytic nevi The RCM pitfall here stems from the fact that the malignant findings may be located focally and, therefore, get missed on RCM imaging within the background context of an otherwise typical RCM melanocytic nevus morphology. To avoid this pitfall requires complete and meticulous examination of the entire lesion via RCM, which can be a time-consuming endeavor.[43]

False-Positive Melanomas

False-positive melanomas are nevi that display RCM morphologic features suggestive of melanoma.

Spitz nevi or heavily pigmented fusiform cellular nevi (Reed nevi)

Although the presence of pagetoid spread of melanocytes within the epidermis is an important clue for melanoma diagnosis, this feature is also observable in Spitz nevi. In Spitz nevi the pagetoid cells are usually sporadically distributed in the suprabasal layers and clustered toward the center of the lesion, whereas in melanoma these cells are randomly distributed in a more diffuse manner. However, in the face of an RCM image displaying pagetoid cells, it is often impossible to differentiate Spitz tumors from melanoma. Spitz nevi can also be an RCM pitfall because, similar to melanoma, they can manifest architectural disarray and cytologic atypia.[44,45] Of course, the depth of penetration of RCM imaging precludes any ability to evaluate the presence of cell maturation in the deeper dermis, which is an important feature of these nevi. Although Spitz nevi can have pagetoid cells, Spitz nevi often display a normal honeycombed pattern on RCM. The globular Spitz nevi present with elongated clods and clusters at the DEJ. These clusters tend to be of uniform size and shape with a tendency toward confluence. They also have a characteristic abrupt border with refractive polygonal aggregates or clods at the lesion's perimeter. In the case of heavily pigmented melanocytic lesions displaying a blue color, RCM enables the distinction between blue veil due to regression and blue veil due to melanocytosis. The former is characterized by plump bright cells on RCM, which corresponds to melanophages and inflammatory infiltrate in the papillary dermis on histology. The latter is characterized by the presence of epidermal and dermal features consistent with diagnosis of melanoma and includes the following features: disarranged pattern, pagetoid cells, cytologic and architectural atypia, nonhomogeneous and cerebriform clusters, and dermal nucleated cells (Fig. 7).

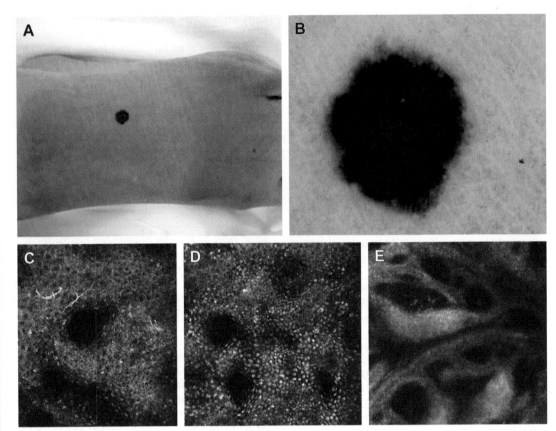

Fig. 7. (*A*) This patient presented with a rapidly growing and heavily pigmented lesion on the dorsum of her foot. (*B*) Symmetric dark brown to black lesion with a superficial black network seen with dermoscopy is fairly characteristic of a Reed's nevus. (*C*) Single RCM image of the superficial epidermis shows a honeycomb pattern with isolated dendritic pagetoid cells. (*D*) Single RCM image along the spinosum epidermal layer shows the typical cobblestone pattern, which is due to the presence of pigmented keratinocytes. (*E*) Single RCM image along the DEJ reveals a meshwork pattern with regular and dense aggregates and junctional thickenings and edged papillae. A few refractile non-nucleated cells within the papillae, corresponding to melanophages, can be seen. DIAGNOSIS: Pigmented fusiform cellular Spitz nevus (Reed nevus).

Nevi with pagetoid infiltration of single cells

RCM enables excellent visualization of melanocytes spreading upward in a pagetoid fashion. The problem is that the simple presence of pagetoid cells does not make a diagnosis of melanoma. For example, pagetoid cells can be seen in Spitz nevi and nevi of special sites such as those on the breast and genital region. Pathologists interpret the significance of pagetoid spread by evaluating the degree of spread within the context of the rest of the lesion when differentiating nevi from melanoma. However, because the entire cellular details, including evaluating cellular maturation as a function of depth, cannot be assessed adequately with RCM, the visualization of pagetoid infiltration on RCM in a nevus usually leads to a false-positive diagnosis of melanoma. Although it has been suggested that the presence of a disarranged pattern in the superficial layers together with numerous large and closely arranged cells extending into the stratum corneum correlates strongly with malignancy, melanoma cannot be excluded simply based on the absence or paucity of pagetoid cells on RCM imaging because at least 10% of melanomas will have no or only a few such cells.[46]

Inflamed or irritated nevi

RCM imaging of inflamed nevi including halo nevi and nevi with eczematouslike inflammation (Meyerson nevus) reveal architectural disarray at the DEJ, bright particles, and plump bright cells (corresponding to melanophages) in the dermal papillae. In addition, these nevi can also show roundish and dendritic pagetoid cells on RCM imaging. Although the dendritic cells noted in these inflamed nevi correspond to intraepidermal melanocytes, more often than not they correspond to

Langerhans cells (presented by Martins da Silva V et al. at the 73rd American Academy of Dermatology [AAD] meeting, San Francisco, unpublished data, 2015). Currently it is impossible to differentiate, with certainty, dendritic melanocytes from Langerhans cells via RCM imaging.[47]

Nevi after ultraviolet radiation exposure

It has been demonstrated that acute and repeated UV radiation (UVR) exposure to nevi can lead to transient melanomalike findings on dermoscopy, RCM, and even histopathology. Several studies have demonstrated melanocytic activation and cell proliferation in nevi after a single dose of UV-B.[48,49] Inflammation-induced changes and melanocytic activation can in fact be observed in vivo, with RCM revealing the presence of intraepidermal dendritic cells and bright particles at DEJ and papillary dermis. If RCM features were evaluated in isolation and without knowledge that the nevus was recently irradiated by UVR, the RCM features would lead to the false diagnosis of melanoma (presented by Takigami MC et al. at the 73rd American Academy, San Francisco, unpublished data, 2015).

SUMMARY

Accurate and thorough RCM evaluation of clinically and dermoscopically equivocal melanocytic lesions allows for improved differentiating of melanoma from nevi. It leads to the recognition of incipient melanomas while at the same time decreasing the unnecessary excision of many nevi. However, although RCM has significantly improved our sensitivity and specificity and impacted our B:M ratio in a positive manner, it is not 100% accurate. The situations responsible for a false-positive diagnosis of melanoma and perhaps more importantly the situations resulting in a false-negative diagnosis of melanoma are important to acknowledge. Obviously, it is imperative that the RCM operator also understands the limitations of RCM, such as its inability to view the deeper component of lesions. As a general rule, correlation should always be sought between the clinical, dermoscopic, and RCM findings for all lesions. This correlation will help minimize the risk of missing melanomas. In other words, RCM should be viewed as a complementary tool that needs to be integrated with other diagnostic data. Although all this information may create noise, the experienced clinician will be able see the signal to help him or her arrive at the correct management decision via abductive reasoning. For example, in the case of flat lesions with significant clinical-dermoscopic concern but with benign features on RCM imaging, short-term digital monitoring would be an acceptable alternative to immediate biopsy. In contrast, suspicious nodular lesions should be biopsied even if no concerning features are seen on RCM imaging.[50]

It should be intuitively obvious that training and experience with RCM image acquisition, RCM image interpretation, and dermatopathology will improve the operator's diagnostic acumen.

REFERENCES

1. Katalinic A, Waldmann A, Weinstock MA, et al. Does skin cancer screening save lives? An observational study comparing trends in melanoma mortality in regions with and without screening [Internet]. Cancer 2012;118(21):5395–402.
2. Aneja S, Aneja S, Bordeaux JS. Association of increased dermatologist density with lower melanoma mortality. Arch Dermatol 2012;148(2):174–8.
3. Argenziano G, Zalaudek I, Hofmann-Wellenhof R, et al. Total body skin examination for skin cancer screening in patients with focused symptoms. J Am Acad Dermatol 2012;66(2):212–9.
4. Goodson AG, Florell SR, Hyde M, et al. Comparative analysis of total body and dermatoscopic photographic monitoring of nevi in similar patient populations at risk for cutaneous melanoma [Internet]. Dermatol Surg 2010;36(7):1087–98.
5. Haenssle HA, Hoffmann S, Holzkamp R, et al. Melanoma thickness: the role of patients' characteristics, risk indicators and patterns of diagnosis. J Eur Acad Dermatol Venereol 2015;29:102–8.
6. Carli P, De Giorgi V, Crocetti E, et al. Improvement of malignant/benign ratio in excised melanocytic lesions in the "dermoscopy era": a retrospective study 1997-2001 [Internet]. Br J Dermatol 2004;150(4):687–92.
7. Salerni G, Carrera C, Lovatto L, et al. Benefits of total body photography and digital dermatoscopy ("two-step method of digital follow-up") in the early diagnosis of melanoma in patients at high risk for melanoma [Internet]. J Am Acad Dermatol 2012;67(1):e17–27.
8. Salerni G, Terán T, Puig S, et al. Meta-analysis of digital dermoscopy follow-up of melanocytic skin lesions: a study on behalf of the International Dermoscopy Society [Internet]. J Eur Acad Dermatol Venereol 2013;27(7):805–14.
9. Vestergaard ME, Macaskill P, Holt PE, et al. Dermoscopy compared with naked eye examination for the diagnosis of primary melanoma: a meta-analysis of studies performed in a clinical setting [Internet]. Br J Dermatol 2008;159(3):669–76.
10. Argenziano G, Cerroni L, Zalaudek I, et al. Accuracy in melanoma detection: a 10-year multicenter survey [Internet]. J Am Acad Dermatol 2012;67(1):54–9.

11. Pellacani G, Guitera P, Longo C, et al. The impact of in vivo reflectance confocal microscopy for the diagnostic accuracy of melanoma and equivocal melanocytic lesions [Internet]. J Invest Dermatol 2007;127(12):2759–65.

12. Segura S, Puig S, Carrera C, et al. Development of a two-step method for the diagnosis of melanoma by reflectance confocal microscopy [Internet]. J Am Acad Dermatol 2009;61(2):216–29.

13. Alarcon I, Carrera C, Palou J, et al. Impact of in vivo reflectance confocal microscopy on the number needed to treat melanoma in doubtful lesions [Internet]. Br J Dermatol 2013;170(4):802–8.

14. Pellacani G, Pepe P, Casari A, et al. Reflectance confocal microscopy as a second-level examination in skin oncology improves diagnostic accuracy and saves unnecessary excisions: a longitudinal prospective study. Br J Dermatol 2014;171(5):1044–51.

15. Stevenson AD, Mickan S, Mallett S, et al. Systematic review of diagnostic accuracy of reflectance confocal microscopy for melanoma diagnosis in patients with clinically equivocal skin lesions [Internet]. Dermatol Pract Concept 2013;3(4):19–27.

16. Tsao H, Bevona C, Goggins W, et al. The transformation rate of moles (melanocytic nevi) into cutaneous melanoma: a population-based estimate [Internet]. Arch Dermatol 2003;139(3):282–8.

17. Scope A, Dusza SW, Halpern AC, et al. The "ugly duckling" sign: agreement between observers [Internet]. Arch Dermatol 2008;144(1):58–64.

18. Argenziano G, Catricalà C, Ardigo M, et al. Dermoscopy of patients with multiple nevi: Improved management recommendations using a comparative diagnostic approach [Internet]. Arch Dermatol 2011;147(1):46–9.

19. Salerni G, Carrera C, Lovatto L, et al. Characterization of 1152 lesions excised over 10 years using total-body photography and digital dermatoscopy in the surveillance of patients at high risk for melanoma [Internet]. J Am Acad Dermatol 2012;67(5):836–45.

20. Lovatto L, Carrera C, Salerni G, et al. In vivo reflectance confocal microscopy of equivocal melanocytic lesions detected by digital dermoscopy follow-up [Internet]. J Eur Acad Dermatol Venereol 2015;29(10):1918–25.

21. Stanganelli I, Longo C, Mazzoni L, et al. Integration of reflectance confocal microscopy in sequential dermoscopy follow-up improves melanoma detection accuracy [Internet]. Br J Dermatol 2015;172(2):365–71.

22. Pellacani G, Farnetani F, Gonzalez S, et al. In vivo confocal microscopy for detection and grading of dysplastic nevi: a pilot study [Internet]. J Am Acad Dermatol 2012;66(3):e109–21.

23. Carrera C. High-risk melanoma patients: can unnecessary naevi biopsies be avoided? [Internet]. Br J Dermatol 2015;172(2):313–5.

24. Debarbieux S, Dalle S, Depaepe L, et al. Second primary melanomas treated with BRAF blockers: study by reflectance confocal microscopy [Internet]. Br J Dermatol 2013;168(6):1230–5.

25. Perier-Muzet M, Thomas L, Poulalhon N, et al. Melanoma patients under vemurafenib: prospective follow-up of melanocytic lesions by digital dermoscopy [Internet]. J Invest Dermatol 2014;134(5):1351–8. Available at: http://www.nature.com/doifinder/10.1038/jid.2013.462.

26. Carrera C, Puig-Butillè JA, Tell-Marti G, et al. Multiple BRAF wild-type melanomas during dabrafenib treatment for metastatic BRAF -mutant melanoma [Internet]. JAMA Dermatol 2015;151(5):544.

27. Potrony M, Badenas C, Aguilera P, et al. Update in genetic susceptibility in melanoma [Internet]. Ann Transl Med 2015;3(15):210. Available at: http://www.pubmedcentral.nih.gov/articlerender.fcgi?artid=4583600&tool=pmcentrez&rendertype=abstract.

28. Bradford PT, Goldstein AM, Tamura D, et al. Cancer and neurologic degeneration in xeroderma pigmentosum: long term follow-up characterises the role of DNA repair [Internet]. J Med Genet 2011;48(3):168–76. Available at: http://www.pubmedcentral.nih.gov/articlerender.fcgi?artid=3235003&tool=pmcentrez&rendertype=abstract.

29. Argenziano G, Fabbrocini G, Carli P, et al. Epiluminescence microscopy for the diagnosis of doubtful melanocytic skin lesions. Comparison of the ABCD rule of dermatoscopy and a new 7-point checklist based on pattern analysis [Internet]. Arch Dermatol 1998;134(12):1563–70.

30. Ferrari B, Pupelli G, Farnetani F, et al. Dermoscopic difficult lesions: an objective evaluation of reflectance confocal microscopy impact for accurate diagnosis [Internet]. J Eur Acad Dermatol Venereol 2015;29(6):1135–40.

31. Pupelli G, Longo C, Veneziano L, et al. Small-diameter melanocytic lesions: morphological analysis by means of in vivo confocal microscopy [Internet]. Br J Dermatol 2013;168(5):1027–33.

32. Losi A, Longo C, Cesinaro AM, et al. Hyporeflective pagetoid cells: a new clue for amelanotic melanoma diagnosis by reflectance confocal microscopy [Internet]. Br J Dermatol 2014;171(1):48–54.

33. Curchin C, Wurm E, Jagirdar K, et al. Dermoscopy, reflectance confocal microscopy and histopathology of an amelanotic melanoma from an individual heterozygous for MC1R and tyrosinase variant alleles [Internet]. Australas J Dermatol 2012;53(4):291–4.

34. Carrera C, Palou J, Malvehy J, et al. Early stages of melanoma on the limbs of high-risk patients: clinical, dermoscopic, reflectance confocal microscopy and histopathological characterization for improved recognition [Internet]. Acta Derm Venereol 2011;91(2):137–46.

35. Moscarella E, Rabinovitz H, Oliviero MC, et al. The role of reflectance confocal microscopy as an aid in the diagnosis of collision tumors [Internet]. Dermatology 2013;227(2):109–17.

36. Debarbieux S, Depaepe L, Poulalhon N, et al. Reflectance confocal microscopy accurately discriminates between benign and malignant melanocytic lesions exhibiting a "dermoscopic island" [Internet]. J Eur Acad Dermatol Venereol 2013;27(2):e159–65.

37. Moscarella E, Zalaudek I, Agozzino M, et al. Reflectance confocal microscopy for the evaluation of solitary red nodules [Internet]. Dermatology 2012;224(4):295–300.

38. Longo C, Moscarella E, Pepe P, et al. Confocal microscopy of recurrent naevi and recurrent melanomas: a retrospective morphological study. Br J Dermatol 2011;165:61–8.

39. Coco V, Farnetani F, Cesinaro AM, et al. False-negative cases on confocal microscopy examination: a retrospective evaluation and critical reappraisal [Internet]. Dermatology 2016;232(2):189–97. Available at: http://www.karger.com/Article/FullText/443637.

40. Segura S, Pellacani G, Puig S, et al. In vivo microscopic features of nodular melanomas: dermoscopy, confocal microscopy, and histopathologic correlates [Internet]. Arch Dermatol 2008;144(10):1311–20.

41. Longo C, Farnetani F, Ciardo S, et al. Is confocal microscopy a valuable tool in diagnosing nodular lesions? A study of 140 cases [Internet]. Br J Dermatol 2013;169(1):58–67.

42. Oliveira A, Arzberger E, Massone C, et al. Verrucous melanoma simulating melanoacanthoma: dermoscopic, reflectance confocal microscopic and high-definition optical coherence tomography presentation of a rare melanoma variant [Internet]. Australas J Dermatol 2016;57(1):72–3.

43. Longo C, Rito C, Beretti F, et al. De novo melanoma and melanoma arising from pre-existing nevus: in vivo morphologic differences as evaluated by confocal microscopy [Internet]. J Am Acad Dermatol 2011;65(3):604–14.

44. Pellacani G, Bassoli S, Longo C, et al. Diving into the blue: In vivo microscopic characterization of the dermoscopic blue hue [Internet]. J Am Acad Dermatol 2007;57(1):96–104. Available at: http://linkinghub.elsevier.com/retrieve/pii/S0190962206040217.

45. Pellacani G, Longo C, Ferrara G, et al. Spitz nevi: in vivo confocal microscopic features, dermatoscopic aspects, histopathologic correlates, and diagnostic significance [Internet]. J Am Acad Dermatol 2009;60(2):236–47.

46. Pellacani G, Cesinaro AM, Seidenari S. Reflectance-mode confocal microscopy for the in vivo characterization of pagetoid melanocytosis in melanomas and nevi. J Invest Dermatol 2005;125:532–7.

47. Hashemi P, Pulitzer MP, Scope A, et al. Langerhans cells and melanocytes share similar morphologic features under in vivo reflectance confocal microscopy: a challenge for melanoma diagnosis [Internet]. J Am Acad Dermatol 2012;66(3):452–62.

48. Carrera C, Puig-Butillè JA, Aguilera P, et al. Impact of sunscreens on preventing UVR-induced effects in nevi: in vivo study comparing protection using a physical barrier vs sunscreen [Internet]. JAMA Dermatol 2013;149(7):803–13.

49. Hofmann-Wellenhof R, Soyer HP, Wolf IH, et al. Ultraviolet radiation of melanocytic nevi: a dermoscopic study [Internet]. Arch Dermatol 1998;134(7):845–50.

50. Scope A, Longo C. Recognizing the benefits and pitfalls of reflectance confocal microscopy in melanoma diagnosis. Dermatol Pract Concept 2013;4(3):67–71.

Melanomas

Caterina Longo, MD, PhD[a],*, Giovanni Pellacani, MD[b]

KEYWORDS

- Melanoma • Reflectance confocal microscopy • Pagetoid cells • Cytologic atypia • Atypical nesting

KEY POINTS

- The melanoma family encompasses a wide range of tumors that differ in their epidemiology, morphology, genetic profile, and biological behavior. According to histologic classification, melanomas can be grouped as superficial spreading melanoma (SSM), lentigo maligna (LM), and nodular melanoma (NM).
- On reflectance confocal microscopy, SSM typically shows the presence of atypical melanocytes with rounded, large body cells that are arranged in pagetoid fashion.
- LM is typified by the presence of dendritic melanocytes that are preferentially located around and along the adnexal openings.
- The hallmark of NM is represented by the presence of the so-called cerebriform nests that are solid and dark aggregates of melanocytes demarcated by bright fibrous collagen bundles.

INTRODUCTION

Reflectance confocal microscopy (RCM) is recognized as a useful tool for the evaluation of skin lesions that are dermoscopically doubtful by increasing diagnostic accuracy and specificity.[1–7] However, this level of improvement is contingent on gaining expertise in its use as per any technology (ie, reading computed tomography [CT] scan or MRI). Although, the use of RCM has been mainly to help clinicians in detecting more melanomas at an early stage, it is useful to reduce the number of unnecessary biopsies of benign lesions that might be dermoscopically regarded as melanoma simulators.[8] This, in turn, results in an improved malignant biopsy to benign biopsy ratio. In fact, a main challenge in dermato-oncology remains differentiating atypical nevi from melanoma. To accomplish this task, it is important to recognize the benign patterns commonly seen in nevi that are overwhelmingly present compared with melanoma. Several studies have demonstrated that melanocytic nevi tend to manifest 1 or 2 benign architectural patterns that exhibit symmetry in their silhouette and the absence or paucity of cytologic atypia. Conversely, melanomas tend to manifest architectures that deviate from the benign nevus patterns. In fact, melanomas manifest a wide range of confocal features and these are obviously linked to specific factors such as the histopathological subtype, anatomic location, tumor thickness, and possibly even the specific genetic mutations carried by the tumor. Thus, it is intuitively obvious that melanoma may express a variable combination of RCM features that can be theoretically infinite.[9] With that said, what many melanomas have in common is that they deviate from the benign nevus pattern and they often reveal at least 1 or 2 of the melanoma-specific structures summarized in **Table 1**. RCM is not currently explored in vivo for the diagnosis of acral melanomas and nail melanoma because of the intrinsic limitation of the device.

The authors have no conflict of interest to declare.

Funding Source: This study was partially funded by Italian Ministry of Health (Research Project NET-2011-02347213).

[a] Skin Cancer Unit, Arcispedale S. Maria Nuova-IRCCS, Viale Risorgimento, 80, Reggio Emilia 42100, Italy;
[b] Dermatology Unit, UniMore, via del Pozzo, 71, Modena 41121, Italy
* Corresponding author.
E-mail address: longo.caterina@gmail.com

Table 1
Melanoma specific structures on confocal microscopy

	RCM Criterion	Definition
Epidermis	Pagetoid cells	Pagetoid cells are considered when large nucleated cells, twice the size of keratinocytes, with a dark nucleus and bright cytoplasm, are observable within superficial layers. They can be differentiated based on the shape (roundish, dendritic, or pleomorphic) when both shapes are present. Pagetoid cells, especially the roundish ones, represent the most accurate pattern for melanoma diagnosis.
	Broadened honeycombed pattern	Broadened honeycombed corresponds to a honeycombed pattern with bright enlarged and broadened intercellular spaces, frequently observable in nodular lesions, such as nodular melanomas and nodular nonmelanocytic skin cancers.
	Irregular keratinocytes	The overall epidermal pattern is constituted by irregular keratinocytes when irregularity in size of the cells and thickness of the contour are present.
	Disarranged pattern	It is characterized by disarray of the normal architecture of the superficial layers with unevenly distributed bright granular particles and cells, in the absence of honeycombed or cobblestone pattern.
Dermoepidermal junction	Atypical cells	Atypical cells correspond to irregular in size, shape, and reflectivity, round to oval or stellate cells, occasionally with branching dendritic structures. They show a bright cytoplasm with clearly outlined borders and sharply contrasted dark nucleus inside.
	Nonspecific pattern at dermoepidermal junctional	A nonuniform architecture constituted by unevenly distributed dermal papillae, irregular in size and shape, usually without a demarcated rim of bright cells (nonedged papillae), and separated by series of large reflecting cells, is typically observed in melanomas.
	Nonedged papillae	Dermal papillae usually show a not clearly outlined contour, without a demarcated rim of bright cells but separated by a series of large reflecting cells or by nondiscrete aggregates of melanocytes at the dermoepidermal junction.
Upper Dermis	Atypical cells within the papillae	Single nucleated cells correspond to round to oval, not aggregated cells, with well-demarcated refractive cytoplasm and well-demarcated dark nucleus infiltrating dermal papilla.
	Atypical dense and sparse nests	Dense and sparse nests constituted by aggregates of pleomorphic cells, nonhomogeneous in size, shape, and reflectivity, observable in melanomas.
	Cerebriform nests	Cerebriform clusters correspond to cellular clusters consisting of confluent amorphous aggregates of low-reflecting cells exhibiting granular cytoplasm without evident nuclei and ill-defined borders, being the aggregates brain-like in appearance, showing a fine hyporeflective fissure-like appearance. Although their observation is infrequent, cerebriform nests are specific for invasive melanomas and they are usually located within the nodular component of the tumor.
	Inflammation	Plump bright cells are described as plump, irregular, bright cells with ill-defined borders and usually no visible nucleus. Sometimes they are crowded within the papilla. Bright spots and small bright particles are small cells with very bright hyper-reflecting cytoplasm, sometimes visible nuclei, corresponding to leukocyte infiltration.
	Fibrosis	Fibrosis is composed by coarse collagen structures which appear as an amorphous fibrillary material. Their distribution could be reticulated, forming coarse web-like structures in the dermis, or in bundles, gathered into large fasciae.

Furthermore, there still remain melanomas that are featureless on dermoscopy and RCM. To not miss these lesions, careful periodic digital dermoscopic surveillance should be always considered.[10]

This article provides a comprehensive overview of the different confocal main morphologies of distinct melanoma types as a function of the anatomic location of the tumor.

REFLECTANCE CONFOCAL MICROSCOPY FEATURES OF MELANOMAS

It must be admitted that the term cutaneous melanoma encompasses a heterogeneous subset of malignant melanocytic proliferations that differ significantly with respect to their epidemiology, morphology, growth dynamics, genetics, and potential to metastasize. Even though the classification of cutaneous melanoma is an evolving science and, as a result, different schemes can be applied for the classification of melanoma, melanomas can be assigned into 3 main groups: superficial spreading melanoma (SSM), lentigo maligna (LM), and nodular melanoma (NM) (Table 2). Mucosal melanoma should be considered as a special body site tumor.

SUPERFICIAL SPREADING MELANOMA

Most melanomas developing on nonglabrous skin are of the SSM subtype. Dermoscopically, they show colors that may range from brown to black with red, white, and/or blue-gray structures, and a variable combination of the melanoma-specific structures (ie, atypical network, irregular dots or globules, streaks, and regression).

Considering the different aspects at distinct skin level, RCM characteristic features of the epidermis include the presence of pagetoid spread.[11,12]

Remarkably, pagetoid cells show up as large nucleated, rounded cells in SSM (Fig. 1). Those melanocytes are mostly rounded with variably short and thick dendrites and a dark eccentric nucleus. Additionally, dendritic melanocytes could be detected, although this melanoma subtype is mainly typified by the presence of roundish atypical melanocytes. One of the most frequently asked questions is whether pagetoid cells could be differentiated from the neighboring keratinocytes. By definition, pagetoid cells have a large size, at least double of the surrounding keratinocytes. Furthermore, keratinocytes are polygonal with brighter cell outline and grainy dark cytoplasm without a detectable nucleus. Pagetoid melanocytes are large, variably rounded, and scattered within the suprabasal epidermal layer without any cell connection with the neighboring keratinocytes, generating the impression of floating cells.

Recognition of pagetoid spread is fundamental to the diagnosis of melanoma on RCM images. This criterion is variably expressed according to tumor phase of growth. In situ melanomas would present few or localized pagetoid cells compared with invasive tumors in which a florid pagetoid infiltration could be observed throughout the entire area and at all epidermal layers, even in the stratum corneum.

Under RCM, 3 main tumor architectures can be detected: irregular ringed, meshwork, and clod, as well as variable combinations of all of them. Furthermore, some tumors might not display any of those but rather a nonspecific pattern in which rings, mesh, or nests are no longer visible.

From a cytologic point of view, atypical melanocytes in SSM tend to be roundish with bright cytoplasm and dark internal nucleus in pigmented lesions; conversely, hypo and amelanotic melanomas are typified by rounded melanocytes that appear hyporeflective because of paucity of

	SSM	LM	NM	Mucosal melanomas
Epidermis	Normal or hyperplastic	Atrophic	Atrophic or ulcerated	Hyperplastic
Pagetoid spread	Present	Present	Focal or absent	Present
Usual cell type	Rounded melanocytes	Dendritic melanocytes	Pleomorphic	Rounded or dendritic
Papillary dermis	Nests (dense & sparse, sheet)	Junctional nests (caput medusae)	Sheet-like cerebriform	Not present (few data)
Nevus-associated	Yes	No	No	No

Table 2
Reflectance confocal microscopy features of distinct melanoma subtypes

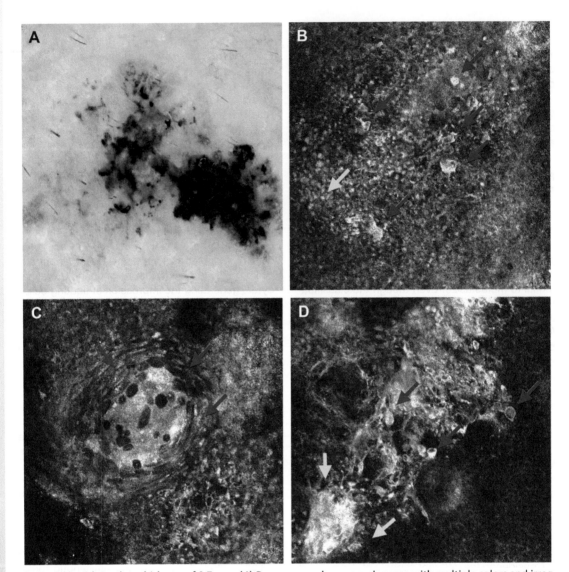

Fig. 1. SSM with Breslow thickness of 0.7 mm. (*A*) Dermoscopy shows a melanoma with multiple colors and irregularly distributed globules. (*B*) RCM image at suprabasal epidermal layer reveals the presence of several large pagetoid cells (*red arrows*), rounded with short dendrites. A keratinocyte with a smaller size and polygonal compared with the surrounding pagetoid cells (*yellow arrow*). (*C*) Dense nest (*red arrows*) with atypical large melanocytes. (*D*) Atypical melanocytes in the dermis loosely arranged to form sheet-like structures (*red arrows*) and dense and sparse nest (*yellow arrows*).

melanin.[13–15] Interestingly, the morphology of melanocytes is similar either when scattered in the suprabasal epidermal layer (pagetoid spread) or at the dermoepidermal junction.

Different nest types can be observed. Typically, they are irregularly located within the lesion and reveal atypical cells within the nests.[16,17] Distinct nest types can be observed according to the growth phase of the tumor: dense nests are found in early phase whereas dense and sparse and sheet-like structures are linked to dermal invasion (see **Fig. 1**).

SSM could arise in association with a preexisting nevus. RCM helps to detect the remnant of the nevus and its location in relation to the tumor.[18] The presence of abrupt transition, junctional atypical cells with focal distribution and dense dermal nests indicate that the tumor arose from a nevus. The main point that needs to be underlined is that RCM imaging should always be performed in the most dermoscopically atypical areas to avoid the risk of missing the malignant part in favor of the nevus component.

Differential diagnoses of SSM include mostly acquired nevi; congenital nevi; traumatized nevi, spitzoid lesions; and, rarely, nonmelanocytic entities. The diagnosis is based on the complex analysis of patients' factors, lesion clinical aspects, dermoscopic features, and specific RCM criteria that serve as supporting data for the initial provisional diagnosis.

LENTIGO MALIGNA

The most common subtype of melanoma presenting on the face is LM, which characteristically displays a different set of dermoscopic structures than those commonly observed in SSM. Typically, early clinical recognition of LM on the face can be extremely challenging because it often arises in the context of multiple solar lentigines with clinical features overlapping with early LM. Dermoscopically, the presence of gray color arranged to form slate-gray dots or granules surrounding adnexal openings, and pigment surrounding follicular openings in an asymmetric zig-zag pattern, are considered key features for early diagnosis. As the LM progresses, the pigment invades the interfollicular space, creating polygonal lines, rhomboidal structures, and homogeneous darkly pigmented areas.

On RCM, the characteristic morphologic appearance of LM is dendritic melanocytes dispersed as individual units, initially confined to the basal layer of the epidermis in a discontinuous lentiginous fashion[2,19] (Fig. 2). These atypical melanocytes extend along the outer root sheath epithelium of hair follicles. Overall, the epidermis in this tumor subtype is typically atrophic, manifesting thinning (rapid transition from epidermis to dermis), loss of the rete-ridges overlying coarse collagen, and curled fibers referable to elastotic dermis. As the lesion progresses, even if still in situ, continuity of single-cell basilar melanocytic proliferation is observed, followed by a nested junctional pattern. Nests appear as elongated aggregates of dendritic melanocytes connected to the hair follicles, generating a sort of caput medusae (see Fig. 2).

Similarly to histopathology, the presence of florid pagetoid spread and nesting pattern are the harbingers of the next phase of tumor evolution, namely dermal invasion.

Differential diagnosis often includes lichenoid keratosis in which epidermal cords associated with melanophages should be considered clues for benignity. To complicate the matter, some pigmented actinic keratoses[20] could simulate LM because of the presence of dendritic cells in the epidermal layers. However, those cells are usually interspersed and not located around and along hair follicles and no nesting is seen.

NODULAR MELANOMA

NM is a vertically growing tumor with only minimal horizontal spread, and with intraepidermal growth not extending beyond the width of 3 rete ridges in any section. The peculiar morphologic aspect of NM led to the hypothesis that it could originate in the dermis and, as a consequence, the initial proliferation is hidden. Furthermore, the dermoscopic aspect of this tumor that can lack or have minimal epidermal involvement is different from SSM or LM; it can mimic any other benign or malignant skin neoplasms. Dermoscopically, most tumors show a homogeneous, disorganized, asymmetrical pattern or a featureless pattern with atypical vessels. Pigmented NM might reveal a nonspecific global dermoscopic pattern, globules, blue-white veil, atypical vessels, and structureless areas as well as the presence of blue-black color (BB rule).

On RCM, NM reveals an epidermis that is commonly spared any pagetoid infiltration[21-24] (Fig. 3). When present, pagetoid cells are focally detected unless the tumor presents epidermal consumption. Ulceration, partial or fully developed, is another common occurrence in this aggressive tumor. In pigmented NM, black blotches result from the epidermis being totally filled by upward-migrating melanocytes as nests and pagetoid cells or clusters, whereas black dots or globules correspond to the epidermis having spared areas in between the upward-migrating nests and pagetoid cells or clusters.[22] Epidermal consumption is associated with upward-bulging dermal masses of atypical melanocytes covered only by an extremely attenuated layer of epidermis. The dermoepidermal junction is completely disrupted and the dermal compartment is filled with a solid proliferation of melanocytes with variable shape and size arranged as single cells or clustered. Nest types include the so-called sheet-like structures that represent dyscohesive atypical melanocytes with prominent nuclei that are juxtaposed to enlarged and tortuous vessels. Remarkably, cerebriform nests are typically found in NM and also in melanoma skin metastasis. Those nests show up as dark hyporeflective clusters of melanocytes that are outlined by brighter collagen fibers. Their detection could be rather difficult. A simple rule is to carefully check the hot spot around vessels that are readily detectable during live imaging. In fact, tumor clusters are commonly found in proximity to these newly formed vessels.

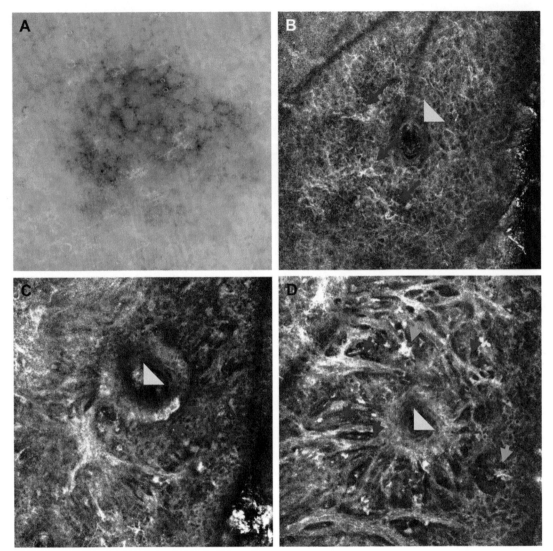

Fig. 2. LM. (*A*) Dermoscopy shows brown lesion with gray arranged to form polygon structures. (*B*) Pagetoid dendritic cells (*red arrows*) located around the hair follicle. (*C*) Atypical melanocytes (*red arrows*) descending along the outer root of the hair follicle. (*D*) Junctional nesting (*red arrows*) with atypical dendritic melanocytes (*blue arrows*) arranged to form the so-called caput medusae. (*B–D*) Hair follicle (*arrowheads*) in the middle of the structure.

Differential diagnosis of NM includes a variety of benign and malignant neoplasms, including basal cell carcinoma, clear cell acanthoma, dermal nevus, and seborrheic keratosis.

It may be argued that RCM is not a suitable tool to explore nodules because of its limited laser depth penetration. However, most nodules display at least 1 or 2 diagnostic features that permit a correct diagnosis. Furthermore, the presence of a thin or atrophic epidermis could be of help in detecting dermal diagnostic features.[25] Subcutaneous nodules, blue nevi, deep dermal metastasis, or fully ulcerated tumors represent exceptions to the rule.

To avoid the risk of missing NM, a careful patient history and clinical and dermoscopic examination should always be part of the workup that includes, as a final step, the RCM imaging.

MUCOSAL MELANOMA

By definition, mucosal melanomas include those located on the glabrous portion of the lips, oral cavity, and anogenital areas. On dermoscopy, mucosal melanomas often reveal a multicomponent pattern composed of irregular brown-black dots, blue-white veil, atypical vessels, and/or

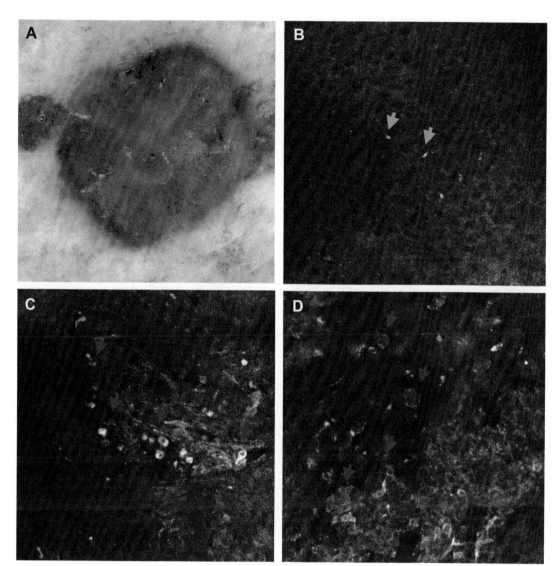

Fig. 3. NM with Breslow thickness of 3 mm. (*A*) Dermoscopy reveals a homogeneous structureless bluish area with few eccentric black dots. (*B*) Epidermis is typified by a normal honeycombed pattern without pagetoid cells and with few bright dots corresponding to free melanin pigment. (*C*) Pleomorphic cells with visible nucleus and different size located in the dermis and arranged as linearly, indicating tumor invasion. (*D*) Solid dermal proliferation of giant atypical melanocytes with few tendencies to cluster.

negative network globules, parallel structures or ring-like structures. It has been suggested that the presence of multiple patterns and colors are associated with more advanced melanomas, whereas structureless areas and gray color are more frequently seen in early melanomas. However, the distinction between melanosis and melanoma could be challenging because melanoses may exhibit overlapping features such as the presence of gray color associated with a structureless pattern.

Few data are currently available on the RCM diagnostic features for this melanoma subtype.[26,27] Overall, the presence of roundish cells, a high density of dendritic cells with atypia, and intraepithelial bright cells have been identified as clues for malignancy. Further study is strongly encouraged to better define the diagnostic RCM criteria and their value in clinical practice.

FINAL REMARKS

The use of RCM in clinical practice is becoming more widely diffused as a tool for detection of skin cancer. Diagnostic RCM clues for melanoma diagnosis have been discovered and tested for their accuracy although more studies are needed to further explore the varied morphologic features of melanoma that may demonstrate different combinations of features. Furthermore, a dedicated teaching program should be considered as fundamental for clinicians to learn how to image, interpret, and diagnose a given lesion by means of RCM.

Besides offering an improvement of diagnostic accuracy for melanoma detection, RCM should be considered as a research tool that could theoretically permit linking of in vivo morphologic dynamic information with biomolecular signatures of distinct tumor subtypes that might serve to better stratify patients' diagnoses.

REFERENCES

1. Pellacani G, Guitera P, Longo C, et al. The impact of in vivo reflectance confocal microscopy for the diagnostic accuracy of melanoma and equivocal melanocytic lesions. J Invest Dermatol 2007;127(12): 2759–65.

2. Guitera P, Pellacani G, Crotty KA, et al. The impact of in vivo reflectance confocal microscopy on the diagnostic accuracy of lentigo maligna and equivocal pigmented and nonpigmented macules of the face. J Invest Dermatol 2010;130(8):2080–91.

3. Guitera P, Menzies SW, Longo C, et al. In vivo confocal microscopy for diagnosis of melanoma and basal cell carcinoma using a two-step method: analysis of 710 consecutive clinically equivocal cases. J Invest Dermatol 2012;132(10):2386–94.

4. Pellacani G, Pepe P, Casari A, et al. Reflectance confocal microscopy as a second-level examination in skin oncology improves diagnostic accuracy and saves unnecessary excisions: a longitudinal prospective study. Br J Dermatol 2014;171(5):1044–51.

5. Alarcon I, Carrera C, Palou J, et al. Impact of in vivo reflectance confocal microscopy on the number needed to treat melanoma in doubtful lesions. Br J Dermatol 2014;170(4):802–8.

6. Scope A, Longo C. Recognizing the benefits and pitfalls of reflectance confocal microscopy in melanoma diagnosis. Dermatol Pract Concept 2014; 4(3):67–71.

7. Longo C, Zalaudek I, Argenziano G, et al. New directions in dermatopathology: in vivo confocal microscopy in clinical practice. Dermatol Clin 2012; 30(4):799–814, viii.

8. Pellacani G, Farnetani F, Gonzales S, et al. In vivo confocal microscopy for detection and grading of dysplastic nevi: a pilot study. J Am Acad Dermatol 2012;66(3):e109–21.

9. Pellacani G, De Pace B, Reggiani C, et al. Distinct melanoma types based on reflectance confocal microscopy. Exp Dermatol 2014;23(6):414–8.

10. Stanganelli I, Longo C, Mazzoni L, et al. Integration of reflectance confocal microscopy in sequential dermoscopy follow-up improves melanoma detection accuracy. Br J Dermatol 2015;172(2):365–71.

11. Farnetani F, Scope A, Braun RP, et al. Skin cancer diagnosis with reflectance confocal microscopy: reproducibility of feature recognition and accuracy of diagnosis. JAMA Dermatol 2015;151(10): 1075–80.

12. Pellacani G, Cesinaro AM, Seidenari S. Reflectance-mode confocal microscopy for the in vivo characterization of pagetoid melanocytosis in melanomas and nevi. J Invest Dermatol 2005;125(3):532–7.

13. Maier T, Sattler EC, Braun-Falco M, et al. Reflectance confocal microscopy in the diagnosis of partially and completely amelanotic melanoma: report on seven cases. J Eur Acad Dermatol Venereol 2013;27(1):e42–52.

14. Longo C, Moscarella E, Argenziano G, et al. Reflectance confocal microscopy in the diagnosis of solitary pink skin tumors: review of diagnostic clues. Br J Dermatol 2015;173(1):31–41.

15. Losi A, Longo C, Cesinaro AM, et al. Hyporeflective pagetoid cells: a new clue for amelanotic melanoma diagnosis by reflectance confocal microscopy. Br J Dermatol 2014;171(1):48–54.

16. Pellacani G, Cesinaro AM, Seidenari S. In vivo confocal reflectance microscopy for the characterization of melanocytic nests and correlation with dermoscopy and histology. Br J Dermatol 2005;152(2): 384–6.

17. Benati E, Argenziano G, Kyrgidis A, et al. Melanoma and naevi with a globular pattern: confocal microscopy as an aid for diagnostic differentiation. Br J Dermatol 2015;173(5):1232–8.

18. Longo C, Rito C, Beretti F, et al. De novo melanoma and melanoma arising from pre-existing nevus: in vivo morphologic differences as evaluated by confocal microscopy. J Am Acad Dermatol 2011; 65(3):604–14.

19. Wurm EM, Curchin CE, Lambie D, et al. Confocal features of equivocal facial lesions on severely sun-damaged skin: four case studies with dermatoscopic, confocal, and histopathologic correlation. J Am Acad Dermatol 2012;66(3):463–73.

20. Moscarella E, Rabinovitz H, Zalaudek I, et al. Dermoscopy and reflectance confocal microscopy of pigmented actinic keratoses: a morphological study. J Eur Acad Dermatol Venereol 2015;29(2):307–14.

21. Segura S, Pellacani G, Puig S, et al. In vivo microscopic features of nodular melanomas: dermoscopy, confocal microscopy, and histopathologic correlates. Arch Dermatol 2008;144(10):1311–20.

22. Longo C, Farnetani F, Moscarella E, et al. Can noninvasive imaging tools potentially predict the risk of ulceration in invasive melanomas showing blue and black colors? Melanoma Res 2013;23(2):125–31.

23. Longo C, Gambara G, Espina V, et al. A novel biomarker harvesting nanotechnology identifies

Bak as a candidate melanoma biomarker in serum. Exp Dermatol 2011;20(1):29–34.

24. Beretti F, Manni P, Longo C, et al. CD271 is expressed in melanomas with more aggressive behaviour, with correlation of characteristic morphology by in vivo reflectance confocal microscopy. Br J Dermatol 2015;172(3):662–8.

25. Longo C, Farnetani F, Ciardo S, et al. Is confocal microscopy a valuable tool in diagnosing nodular lesions? A study of 140 cases. Br J Dermatol 2013; 169(1):58–67.

26. Debarbieux S, Perrot JL, Erfan N, et al, Groupe d'Imagerie Cutanée Non Invasive de la Société Française de Dermatologie. Reflectance confocal microscopy of mucosal pigmented macules: a review of 56 cases including 10 macular melanomas. Br J Dermatol 2014;170(6): 1276–84.

27. Cinotti E, Couzan C, Perrot JL, et al. In vivo confocal microscopic substrate of grey colour in melanosis. J Eur Acad Dermatol Venereol 2015; 29(12):2458–62.

Lentigo Maligna, Macules of the Face, and Lesions on Sun-Damaged Skin
Confocal Makes the Difference

Phoebe Star, MBBS, BSc, BA[a], Pascale Guitera, MD, PhD, FACD[b],*

KEYWORDS

• Lentigo maligna • Melanoma • Benign facial macules • Solar damage • Confocal microscopy

KEY POINTS

• Lentigo maligna (LM) and lentigo maligna melanoma (LMM) often resemble one another and are difficult to distinguish from solar-induced macules of the face, clinically, and on dermoscopy and histopathology.

• LM/LMM has the highest recurrence rate of all melanoma subtypes despite treatment, reflecting the diagnostic and treatment ambiguities this lesion presents.

• In vivo reflectance confocal microscopy addresses many of the complexities and challenges of LM/LMM, enhancing patient care at all stages of diagnosis and management.

INTRODUCTION

Lentigo maligna (LM) is defined as a form of melanoma in situ that presents as a slowly growing variably pigmented macule typically on the sun-damaged skin of the elderly, most commonly on the head and neck.[1] LM involves the proliferation of atypical malignant melanocytes along the basal layer of the epidermis. Lentigo maligna melanoma (LMM) is defined as the invasive progression of LM, whereby atypical melanocytes are no longer confined to the epidermis.[2]

The incidence of LM is estimated to be approximately 13.7 per 100,000 person-years but is difficult to confirm due to incomplete data collection for in situ melanoma in most cancer registries.[3] Evidence suggests that LM/LMM is underestimated, and LM rates are likely to increase with an aging population in most high-income countries.[3–5] Although LM grows slowly, once invasive, it has the same prognosis as other malignant melanoma in terms of metastatic potential, when adjusted for Breslow thickness.[6]

Due to shared aetiology of UV exposure and age, LM typically copresents with general solar and aged-induced macules and lesions, which include solar lentigines (SL), pigmented actinic keratosis (PAK), seborrheic keratosis (SK), lichen planus-like keratosis (LPLK), as well as freckles and generalized UV-induced pigmentation.[7] The borders of LM are frequently obscured by their collision with these lesions and emergence on photo-damaged skin.

Distinguishing melanocytic hyperplasia in actinically damaged skin from atypical melanocytes, especially in the peripheries of LM, is difficult on histopathology.[8] There is significant controversy

Conflicts of Interest: None.
[a] Department of Dermatology, Melanoma Institute Australia, 40 Rocklands Road, North Sydney, New South Wales 2060, Australia; [b] Dermatology, Sydney Melanoma Diagnostic Centre (SMDC), Royal Prince Alfred Hospital, Melanoma Institute Australia, Central Clinical School, Sydney University, Missenden Road, Camperdown, New South Wales 2050, Australia
* Corresponding author.
E-mail address: pascale.guitera@melanoma.org.au

Dermatol Clin 34 (2016) 421–429
http://dx.doi.org/10.1016/j.det.2016.05.005
0733-8635/16/$ – see front matter © 2016 Elsevier Inc. All rights reserved.

about what constitutes a negative margin.[7,8] This controversy is reflected in high discordance rates between pathologists in interpreting excision margins.[9,10] The high recurrence rate of LM after conventional surgery, estimated to be between 8% and 31%, indicates more accurate margin assessment is needed.[11–13]

Dermoscopy has made significant progress in distinguishing LM/LMM from benign pigmented macules of the face.[14,15] Schiffner and colleagues[16] demonstrated the 4 main dermatoscopic criteria enabling 93% of lesions to be correctly identified as LM (sensitivity of 89% and specificity of 96%), while the vascular features on dermoscopy added by Pralong and colleagues[17] are particularly beneficial in assessing amelanotic LM/LMM peripheries, devoid of pigment.

There are several other studies producing dermatoscopic criteria against which the ability to distinguish LM from pigmented macules of the face are tested.[18–22] However, dermoscopy is limited by the overlap of features between benign and malignant lesions.[23,24] For example, the dermatoscopic features including gray color, gray circles, and annular granular structures can be seen in PAK and LM. Similarly, the hyperpigmented rim of follicular openings of LM/LMM can be mistaken for pseudofollicular openings of SK.[19]

There are multiple controversial issues with the time line of the disease and its progression from benign solar damage to fully invasive LMM. Early LM is extremely subtle and may involve a gradual increase in the number of individual melanocytes at the dermoepidermal junction (DEJ). Some atypical cells may be present. However, these features are also seen in severely sun-damaged skin.[8] Reflectance confocal microscopy (RCM) is well suited to assessing the morphology and subtle or complex features of a macule such as LM. It also enables the visualization of cellular features that differentiate LM/LMM from its pigmented counterparts.[25,26] RCM generates a horizontal (enface) view of at least 8 × 8 mm from stratum corneum to the level of the upper dermis at cellular resolution, an approximate depth of 250 µm, which is appropriate for assessing the radial spread of LM throughout the epidermis, often over very large areas.

CONFOCAL MAKES THE DIFFERENCE THROUGH SEVERAL APPLICATIONS
Differentiating Lentigo Maligna from Benign Macules of the Face and Solar Damage

It is important to differentiate LM/LMM from benign macules and solar damage. Diagnostic ambiguities can lead to unnecessary excisions of LM-like benign macules, which can carry surgical morbidly in the elderly patient and cosmetic issues on sensitive areas of the face.[18] Similarly, erroneous diagnosis of LM as a benign macule can lead to inappropriate management and delayed melanoma diagnosis.[27]

There are numerous case series examining the RCM features of benign lesions and solar damage in correlation with histopathology and/or dermoscopy, including the following:

- SK[25,28–32] (Fig. 1)
- Actinic keratosis (AK)[18,32–37] (Fig. 2)
- SL[27,38–40] (Fig. 3)
- LPLK[41]
- Chronic UV-induced changes[42–45] (Fig. 4)

Similarly, the features of LM/LMM have been elucidated on RCM[11,27,46–50] (Fig. 5). The proliferation of atypical melanocytes at the DEJ may be visualized on RCM as atypical pleomorphic cells,

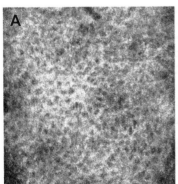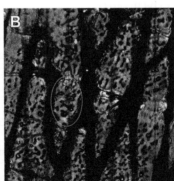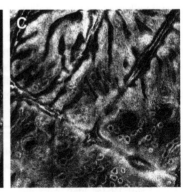

Fig. 1. Seborrheic keratosis. (A) Confocal image, 0.5 × 0.5 mm, of a SK with broadened honeycomb pattern in the epidermis. (B) Confocal images in a 4 × 4-mm mosaic of a SK in the epidermis showing cysts (red arrows), crypts (green arrows), and bulbous projections (circle). (C) Confocal images in a 2 × 2-mm mosaic of a SK in the DEJ showing a ringed pattern (red arrow).

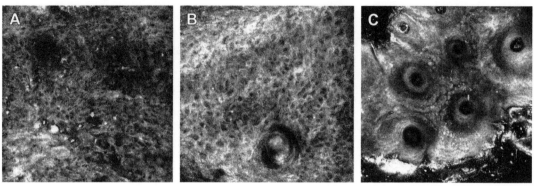

Fig. 2. Actinic keratoswis. (*A*) Confocal images in a 0.5 × 0.5 mm mosaic of an actinic keratinocyte showing detached corneocytes (*red arrow*) and parakeratosis (*green arrow*) in the stratum corneum. (*B*) Confocal images in a 0.5 × 0.5 mm mosaic of an actinic keratinocyte showing architectural disarray and atypical honeycomb pattern at the level of the stratum granulosum. (*C*) Confocal images of 0.5 × 0.5 mm at the DEJ, showing irregularly shaped keratinocytes (*red arrow*) around hair follicles (*green arrow*).

both round and/or dendritic. These atypical cells are twice the size of the adjacent keratinocytes. As LM becomes more extensive, pagetoid spread of large pleomorphic cells with prominent dendritic processes are seen through all layers of the epidermis, causing epidermal disarray. The often asymmetrical periadnexal extension is also striking on horizontal section.[46] LMM is typified by pagetoid cells, confluence of cells, and formation of nests in the dermis, resulting in global disruption of the junction.

Preliminary reports showed that RCM could be used to differentiate LM from other pigmentations of the face.[18,27,47,48] Guitera and colleagues[11] assessed the sensitivity and specificity of 64 RCM features of LM in a series of clinically equivocal macules of the face (81 LM and 203 benign macules) and developed an LM score to distinguish LM from benign lesions. The score consists of 2 major and 4 minor criteria (**Table 1**). An LM score of greater than 2 resulted in a sensitivity of 85% and specificity of 76% for the diagnosis of LM (odds ratio [OR] for LM 18.6; 95% confidence interval [CI] 9.3 to 37.1). The algorithm was equally effective in the diagnosis of amelanotic lesions and demonstrated good interobserver reproducibility (87%). In a test set of 29 LMs and 44 benign macules, the OR for LM was 60.7 (CI: 11.9–309) (93% sensitivity, 82% specificity). However, the score cannot be applied to margin assessment, such as in staged excision procedures, where the subtle presence of atypical melanocytes may be the only clue.[51]

Diagnosis of Lentigo Maligna Melanoma, that Is, Invasion, Targeting Biopsy to the Most Affected Area

It is vital to diagnose possible invasive LMM within a lesion. The presence of invasion excludes the possibility of nonsurgical treatment such as radiotherapy or imiquimod. Incisional biopsies

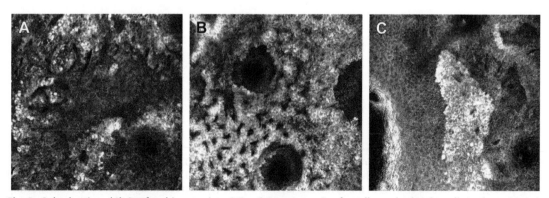

Fig. 3. Solar lentigo. (*A*) Confocal images in a 0.5 × 0.5 mm mosaic of small regular bright cells in the epidermis (*arrows*). (*B*) Confocal images in a 0.5 × 0.5 mm mosaic of bright cells forming a polycyclic pattern at DEJ. (*C*) Confocal images in a 0.5 × 0.5 mm mosaic of small regular bright cells (basal keratinocytes) arranged in clumps rather than polycyclic pattern at DEJ.

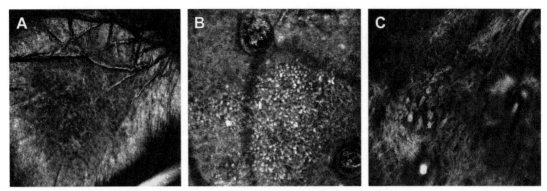

Fig. 4. Photoageing. (*A*) Confocal image of 0.5 × 0.5 mm showing large skin furrows (*red arrow*) in the epidermis. (*B*) Confocal image of 0.5 × 0.5 mm showing irregularly distributed keratinocytes at the granular layer. (*C*) Confocal image of 0.5 × 0.5 mm showing bright collagen bundles in upper dermis: coarse collagen (*red arrow*) and dense collagen (*green arrow*).

are associated with high sampling error and false negative rate due to the heterogeneity of these lesions. A compromise must often be reached between extensive sampling and the cosmetic and function sequelae of biopsies on the face.[52] Agarwal-Antal and colleagues[53] examined 92 cases of biopsy-proven LM undergoing Mohs surgery and found that 16% of patients had an invasive component, indicating the risk of underestimating invasion. Dalton and colleagues[52] demonstrated that 48% of small facial LM incisional biopsy specimens contained a contiguous

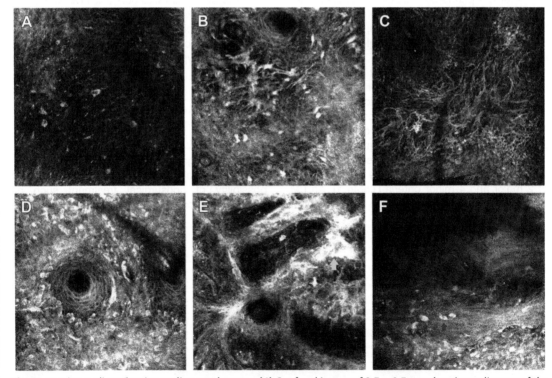

Fig. 5. Lentigo maligna/lentigo maligna melanoma. (*A*) Confocal image of 0.5 × 0.5 mm showing a disarray of the honeycomb pattern at the epidermal layer of an LM. (*B*) Confocal image of 0.5 × 0.5 mm showing pagetoid spread of round atypical cells (*red arrows*) at the epidermal layer of an LM. (*C*) Confocal image of 0.5 × 0.5 mm showing multiple dendritic processes, at the epidermal layer of an LM. (*D*) Confocal image of 0.5 × 0.5 mm showing atypical cells around hair follicles at the DEJ of an LM. (*E*) Confocal image of 0.5 × 0.5 mm showing nonedged papillae (*red arrows*) with a distortion of the junction layer by nests of atypical cells (*green arrow*). (*F*) Confocal image of 0.5 × 0.5 mm showing nucleated cells (*red arrows*) in dermis in an LM melanoma microinvasive.

Table 1
Lentigo maligna score

	Criteria	Points
Major	Nonedged papillae	+2
	Round pagetoid cells >20 μm	+2
Minor	Three or more atypical cells at the DEJ in five 0.5 × 0.5-mm² fields	+1
	Follicular localization of pagetoid cells and/or atypical junctional cells	+1
	Nucleated cells within the dermal papillae	+1
	Broadened honeycomb pattern	−1

Score ≥1, sensitivity of 93% and specificity of 61% for LM. Score ≥2, sensitivity of 85% and specificity of 76% (OR 18.6; 95% CI: 9.3–37.1).

secondary lesion, "collision lesion" such as SL, PAK, SK. Furthermore, skip lesions or areas of discontinuous melanocytic proliferation do occur within the lesion itself.[52]

Confocal microscopy enables the clinician to assess the possible deep invasive components of LMM and target biopsies to the worst area, possibly reducing sampling error. However, the ability of RCM to reduce sampling error in diagnosing invasion is yet to be demonstrated in prospective studies or randomized controlled trials. RCM has also demonstrated superiority to dermoscopy in the diagnosis of collision tumors in a case series examining basal cell carcinoma, squamous cell carcinoma, nevi, and melanoma including LM.[31]

Defining Margins for Treatment

LM is characterized by indistinct poorly delineated margins. Subclinical spread of atypical melanocytes far beyond the clinically visible margins is common, due to an often amelanotic periphery or because of the collision of lesions, leading to underestimation of the extent of the lesion.[53,54] Margins are especially important to estimate correctly to spare tissue on cosmetically and anatomically challenging areas of the face.

Margins are also difficult on pathology because they "melt" into melanocytic hyperplasia on sun-damaged skin. Several studies have attempted to characterize the differences between LM and sun-damaged skin on histopathology through morphometry,[8,55,56] immunostaining,[57] and statistical models examining melanocytic number.[58] However, residual disease after surgical excision is common, indicating failure of margin assessment. In a recent retrospective review of 807 cases

of residual melanoma in wide local excision after complete surgical resection, LM was the subtype at greatest risk for persistent disease despite reportedly clear margins.[59]

RCM is well suited to defining the margins of ill-defined and difficult lesions even when they are lightly colored or amelanotic.[60–62]

The use of RCM to map the extent of LM before surgical intervention is promising and can guide surgeons to more accurately achieve surgical clearance on primary excision or guide the field of treatment for radiotherapy and imiquimod[48,63,64] (**Fig. 6**). Guitera and colleagues[50] used RCM to map the margins in 37 patients with LM. Of the 29 patients who did not have amelanotic lesions, 17 had disease more than 5 mm beyond the dermatoscopically mapped margin. This finding resulted in a major change in the surgical procedure of 11 patients, and 16 were offered radiotherapy or imiquimod treatment based on the RCM findings. Hibler and colleagues[65] published a case report in which RCM was used intraoperatively for real-time assessment of LM of the lower eyelid. Similarly, RCM was integrated into a staged excision technique by Champin and colleagues[51] in managing 33 patients with LM. In all cases, the area mapped was 5 mm greater than clinically visible margins. On 10-month follow-up of 27 patients, there was no recurrence.

Clarifying the Natural History of Lentigo Maligna

Early LM may involve a gradual increase in the number of individual melanocytes at the DEJ. However, these features are also seen in severely sun-damaged skin.[8] Some suggest this is a premalignant stage and a separate entity to LM.[2,66] Others suggest LM exists on a spectrum of disease involving the accumulation

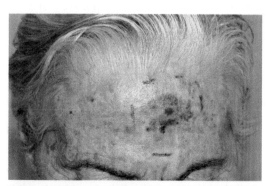

Fig. 6. Mapping the extent of lentigo maligna of the central forehead. Subclinical spread detected on RCM is often beyond the clinically visible margins.

of atypical attributes over time. For example, it has been suggested that solar lentigo with melanocytic hyperplasia, so-called unstable solar lentigo, could also represent a precursor lesions to LM.[67] The threshold at which a certain number of atypical melanocytes should be diagnosed as LM as opposed to solar damage is unknown,[50,52] making diagnosis particularly difficult for pathologists because there are no clear guidelines to distinguish the stages of the disease.[68] Stolz and colleagues[24] created a 4-stage dermatoscopic model of tumor progression from LM to LMM, but the sensitivity and specificity of this model are yet to be tested on a large number of lesions or in correlation with RCM.

Follow-up Short Margins/Treatment Failure of Radiotherapy and Imiquimod

Postoperative follow-up can be assisted by RCM. Short margins after surgical excision are often reported on histopathology. RCM can enable the clinician to assess residual disease at excision sites and map the area for further surgical excision or medical treatment, if there is no invasive element. In one of the author's experience (P.G.), it is important to wait at least 3 months after surgery to assess with RCM so as not to be distracted by inflammation and early scarring.

RCM can be used for serial imaging during imiquimod or radiotherapy treatment to evaluate response to therapy over time and to evaluate the field of treatment on follow-up.[49] It has also been used to assess the response to field imiquimod treatment for AKs.[33]

Diagnostic criteria for assessing treatment failure using RCM based on the LM score have been developed in a retrospective study of 98 patients after nonsurgical intervention with radiotherapy and imiquimod.[49] The diagnosis of treatment failure was difficult with dermoscopy, with a sensitivity of 80% and specificity of 56%. Whereas the RCM-assessed LM score had a specificity of 94% and sensitivity of 100%.

Detecting Recurrence Long Term

LM represents a therapeutic challenge to achieve long-term control without being too aggressive in aging patients, often with multiple comorbidities. LM has the highest recurrence rate of all melanoma subtypes after conventional surgery, whereas staged excision and Mohs surgery demonstrate much lower rates of recurrence.[13] Similarly, recurrence after imiquimod treatment is estimated to be 18% and after radiotherapy to be 1% to 19%.[69]

There are several difficulties in detecting recurrence in LM. LM/LMM is known to have amelanotic or lightly pigmented nonspecific recurrences, the diagnosis of which is only complicated by the presence of scar, if surgery has occurred.[49] In these settings, vessels are often distorted by treatment, making the Pralong criteria for dermatoscopic assessment limited.[49] After radiotherapy and imiquimod, treatment-induced inflammation can cause nonspecific pigmentation, which can also complicate the assessment of recurrence.[50] In particular the melanocytes of pigment incontinence can resemble atypical melanocytes of recurrence.[70]

RCM can be used to detect subtle pigmentation, similar to the assessment of amelanotic margins as described above as well as distinguish melanophages of pigment incontinence from atypical melanocytes.[26]

LIMITATIONS AND TECHNICAL ISSUES

Because of several practical impediments, RCM is currently used in practice as an adjunct or secondary evaluation tool.[62,71] Some limitations include the cost of the equipment, the time required to assess each lesion, the significant training and experience needed to accurately map the extent of a lesion, and the difficulty reaching small or delicate anatomic areas, such as the eyelid, ear, and nose. Because of its reliance on the reflected light from tissues, the presence of scale on the surface of a lesion can obscure assessment. Similarly, lesions in the deep dermis are beyond the visibility of RCM. It can also be difficult to orientate the visual image to the particular horizontal level (junctional vs dermal) when the DEJ is particularly distorted by atypical cells and may lead to over-diagnosis of microinvasion.[50] Furthermore, in correlation studies, discrepancy can result between RCM and pathology findings due to the difficulty in targeting the biopsy to the exact site of RCM.

Confocal microscopy presents ambiguity in morphologic assessment of some cellular features. The pagetoid spread of melanocytes on RCM is strongly associated with melanoma.[72] However, intraepidermal Langerhans cells, which are benign immune system cells, can resemble pagetoid spread of malignant melanocytes on RCM. A study by Hashemi and colleagues[73] found that the presence of bright cells in pagetoid spread on RCM led to false positive melanoma diagnosis in 24 of 39 assessed. There is also much debate around the significance of dendritic cells on RCM. Both melanocytes and Langerhans cells can have dendritic extensions. Large dendritic cells can represent melanocytic hyperplasia in

AK, SL, and inflammation but are also visualized in LM.[25] Guitera and colleagues[62] found that round pagetoid cells greater than 20 μm were more specific (OR 7.8) than dendritic cells in correctly diagnosing LM on RCM. Some confocalists suggest there is a threshold in the number of cells or the size of the body of the cells as a differentiating factor, but no convincing criteria have been established yet. Others consider single large dendritic cells at the margins to be significant enough to warrant wider excision.[51]

PAK are also difficult sometimes to distinguish from LM due to the distortion of pigmented keratinocytes that can resemble atypical pagetoid cells with RCM. Finally, the subtle changes of early LM can be misclassified as benign solar damage with RCM similar to the difficulties faced in histopathology.[62]

SUMMARY

RCM is becoming an important part of dermatologic care in all stages of the multidisciplinary management of patients with LM. It enhances the diagnostic confidence of the classic tools, dermoscopy and hisopathology, but over and above this, has a unique role in addressing the complex features of LM/LMM and other melanocytic lesions of the face.

REFERENCES

1. LeBoit PE, Burg G, Weedon D, et al, editors. WHO classification of tumours. Pathology and genetics of skin tumours. Lyon (France): IARC Press; 2006.
2. Tannous ZS, Lerner LH, Duncan LM, et al. Progression to invasive melanoma from malignant melanoma in situ, lentigo maligna type. Hum Pathol 2000;31(6):705–8.
3. Mirzoyev SA, Knudson RM, Reed KB, et al. Incidence of lentigo maligna in Olmsted County, Minnesota, 1970 to 2007. J Am Acad Dermatol 2014;70(3):443–8.
4. Mocellin S, Nitti D. Cutaneous melanoma in situ: translational evidence from a large population-based study. Oncologist 2011;16(6):896–903.
5. Higgins HW, Lee KC, Galan A, et al. Melanoma in situ: part I. Epidemiology, screening, and clinical features. J Am Acad Dermatol 2015;73(2):181–90.
6. Florell SR, Boucher KM, Leachman SA, et al. Histopathological recognition of involved margins of lentigo maligna excised by staged excision: an interobserver comparison study. Arch Dermatol 2003;139:595–604.
7. Zalaudek I, Cota C, Ferrara G, et al. Flat pigmented macules on sun-damaged skin of the head/neck: Junctional nevus, atypical lentiginous nevus, or melanoma in situ? Clin Dermatol 2014;32:88–93.
8. Weyers W, Bonczkowitz M, Weyers I, et al. Melanoma in situ versus melanocytic hyperplasia in sun-damaged skin: assessment of the significance of histopathologic criteria for differential diagnosis. Am J Dermatopathol 1996;18:560–6.
9. Lodha S, Sagger S, Celebi JT, et al. Discordance in the histopathologic diagnosis of difficult melanocytic neoplasms in the clinical setting. J Cutan Pathol 2008;35(4):349–52.
10. Farmer ER, Gronin R, Hanna MP. Discordance in the histopathologic diagnosis of melanoma and melanocytic nevi between expert pathologists. Hum Pathol 1996;27(6):528–31.
11. Guitera P, Pellacani G, Crotty KA, et al. The impact of in vivo reflectance confocal microscopy on the diagnostic accuracy of lentigo maligna and equivocal pigmented and nonpigmented macules of the face. J Invest Dermatol 2010;130:2080–91.
12. MacKenzie Ross AD, Haydu LE, Quinn MJ, et al. The association between excision margins and local recurrence in 11,290 thin (T1) primary cutaneous melanomas: a case-control study. Ann Surg Oncol 2016;23(4):1082–9.
13. Hazan C, Dusza SW, Delgado R, et al. Staged excision for lentigo maligna and lentigo maligna melanoma: a retrospective analysis of 117 Cases. J Am Acad Dermatol 2008;58(1):142–8.
14. Menzies SW. Cutaneous melanoma: making a clinical diagnosis, present and future. Dermatol Ther 2006;19:32–9.
15. Menzies SW, Zalaudek I. Why perform dermoscopy? The evidence for its role in the routine management of pigmented skin lesions. Arch Dermatol 2006;142:1211–2.
16. Schiffner R, Schniffner-Rohe J, Vogt T, et al. Improvement of early recognition of lentigo maligna using dermatoscopy. J Am Acad Dermatol 2000;42:25–32.
17. Pralong P, Bathelier E, Dalle S, et al. Dermoscopy of lentigo maligna melanoma: report of 125 cases. Br J Dermatol 2012;167:280–7.
18. Nascimento MM, Shitara D, Enokihara MMSS, et al. Inner gray halo, a novel dermoscopic feature for the diagnosis of pigmented actinic keratosis: clues for the differential diagnosis with lentigo maligna. J Am Acad Dermatol 2014;71:708–15.
19. Lallas A, Tschandl P, Kyrigidis A, et al. Dermoscopic clues to differentiate facial lentigo maligna from pigmented actinic keratosis. Br J Dermatol 2016;174(5):1079–85.
20. Tschandl P, Rosendahl C, Kittler H. Dermatoscopy of flat pigmented facial lesions. J Eur Acad Dermatol Venereol 2015;29:120–7.
21. Sahin MT, Ozturkcan S, Ermertcan AT, et al. A comparison of dermoscopic features among

lentigo senilis/initial seborrheic keratosis, lentigo maligna and lentigo maligna melanoma on the face. J Dermatol 2004;31:884–9.

22. Takana M, Sawada M, Kobayashi K. Key points in dermoscopic differentiation between lentigo maligna and solar lentigo. J Dermatol 2011;38:53–8.

23. Menzies SW, Ingvar C, Crotty KA, et al. Frequency and morphologic characteristics of invasive melanomas lacking specific surface microscopy features. Arch Dermatol 1996;132(10):1178–82.

24. Stolz W, Schiffner R, Burgdorf WH. Dermoscopy for facial pigmented skin lesions. Clin Dermatol 2002; 20(3):276–8.

25. Busam KJ, Carlos C, Lee G, et al. Morphologic features of melanocytes, pigmented keratinocytes, and melanophages by in vivo confocal scanning laser microscopy. Mod Pathol 2001;14(9):862–8.

26. Guitera P, Scolyer RA, Menzies SW, et al. Morphologic features of melanophages under in vivo reflectance confocal microscopy. Arch Dermatol 2010; 146(5):492–8.

27. Langley RGB, Burton E, Walsh N, et al. In vivo confocal scanning laser microscopy of benign lentigines: comparison to conventional histology and in vivo characteristics of lentigo maligna. J Am Acad Dermatol 2006;55:88–97.

28. Longo C, Farnetani F, Ciardo S, et al. Is confocal microscopy a valuable tool in diagnosing nodular lesions? A study of 140 cases. Br J Dermatol 2013;169:58–67.

29. Ahlgrimm-Siess V, Cao T, Olivero M, et al. The vasculature of nonmelanocyteic skin tumors in reflectance confocal microscopy, II: vascular features of seborrheic keratosis. Arch Dermatol 2010; 146(6):694–5.

30. Segura S, Puig S, Carrera C, et al. Development of a two-step method for the diagnosis of melanoma by reflectance confocal microscopy. J Am Acad Dermatol 2009;61:216–29.

31. Moscarella E, Rabinovitz H, Olivero MC, et al. The role of reflectance confocal microscopy as an aid in the diagnosis of collision tumors. Dermatology 2013;227:109–17.

32. Koehler MJ, Speicher M, Lange-Asschenfeldt S, et al. Clinical application of multiphoton tomography in combination with confocal laser scanning microscopy for in vivo evaluation of skin diseases. Exp Dermatol 2011;20(7):589–94.

33. Ulrich M, Krueger-Corcoran D, Roewert-Huber J, et al. Reflectance confocal microscopy for noninvasive monitoring of therapy and detection of subclinical actinic keratosis. Dermatology 2010;220:15–24.

34. Ulrich M, Maltusch A, Rowert-Huber J, et al. Actinic keratosis: non-invasive diagnosis for field cancerization. Br J Dermatol 2007;156(Suppl 3):13–7.

35. Ulrich M, Forschner T, Rowert-Huber J, et al. Differentiation between actinic keratosis and disseminated superficial actinic porokeratoses with reflectance confocal microscopy. Br J Dermatol 2007;156(Suppl 3):47–52.

36. Horn M, Gerger A, Ahlgrimm-Siess V, et al. Discrimination of actinic keratosis from normal skin with reflectance mode confocal microscopy. Dermatol Surg 2008;34(5):620–5.

37. Astner S, Gonzalez S, Ulrich M. Actinic keratosis. In: Gonzalez S, editor. Reflectance confocal microscopy in dermatology: fundamentals and clinical applications. Madrid, Spain: Grupo Aula Medica; 2012. p. 69–71.

38. Pollefliet C, Corstjens H, Gonzalez S, et al. Morphological characterization of solar lentigines by in vivo reflectance confocal microscopy: a longitudinal approach. Int J Cosmet Sci 2013;35:149–55.

39. Richtig E, Hofmann -Wellenhof R, Kopera D, et al. In vivo analysis of solar lentigines by reflectance confocal microscopy before and after Q-switched ruby laser treatment. Acta Derm Venereol 2011;91: 164–8.

40. Nakajima A, Funasaka Y, Kawana S. Investigation by in vivo reflectance confocal microscopy: melanocytes at the edges of solar lentigines. Exp Dermatol 2012;21(Suppl 1):18–21.

41. Bassoli S, Rabinovitz HS, Pellacani G, et al. Reflectance confocal microscopy criteria of lichen planus-like keratosis. J Eur Acad Dermatol Venereol 2012;26:578–90.

42. Wurm EMT, Curchin CES, Lambie D, et al. Confocal features of equivocal facial lesions on severely sun-damaged skin: four case studies with dermatoscopic, confocal and histopathologic correlation. J Am Acad Dermatol 2012;66:463–73.

43. Longo C, Casari A, Beretti F, et al. Skin aging: in vivo microscopic assessment of epidermal and dermal changes by means of confocal microscopy. J Am Acad Dermatol 2013;68(3):e73–82.

44. Koller S, Inzinger M, Rothmund M, et al. UV-induced alteration of the skin evaluated over time by reflectance confocal microscopy. J Eur Acad Dermatol Venereol 2014;28:1061–8.

45. Wurm EMT, Longo C, Curchin C, et al. In vivo assessment of chronological ageing and photoageing in forearm skin using reflectance confocal microscopy. Br J Dermatol 2012;167:270–9.

46. Pupelli G, Ferrari B, Farnetani F, et al. Melanoma. In: Gonzalez S, editor. Reflectance confocal microscopy in dermatology: fundamentals and clinical applications. Madrid, Spain: Grupo Aula Medica; 2012. p. 47–51.

47. Ahlgrimm-Siess V, Massone C, Scope A, et al. Reflectance confocal microscopy of facial lentigo maligna and lentigo maligna melanoma: a preliminary study. Br J Dermatol 2009;161(6): 1307–16.

48. Tannous ZS, Mihm MC, Flotte TJ, et al. In vivo examination of lentigo maligna and malignant melanoma in situ, lentigo maligna type by near-infrared reflectance confocal microscopy: comparison of in vivo

confocal images with histologic sections. J Am Acad Dermatol 2002;46:260–3.

49. Guitera P, Haydu LE, Menzies SW, et al. Surveillance for treatment failure of lentigo maligna with dermoscopy and in vivo confocal microscopy: new descriptors. Br J Dermatol 2014;170:1305–12.

50. Guitera P, Moloney FJ, Menzies SW, et al. Improving management and patient care in lentigo maligna by mapping with in vivo confocal microscopy. JAMA Dermatol 2013;149(6):692–8.

51. Champin J, Perrot JL, Cinotti E, et al. In vivo reflectance confocal microscopy to optimize the spaghetti technique for defining surgical margins of lentigo maligna. Dermatol Surg 2014;40:247–56.

52. Dalton SR, Gardner TL, Libow LF, et al. Contiguous lesions in lentigo maligna. J Am Acad Dermatol 2005;52(5):859–62.

53. Agarwal-Antal N, Bowen GM, Gerwels JW. Histologic evaluation of lentigo maligna with permanent sections: Implications regarding current guidelines. J Am Acad Dermatol 2002;47:743–8.

54. Kunishige JH, Brodland DG, Ziteli JA. Surgical margins for melanoma in situ. J Am Acad Dermatol 2012;66(3):438–44.

55. Acker SM, Nicholson JH, Rust PF, et al. Morphometric discrimination of melanoma in situ of sun-damaged skin from chronically sun-damaged skin. J Am Acad Dermatol 1998;39:239–45.

56. Cohen LM. The starburst giant cell is useful for distinguishing lentigo maligna from photodamaged skin. J Am Acad Dermatol 1996;35(6):962–8.

57. Black WH, Thareja SK, Blake BP, et al. Distinction of melanoma in situ from solar lentigo on sun-damaged skin using morphometrics and MITF immunohistochemistry. Am J Dermatopathol 2011;33(6):573–8.

58. Gorman M, Khan MA, Johnson PC, et al. A model for lentigo maligna recurrence using melanocyte count as a predictive marker based upon logistic regression analysis of a blinded retrospective review. J Plast Reconstr Aesthet Surg 2014;67(10):1322–32.

59. Bolshinsky V, Lin MJ, Kelly JW, et al. Frequency of residual melanoma in wide local excision (WLE) specimens after complete excisional biopsy. J Am Acad Dermatol 2016;74(1):102–7.

60. Curiel-Lewandrowski C, Williams CM, Swindells KJ, et al. Use of in vivo confocal microscopy in malignant melanoma. An aid in diagnosis and assessment of surgical and nonsurgical therapeutic approaches. Arch Dermatol 2004;140(9):1127–32.

61. Alani A, Ramsay B, Ahmad K. Diagnosis of amelanotic lentigo maligna by using in vivo reflectance confocal microscopy. Acta Derm Venerol 2016; 96(3):406–7.

62. Pellacani G, Guitera P, Longo C, et al. The impact of in vivo reflectance confocal microscopy for the diagnostic accuracy of melanoma and equivocal melanocytic lesions. J Invest Dermatol 2007;127:1259–65.

63. Chen CSJ, Elias M, Busam K, et al. Multimodal in vivo optical imaging, including confocal microscopy, facilitates pre-surgical margin mapping for clinically complex lentigo maligna melanoma. Br J Dermatol 2005;153:1031–6.

64. Kai AC, Richards T, Coleman A, et al. Five-year recurrence rate of lentigo maligna after treatment with imiquimod. Br J Dermatol 2016;174:165–8.

65. Hibler BP, Wong RJ, Rossi AM. Intraoperative real-time reflectance confocal microscopy for guiding surgical margins of lentigo maligna melanoma. Dermatol Surg 2015;41(8):981–3.

66. Flotte TJ, Mihm MC Jr. Lentigo maligna and malignant melanoma in situ, lentigo maligna type. Hum Pathol 1999;30:533–6.

67. Byrom L, Barksdale S, Weedon D, et al. Unstable solar lentigo: a defined separate entity. Australas J Dermatol 2016. [Epub ahead of print].

68. Joyce KM, Joyce CW, Jones DM, et al. An assessment of histological margins and recurrence of melanoma in situ. Plast Reconstr Surg Glob Open 2015; 3(2):e301.

69. Gautschi M, Oberholzer PA, Baumgartner M, et al. Prognostic markers in lentigo maligna patients treated with imiquimod cream: a long-term follow-up study. J Am Acad Dermatol 2016;74:81–7.

70. Cotter MA, McKenna JK, Bowen GM. Treatment of lentigo maligna with imiquimod before staged excision. Dermatol Surg 2008;34:147–51.

71. Guitera P, Pellacani G, Longo C, et al. In vivo reflectance confocal microscopy enhances secondary evaluation of melanocytic lesions. J Invest Dermatol 2009;129:131–8.

72. Pellacani G, Cesinaro AM, Seidenari S. Reflectance-mode confocal microscopy for the in vivo characterization of pagetoid melanocytosis in melanomas and nevi. J Invest Dermatol 2005;125(3):532–7.

73. Hashemi P, Pulitzer MP, Scopoe A, et al. Langerhans cells and melanocytes share similar morphologic features under in vivo reflectance confocal microscopy: a challenge for melanoma diagnosis. J Am Acad Dermatol 2012;66(3):452–62.

Glowing in the Dark
Use of Confocal Microscopy in Dark Pigmented Lesions

Susana Puig Sardá, MD, PhD[a,b,]*, Rodolfo Suárez, MD[a],
Josep Malvehy Guilera, MD, PhD[a,b]

KEYWORDS

• Reflectance confocal microscopy • Melanoma • Basal cell carcinoma • Blue nevus

KEY POINTS

- Black color in melanoma is associated with melanin in upper epidermis.
- Under reflectance confocal microscopy (RCM), multiple bright atypical pagetoid cells or atypical cobblestone are visible in upper layers of the epidermis.
- Blue color in dermoscopy corresponds with pigment deep in the dermis.
- Blue color may correspond with bright nests or sheets of atypical cells in melanoma, spindle cells in blue nevus, or a tumor island wrapped by dendrites in pigmented basal cell carcinomas.
- Exogenous pigmentation can also be evaluated by RCM.

INTRODUCTION

In vivo reflectance confocal microscopy (RCM) is a noninvasive imaging technique[1–3] that provides images of the superficial layers of the skin at nearly histologic resolution generated thanks to backscatter of light by several structures. Melanosomes, which are highly reflective,[4] are among the structures that generate white images in RCM. Thus, clinically dark lesions are easily visible by RCM because of melanin. In the RCM, light penetrates to a subsurface focus of the laser and reflects back from that focus out of the skin and into a detector in the microscope. Light that reflects superficial to the focus is eliminated, so if the focus is too deep, there will be no signal. For the same reason, if much melanin exists in superficial layers, like in black lamella (Fig. 1), no signal is generated from the deep epidermis or dermoepidermal layer. RCM can also detect pagetoid melanocytes in the epidermis, which correlate with black dots or dark blotches in dermoscopy.

The depth penetration of RCM is limited to 100 to 200 μm in human skin at the 830 nm laser wavelength used in the commercial system. The variability in the imaging penetration depth also depends on natural variations in the concentration of other reflective components comprising skin, such as keratin or collagen in addition to melanin.[5] RCM criteria found in more superficial anatomic layers may be more readily identified, because there is decay in laser light intensity with increasing imaging depth and hence decrease in optical resolution. Because of the limitation in the penetration, those dark blue lesions, in which melanin is deep in dermis, are not always visible by RCM.[6] Finally, some lesions can be clinically dark owing to substances or structures other than melanin structures, such us hemoglobin[7] or exogenous materials.[8] According to the reflective properties of the material, the images generated will be different. In the present article, the RCM criteria of several dark lesions are reviewed (Table 1).

[a] Melanoma Unit, Dermatology Department, Hospital Clinic Barcelona, IDIBAPS, University of Barcelona, Villarroel 170, Barcelona 08036, Spain; [b] CIBER de Enfermedades Raras, Barcelona, Spain
* Corresponding author. Dermatology Department, Hospital Clinic, Villarroel 170, Barcelona 08036, Spain.
E-mail addresses: susipuig@gmail.com; spuig@clinic.ub.es

Dermatol Clin 34 (2016) 431–442
http://dx.doi.org/10.1016/j.det.2016.05.006
0733-8635/16/$ – see front matter © 2016 Elsevier Inc. All rights reserved.

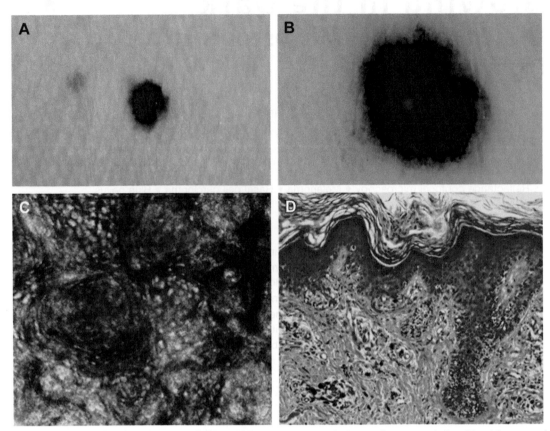

Fig. 1. Black melanoma. (A) Clinical image of a small melanoma on the knee of a woman in her 60s with personal and familial history of melanoma and carrier of a G101W mutation in *CDKN2A*. (B) Under dermoscopy, the lesion is showing a multicomponent pattern with presence of peripheral pigment network, focal globules, and central blotch. Predominant colors are black and blue. (C) Reflectance confocal microscopy (RCM) only reaches superficial layers of the epidermis showing a typical cobblestone pattern and presence of keratin. (D) Hematoxylin and eosin staining (original magnification, ×20) showing an atypical proliferation of melanocytes in the dermoepidermal junction with some nests and focal pagetoid growing. Hyperkeratosis with presence of pigmented corneocytes correlates with the typical cobblestone pattern seen in RCM.

Table 1
Most common cutaneous dark lesions with reported criteria with reflectance confocal microscopy

	Melanocytic	Non Melanocytic
Benign	Black nevus Blue nevus Spitz	Seborrheic keratosis Ink spot lentigo Angioma Angiokeratoma Pilomatricoma Ocronosis, argiria Tattoos
Malignant	Melanoma Seborrhoeic-like melanoma Malignant blue nevus Blue nevus like cutaneous metastasis	Basal cell carcinoma

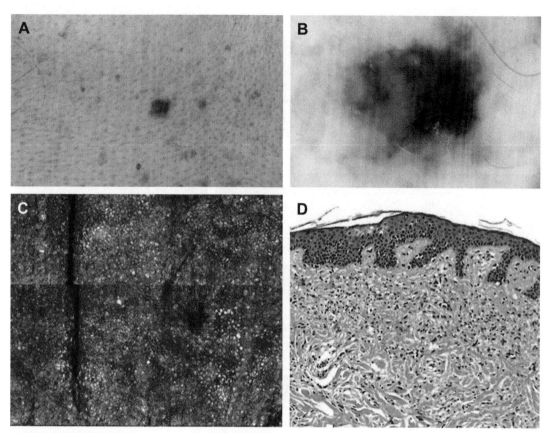

Fig. 2. Black and blue melanoma. (*A*) Clinical image of a dark brown–blue lesion located on the trunk. (*B*) Dermoscopy shows an asymmetric lesion with multicomponent pattern with atypical pigment network, black dots/globules and blue-gray dots. (*C*) Reflectance confocal microscopy (RCM) of the upper epidermis is showing the presence of bright atypical cells (roundish and large) and the presence of atypical cobblestone pattern. (*D*) Hematoxylin and eosin staining (original magnification, ×20) showing an atypical proliferation of melanocytes in the dermoepidermal junction with pagetoid growing.

DARK MELANOCYTIC LESIONS

Even though most melanocytic lesions are brown, from light brown in fair skin to dark brown in dark skin, the presence of black color is less frequent and associated to specific diagnosis: melanoma, pigmented Spitz/Reed nevus, and black nevus (nevus with black lamella in dark skinned patients or after exposure to ultraviolet light). We also consider dark color the presence of dark blue, again, in the context of melanocytic lesions associated to few diagnosis, melanoma and blue nevus.

- Black color in melanoma: The presence of black color in melanoma is associated to the presence of melanin in upper epidermis, under RCM multiple bright atypical pagetoid cells (**Figs. 2** and **3**) are visible in upper layers of the epidermis. Occasionally, in lesions with hyperkeratosis and transepidermal elimination of pigment in keratinocytes, a bright cobblestone is visible obscuring the dermoepidermal layers (see **Fig. 3**). If melanin is in atypical melanocytes in upper epidermis, then atypical cobblestone is present (with larger cells and the presence of large nuclei; **Fig. 4**), but if melanin is only present in keratinocytes of the upper layers of the epidermis, typical cobblestone can be present (see **Fig. 1**), obscuring deeper layers of the epidermis. In those cases, if we cannot see the dermoepidermal junction, melanoma cannot be ruled out by RCM.
- Blue color in melanoma: The presence of dark blue color in melanoma is associated with the presence of deeply located pigmented tumor.

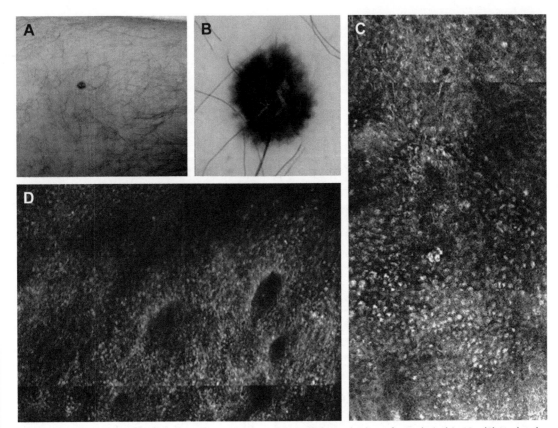

Fig. 3. Spitzoid melanoma. (*A*) Dark palpable fast growing lesion on the leg of a male in his 40s. (*B*) Under dermoscopy, the lesion is showing a star burst pattern with peripheral streaks and paracentral dark blotch and blue white area. (*C*) Reflectance confocal microscopy (RCM) of the upper epidermis is showing pleomorphic pagetoid cells (roundish and dendritic) and an atypical cobblestone pattern with the presence of small round bright nucleated cells. (*D*) RCM of the dermoepidermal junction showing nonedge papilla, atypical basal cells and the obscuring of the basal layer.

If ortokeratosis is also present, then a whitish color is overlying the deep blue (**Figs. 5** and **6**). Under RCM, large bright nests (see **Fig. 4**) or sheets of atypical cells in the dermoepidermal junction (see **Fig. 6**) can be seen.

- Dark pigmented Spitz/Reed nevus. Starburst pattern in dermoscopy (see **Fig. 3**; **Fig. 7**) can be present in Reed/pigmented Spitz nevus but also in melanoma. Recently, Guida and coworkers[9] analyzed the RCM findings present in both entities to identify those criteria that can be used to differentiate between them. In this study, striking cell pleomorphism within epidermis, widespread atypical cells at the dermoepidermal junction (see **Fig. 3**) and marked pleomorphism within nests were significantly associated with the diagnosis of malignant melanoma, whereas spindled cell (**Fig. 8**) and peripheral clefting were exclusively found and pathognomonic of spitz nevi (SNs).

- Black nevus: In these nevi, melanin is present in keratinocytes of the upper layers of the epidermis showing in RCM typical cobblestone. In the dermoepidermal layers, if visible, a ringed pattern is present. In some cases, after exposure to ultraviolet radiation, many dendritic cells can be visible in upper epidermis (see **Fig. 8**). These lesions can show some of the criteria previously described in small melanomas.[10]

- Blue nevi are characterized by the presence of dendritic melanocytes in dermis that produce melanin, even deep in the dermis. In some cases, a superficial component is present being the lesions dark blue. Under dermoscopy, blue homogeneous color without any other structures is present but, when cross-polarized dermoscopy is used, the blue can be less homogeneous and some irregularities visible inside. In those blue nevi with a preserved papillary dermis,

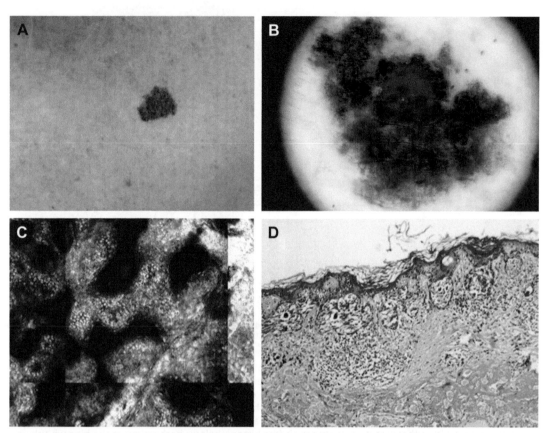

Fig. 4. Superficial spreading melanoma with a black blotch. (*A*) Dark, slightly palpable lesion on the trunk of an elderly man. (*B*) Under dermoscopy the lesion is showing a multicomponent pattern with atypical pigment network, focal presence of dark brown/black dots, dark blotch and gray dots. (*C*) Reflectance confocal microscopy (RCM) of the upper epidermis is showing a warty architecture with the presence of bright cords separated by black holes (sulci). The epidermal pattern is atypical cobblestone with the presence of roundish atypical cells. (*D*) Hematoxylin and eosin staining (original magnification, ×20) showing an atypical proliferation of melanocytes in the dermoepidermal junction with pagetoid growing and large atypical nests in the junction.

RCM is not able to reach the lesion, but, if some nests are present at the papillary dermis, RCM shows a characteristic pattern[11,12] with nests of bright dendritic cells (**Fig. 9**).

DARK NONMELANOCYTIC LESIONS
Basal Cell Carcinoma

Pigmented basal cell carcinoma may clinically mimic melanoma (**Fig. 10**). In a dark-skinned population,[13] pigmented basal cell carcinoma is more frequent than nonpigmented basal cell carcinoma, and may present diagnostic difficulties. Dermoscopy is an easy, noninvasive technique that increases the specificity in the diagnosis of both tumors[14]; however, RCM adds valuable criteria for the diagnosis of pigmented basal cell carcinoma,[6,15,16] with the presence of tumor islands wrapped by bright dendrites and surrounded by clefting. These structures are visible at the dermoepidermal layer or papillary dermis. If the examination with RCM is too superficial, the presence of multiple dendritic cells in the upper layers of the epidermis may induce a misdiagnosis with melanoma. Segura and colleagues[17] demonstrated that dendritic cells in the upper layers of the epidermis in pigmented basal cell carcinomas are Langerhans cells, whereas dendrites in the tumor island correspond with melanocytes colonizing the tumor cords or nests.

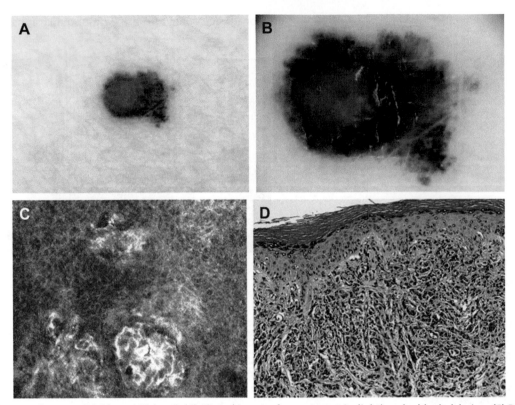

Fig. 5. Melanoma with blue whitish veil. (A) Clinical image of an asymmetric slightly palpable dark lesion. (B) Dermoscopy shows a melanocytic lesion with a multicomponent pattern, with atypical pigment network, streaks, and blue whitish veil. (C) Reflectance confocal microscopy of the dermoepidermal layer is showing nonedged papilla, atypical nests of large cells and atypical cells in the basal layer. (D) Hematoxylin and eosin staining (original magnification, ×20) in the blue whitish area showing an atypical proliferation of very pigmented melanocytes in the dermis with orthokeratotic hyperkeratosis (the histopathologic background of the blue whitish veil).

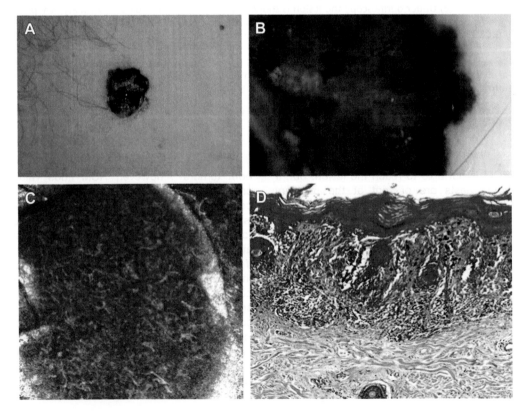

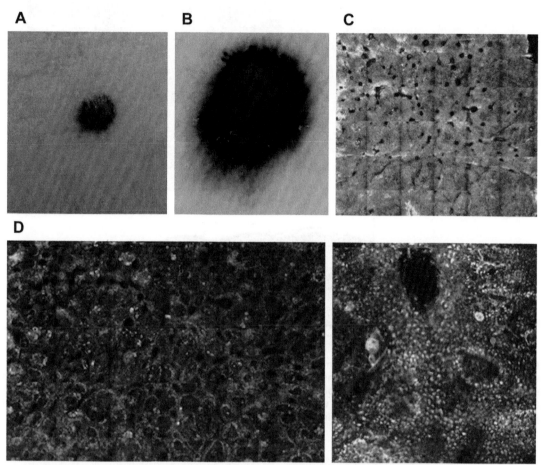

Fig. 7. Pigmented Spitz/Reed nevus. (A) Clinical image of a symmetric, elevated, and pigmented new lesion on the limb of a young man. (B) Dermoscopy shows a star burst pattern with peripheral pseudopods and projections, black dots and globules, atypical pigment network, black blotch and blue hue. (C) Reflectance confocal microscopy mosaic at upper epidermal layers showing a cobblestone pattern with presence of black holes. A detail of this mosaic is shown in the right lower corner showing an atypical cobblestone, dendritic pagetoid cells and small suprabasal nests at the periphery of the lesion. (D) Reflectance confocal microscopy mosaic at the dermoepidermal junction showing visible papilla, atypical bright cells, multiple nests and plump cells in papillary dermis.

Seborrheic Keratosis

Pigmented seborrheic keratosis can be also difficult to differentiate from melanoma. Using dermoscopy as an additional tool, RCM also offers valuable criteria for the correct diagnosis. Under RCM, a typical cobblestone in upper layers of the epidermis (**Fig. 11**) is shown together with the presence of follicular openings (black holes), follicular plugs (concentric bright keratin) and cysts (bright roundish structures) helps in the differential diagnosis.

Fig. 6. (A) Clinical image of an elevated and ulcerated tumor with recent bleeding. (B) Dermoscopy of the non-ulcerated area is showing blue whitish veil. (C) Reflectance confocal microscopy of the nonulcerated area is showing a sheet of atypical cells. (D) Hematoxylin and eosin staining (original magnification, ×20) corresponding with the peripheral area of the tumor, showing an atypical proliferation of melanocytes in the dermoepidermal junction with pagetoid growing and presence of pigment in dermis and overlying orthokeratotic hyperkeratosis (the histopathological background of the blue whitish veil).

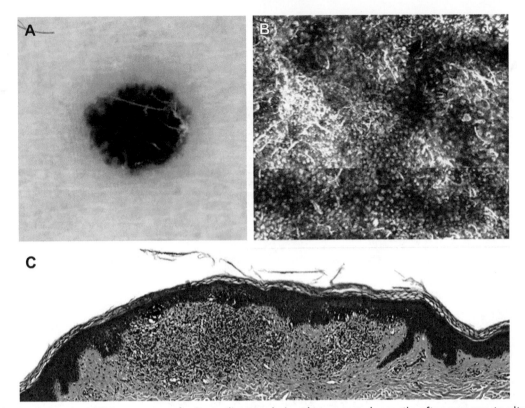

Fig. 8. Black nevus. (*A*) Dermoscopy of a 2-mm diameter lesion that appeared recently, after exposure to ultra-violet light, showing an atypical pigment network. (*B*) Reflectance confocal microscopy of upper epidermis is showing a pleomorphic proliferation of atypical cells, roundish and dendritic. (*C*) Hematoxylin and eosin staining (original magnification, ×20) corresponding with an atypical proliferation of melanocytes in the dermoepidermal junction with heavily pigmented nests and inflammation in dermis.

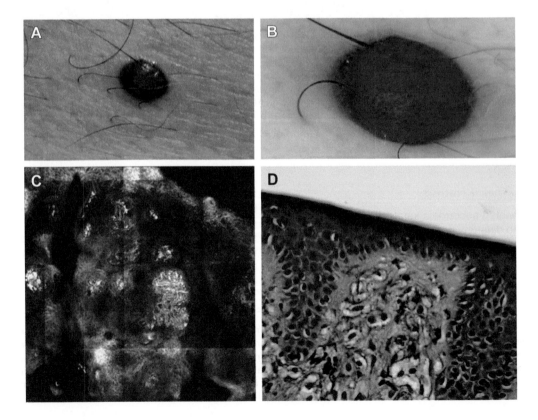

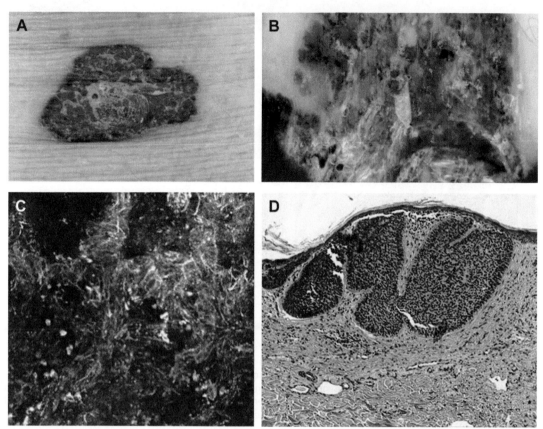

Fig. 10. Pigmented basal cell carcinoma. (*A*) Clinical image of a 4-cm black lesion on the lumbar area. (*B*) Dermoscopy shows a central area with blue whitish veil and some black globules and few erosions, and at the periphery the presence of maple leaf like areas (close to the *B*). (*C*) Reflectance confocal microscopy at the dermoepidermal junction shoving tumor cords wrapped with bright dendrites, palisading, peripheral clefting and presence of plump cells (inflammatory cells and melanophages) in the dermis. (*D*) Basaloid tumor island in superficial dermis showing palisading and clefting.

Ink Spot Lentigo

In these dark lesions, RCM shows a cobblestone pattern in the epidermis and a ringed pattern in the dermoepidermal junction.

Angiokeratomas and Thrombosed Hemangiomas

In these lesions, the dark color is not owing to the presence of melanin, but to the presence of blood in dermis and superficial hyperkeratosis. On RCM,[7] this lesion shows at the epidermal level highly reflective superficial scale with abnormal architecture at the dermoepidermal junction that displays epidermal cells forming septa surrounding the prominent ecstatic vascular lacunae (**Fig. 12**).

EXOGENOUS PIGMENTATION

Ochronosis was the first exogenous pigmentation described with RCM[8] showing dark curved silhouettes corresponding to the classical banana bodies described in histopathology. Later, silver deposits[18] were also characterized by RCM.

Fig. 9. Blue nevus. (*A*) Clinical image of a nodular lesion on the abdomen. (*B*) Blue homogeneous pattern under dermoscopy. (*C*) Reflectance confocal microscopy is showing a nested proliferation of dendritic bright melanocytes in dermal papilla. (*D*) Hematoxylin and eosin staining (original magnification, ×40) showing a proliferation of dendritic and pigmented melanocytes in the dermal papilla.

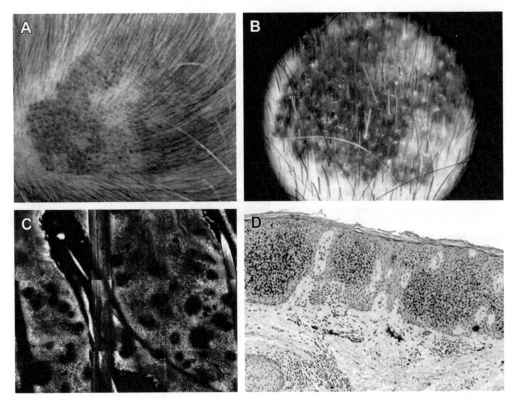

Fig. 11. Clonal seborrheic keratosis. (*A*) Clinical image of a large pigmented lesion on the scalp of a man in his 60s. (*B*) Dermoscopy of 1 area of the lesion is showing homogeneous pigmentation with brown, blue, and black coloration. (*C*) Reflectance confocal microscopy is showing in a mosaic at upper epidermis the presence of a typical cobblestone interrupted by multiple follicular openings. (*D*) Hematoxylin and eosin staining (original magnification, ×20) showing a proliferation of deep pigmented keratinocytes.

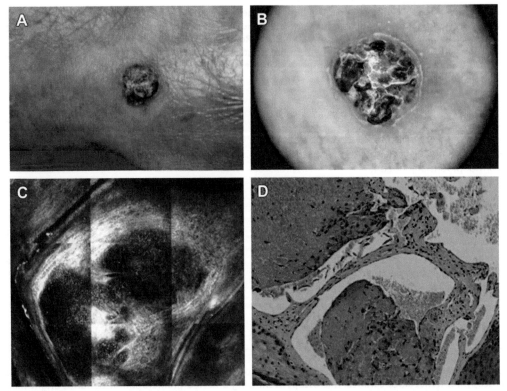

Fig. 12. Angiokeratoma. (*A*) Clinical image of a dark tumor in an acral site. (*B*) Under dermoscopy, the lesion shows black and blue color with the presence of a crust. (*C*) Reflectance confocal microscopy shows a typical honeycomb in the epidermis with the presence of ecstatic vascular structures in papillary dermis. (*D*) Hematoxylin and eosin staining (original magnification, ×20) showing the prominent ecstatic vascular lacunae.

SUMMARY

RCM criteria considered by users as more relevant for melanoma diagnosis may be frequently detected in dark lesions; most dark lesions present melanin that enhances the brightness of confocal criteria. One of the difficulties in the diagnosis of deep pigmented melanomas could be the presence of typical cobblestone pattern in upper epidermis owing to the presence of melanin in keratinocytes that obscure the dermoepidermal layer because decay in laser light intensity.

On RCM, in blue nevi, bright dendritic cells can be visible at the papillary dermis. Pigmented basal cell carcinoma can be recognized easily on RCM if the papillary dermis is reached. There, tumor islands or cords with bright dendrites are recognized easily. If the RCM imaging is too superficial and the tumor in dermis is not reached, the presence of dendritic cells in the epidermis can be misleading towards a diagnosis of melanoma instead of pigmented basal cell carcinoma.

REFERENCES

1. Pellacani G, Vinceti M, Bassoli S, et al. Reflectance confocal microscopy and features of melanocytic lesions: an internet-based study of the reproducibility of terminology. Arch Dermatol 2009;145(10):1137–43. Available at: http://eutils.ncbi.nlm.nih.gov/entrez/eutils/elink.fcgi?dbfrom=pubmed&id=19841401&retmode=ref&cmd=prlinks.

2. Segura S, Puig S, Carrera C, et al. Development of a two-step method for the diagnosis of melanoma by reflectance confocal microscopy. J Am Acad Dermatol 2009;61(2):216–29. Available at: http://eutils.ncbi.nlm.nih.gov/entrez/eutils/elink.fcgi?dbfrom=pubmed&id=19406506&retmode=ref&cmd=prlinks.

3. Pellacani G, Longo C, Malvehy J, et al. In vivo confocal microscopic and histopathologic correlations of dermoscopic features in 202 melanocytic lesions. Arch Dermatol 2008;144(12):1597–608. Available at: http://eutils.ncbi.nlm.nih.gov/entrez/eutils/elink.fcgi?dbfrom=pubmed&id=19075142&retmode=ref&cmd=prlinks.

4. Huzaira M, Rius F, Rajadhyaksha M, et al. Topographic variations in normal skin, as viewed by in vivo reflectance confocal microscopy. J Invest Dermatol 2001;116(6):846–52.

5. Leachman SA, Cassidy PB, Chen SC, et al. Methods of Melanoma Detection. Cancer Treat Res 2016;167:51–105.

6. Casari A, Pellacani G, Seidenari S, et al. Pigmented nodular Basal cell carcinomas in differential diagnosis with nodular melanomas: confocal microscopy as a reliable tool for in vivo histologic diagnosis. J Skin Cancer 2011;2011:406859. Available at: http://www.ncbi.nlm.nih.gov/pubmed/21151507/nhttp://www.ncbi.nlm.nih.gov/pmc/articles/PMC2989703/pdf/JSC2011-406859.pdf.

7. Alarcon I, Brito J, Alos L, et al. In vivo characterization of solitary angiokeratoma by reflectance confocal microscopy and high definition optical coherence tomography. J Am Acad Dermatol 2015;72(1):S43–4. Available at: http://linkinghub.elsevier.com/retrieve/pii/S0190962214015618.

8. Gil I, Segura S, Martínez-Escala E, et al. Dermoscopic and reflectance confocal microscopic features of exogenous ochronosis. Arch Dermatol 2010;146(9):1021–5. Available at: http://eutils.ncbi.nlm.nih.gov/entrez/eutils/elink.fcgi?dbfrom=pubmed&id=20855704&retmode=ref&cmd=prlinks.

9. Guida S, Pellacani G, Cesinaro AM, et al. Spitz naevi and melanomas with similar dermoscopic pattern: can confocal microscopy differentiate? Br J Dermatol 2015;174(3):610–6. Available at: http://doi.wiley.com/10.1111/bjd.14286papers3://publication/doi/10.1111/bjd.14286.

10. Pupelli G, Longo C, Veneziano L, et al. Small-diameter melanocytic lesions: morphological analysis by means of in vivo confocal microscopy. Br J Dermatol 2013;168(5):1027–33. Available at: http://doi.wiley.com/10.1111/bjd.12212.

11. Puig S, Di Giacomo T, Serra D, et al. Reflectance confocal microscopy of blue nevus. Eur J Dermatol 2012;22(4):552–3.

12. Collgros H, Vicente A, Díaz AM, et al. Agminated cellular blue naevi of the penis: dermoscopic, confocal and histopathological correlation of two cases. Clin Exp Dermatol 2016. Available at: http://doi.wiley.com/10.1111/ced.12798.

13. Ahluwalia J, Hadjicharalambous E, Mehregan D. Basal cell carcinoma in skin of color. J Drugs Dermatol 2012;11(4):484–6. Available at: http://eutils.ncbi.nlm.nih.gov/entrez/eutils/elink.fcgi?dbfrom=pubmed&id=22453586&retmode=ref&cmd=prlinks.

14. Argenziano G, Soyer HP, Chimenti S, et al. Dermoscopy of pigmented skin lesions: results of a consensus meeting via the Internet. J Am Acad Dermatol 2003;48(5):679–93. Available at: http://eutils.ncbi.nlm.nih.gov/entrez/eutils/elink.fcgi?dbfrom=pubmed&id=12734496&retmode=ref&cmd=prlinks.

15. Chuah SY, Tee SI, Tan WP, et al. Reflectance confocal microscopy is a useful non-invasive tool in the in vivo diagnosis of pigmented basal cell carcinoma in Asians. Australas J Dermatol 2015. [Epub ahead of print].

16. Cuevas J, Goldgeier M, Nori S, et al. Sensitivity and specificity of reflectance-mode confocal microscopy for in vivo diagnosis of basal cell carcinoma: a multicenter study. J Am Acad Dermatol 2004; 51(6):923–30.

17. Segura S, Puig S, Carrera C, et al. Dendritic cells in pigmented basal cell carcinoma: a relevant finding by reflectance-mode confocal microscopy. Arch Dermatol 2007;143(7):883–6.

18. García-Martínez P, López Aventín D, Segura S, et al. In vivo reflectance confocal microscopy characterization of silver deposits in localized cutaneous argyria. Br J Dermatol 2016. Available at: http://doi.wiley.com/10.1111/bjd.14571.

Enlightening the Pink
Use of Confocal Microscopy in Pink Lesions

Melissa Gill, MD[a,*], Salvador González, MD, PhD[b,c]

KEYWORDS

- Reflectance confocal microscopy (RCM) • Dermoscopy • Amelanotic melanoma • Nevi
- Nonmelanoma skin cancer (NMSC) • Pink skin tumors • Noninvasive diagnostics

KEY POINTS

- The differential diagnosis for a solitary pink lesion is broad, ranging from inflammatory to neoplastic and from benign to malignant. Solitary pink tumors show often vague, nonspecific overlapping clinical and dermoscopic features.
- Reflectance confocal microscopy (RCM) allows for in vivo evaluation of skin lesions at the cellular level, and, as such, allows for noninvasive identification of specific diagnostic features previously only visualized on histopathology.
- Incorporating RCM into the clinical examination of solitary pink tumors provides additional information, which increases the likelihood of achieving an accurate specific diagnosis noninvasively.

INTRODUCTION

Pink lesions are a large, heterogeneous group of skin lesions of neoplastic and/or inflammatory origin that are characterized by a conspicuous absence of pigmentation. They often constitute a difficult diagnostic challenge because of the lack of unique observable features using conventional techniques, for example, dermoscopy. Dermoscopy and other related techniques, despite offering advantages over visual inspection of the lesion, have an elevated rate of misdiagnosis. Rapid accurate diagnosis is particularly crucial in the case of amelanotic melanoma, which requires early diagnosis to increase the probability of therapeutic success.

The gold standard in the assessment of dermatologic disease is histologic analysis of a sample of the lesion. However, this implies the collection of a biopsy specimen, which is invasive and can be aesthetically damaging. Dermoscopy is closer to this standard than visual inspection, but it is still far from it in the case of pink lesions. Other techniques, however, offer better resolution while preserving the noninvasive nature of dermoscopy. One of such techniques is reflectance confocal microscopy (RCM), which takes advantage of light scattering by endogenous skin structures, for example, melanin granules, architectural differences between the skin layers. The differential reflection of the light together with sampling and analysis of the affected area in a noninvasive manner underlies the great promise of RCM in the assessment and management of pink lesions.

In this review, the state-of-the-art regarding the use of RCM for the assessment of pink lesions in the dermatology office is summarized.

Disclosure Statement: M. Gill has no conflicts of interest to disclose. S. González is a consultant for Caliber I.D., New York.
[a] SkinMedical Research and Diagnostics, PLLC, 64 Southlawn Ave., PO Box 42, Dobbs Ferry, NY 10522, USA; [b] Medicine and Medical Specialities Department, Medicine and Health Sciences Faculty, Alcalá University, Univeristy Campus, National road II, 28871- Alcalá de Henares, Madrid, Spain; [c] Dermatology Service, Memorial Sloan-Kettering Cancer Center, 16 E 60th Street, New York, NY 10022, USA
* Corresponding author.
E-mail address: mgill@skinmedicalranddx.com

Dermatol Clin 34 (2016) 443–458
http://dx.doi.org/10.1016/j.det.2016.05.007
0733-8635/16/© 2016 Elsevier Inc. All rights reserved.

A BRIEF CLASSIFICATION OF PINK LESIONS

Pink lesions can be inflammatory in origin or neoplastic. In general, inflammatory pink lesions are clustered or widespread, unlike amelanotic tumors, which are usually solitary and can be either benign or malignant.[1] Examples of benign pink tumors include amelanotic benign nevi, sebaceous hyperplasia (SH), sebaceous adenoma/sebaceoma, trichoepithelioma, seborrheic keratosis (SK), clear cell acanthoma (CCA), dermatofibroma (DF), angioma, and pyogenic granuloma (PG). Examples of malignant pink tumors include amelanotic/hypomelanotic melanoma, mammary and extramammary Paget disease, basal cell carcinoma (BCC), and squamous neoplasia (actinic keratosis [AK], squamous cell carcinoma in situ [SCCIS]/Bowen disease, invasive squamous cell carcinoma [SCC]). Other pink lesions, such as but not limited to, angiosarcoma, Merkel cell carcinoma, and lymphoma as yet have not been well described on dermoscopy or RCM; therefore, these lesions will not be discussed further, but should be considered in lesions that lack features described in this article.

DIAGNOSTIC FLOW OF SKIN LESIONS AT THE DERMATOLOGIST OFFICE

The evolution of imaging techniques such as dermoscopy and RCM has altered the decision and diagnostic trees in the dermatologist's office. Primary visual inspection reveals whether the lesion is inflammatory (usually multifocal) or neoplastic (often solitary), melanotic (contains melanin), or amelanotic/hypomelanotic (not obviously pigmented). Most melanotic lesions are benign nevi, as revealed by dermoscopy and/or RCM. This approach also reveals unique features of malignant melanoma (reviewed elsewhere in this issue); hence, diagnosis has the potential to be efficient and decisive. However, amelanotic/hypomelanotic (pink) lesions are often less easy to distinguish; thus, visual aids and information are required to establish an initial diagnosis. Although the gold standard is histology, a desirable goal (particularly from the patient's point of view) is to obtain information close to the gold standard without resorting to invasive biopsy specimen collection.

THE LIMITS OF DERMOSCOPY IN THE DIAGNOSIS OF SOLITARY PINK LESIONS

Dermoscopy represents a leap over mere visual inspection of solitary pink lesions, particularly in terms of sensitivity. However, it also has severe limitations regarding specificity, which is crucial to determine the course of action to treat the disease. In the following paragraphs, the major dermoscopic observations of a wide range of nonmalignant and malignant pink tumors are outlined with an emphasis on the lack of distinguishing features in many cases.

DERMOSCOPIC FINDINGS OF NONINFLAMMATORY BENIGN PINK TUMORS

Dermoscopy confers a significant advantage over visual inspection alone in the clinical diagnosis of several nonpigmented lesions. Variants of amelanotic nevi include Miescher facial, Unna, Clark (red), and Spitz nevi. The main dermatoscopic feature of Miescher and Unna nevi is the presence of comma-shaped blood vessels, which have great predictive value. Additional features include keratinized crypts. On the other hand, Clark nevi display dotted and comma-shaped vessels arranged regularly against a pink background. Spitz nevi display dotted vessels in a relatively regular arrangement and reticular depigmentation.[2,3]

Dermoscopy varies in its utility for the diagnosis of adnexal tumors. SH is often confused with superficial BCC by visual inspection due to its appearance, which includes yellowish smooth papules on the face. Dermoscopy reveals wreathed and blurred blood vessels and radial telangiectasia. Such radial arrangements are the defining feature that distinguishes SH from BCC, in which telangiectasia are treelike, intense, and very sharp.[4,5] Sebaceous adenoma and sebaceoma show opaque structureless yellow areas surrounded by elongated, radially arranged crown vessels or branching arborizing vessels and a few loosely arranged arborizing vessels.[6] Trichoepithelioma can be very difficult to distinguish from papular variants of BCC clinically and dermoscopically because it also presents as a papule with arborizing telangiectasias. However, because of the characteristic stroma of trichoepithelioma, the tumor lacks the pearliness seen in BCC and has a shiny white background on dermoscopy. Desmoplastic trichoepithelioma closely mimics morpheaform BCC on dermoscopy, appearing as an ivory-white plaque with prominent arborizing telangiectasias.[7]

SK and CCA are benign epithelial tumors that can be confused with SCC or BCC. Dermoscopy of SK reveals lobulated vessels (capillary loops) arranged regularly, but surrounded by whitish halos consistent with keratinized structures. A major distinguishing feature of SK from SCC is that lobulated vessels are irregularly shaped and do not form a pattern in the latter. An exception to this is trauma to the lesion, which may turn the regular distribution of lobulated vessels into an irregular pattern, confusing diagnosis.[8] Regarding CCA, dermoscopy reveals a pattern of coiled vessels forming a necklacelike distribution, which can be reticulated at times. These vessels also display whitish halos, unlike malignant tumors.[9,10]

Dermoscopy can assist in the diagnosis of non-pigmented DF, which usually shows a subtly pigmented area surrounding a whitish scarlike center. However, the vascular tree around the lesion is often not complete,[11] which can lead to confusion with melanoma.

Vascular lesions vary from being fairly straightforward to extremely difficult to distinguish using visual inspection and dermoscopy. Angiomas show variably sized red, purple, or blue lacunae and, if not thrombosed, blanch with contact dermoscopy. PG, however, is more complicated to distinguish from malignancies on dermoscopy, usually showing homogeneous red regions with white collars.[12] The information added by dermoscopy, unfortunately, is not sufficient to exclude nodular amelanotic/hypomelanotic melanoma.

DERMOSCOPY FINDINGS OF MALIGNANT PINK LESIONS

Dermoscopy clearly reveals several findings of amelanotic skin tumors, particularly amelanotic and hypomelanotic melanoma.[13] Some dermoscopy observations include dotted vessels forming an irregular pattern, whitish shiny areas, and ulceration in bona fide amelanotic melanoma.[13–15] Hypomelanotic melanoma can be subdivided into streaked (<30% of the tumor bears 100% pigmentation) and light colored (100% melanoma is lightly pigmented). These melanoma also display irregularly shaped vascularization with scarce pigmentation (peppering) and whitish depigmented areas.[16] Furthermore, the existence of pink (poorly melanotic) regions is a recent novel tool for the dermoscopic identification of melanoma.[17] However, these features are also present in other malignancies; hence, disambiguation often requires histologic examination.

Mammary and extramammary Paget disease commonly show milky red areas, surface scales, and a prominent vascular pattern (most commonly dotted vessels, to a lesser extent glomerular vessels, or polymorphous vessels and rarely linear irregular vessels). Many also show erosions or ulcerations, and a minority shows shiny white lines and/or white structureless areas.[18,19]

Regarding the more frequently encountered BCC, these tumors can be divided into nodular, superficial, infiltrating, and fibroepithelioma of Pinkus variants. Common features of these lesions as observed using dermoscopy include leafing and ulceration. Specific features are as follows: in nodular BCC, bright red arborized vasculature enveloping the lesion; in superficial BCC, thin vascular trees.[20–23] Infiltrating BCC is scarcely described, but one study describes finely arborized trees and scattered telangiectasias.[24] A unique type of BCC is fibroepithelial BCC, or fibroepithelioma of Pinkus. Histologically, Pinkus tumors are characterized by thin branches of atypical basaloid cells extending from the epidermis into the dermis. Dermoscopy reveals bright striae and fine arborized blood vesicles, but less branched than those in other abnormalities. Also, slightly pigmented ulcerations are not uncommon.[2,25]

AK is considered together with SCC, which is the most common type of skin tumor. Dermoscopic observation of the lesion often reveals a pink erythematous network that encircles keratotic hair follicles and abundant yellowish scaling.[26] The vascular system is often twisted in the region of the lesion, appearing as coils in the case of facial AK.[27,28] On the other hand, SCCIS (Bowen disease) reveals scaly pink plaques quite similar to psoriasis plaques and clusters of glomerular vessels,[29,30] similar to the dermoscopic observation of invasive SCC, except the latter displays white halos around the glomerular vessels and the background is white, not pink.[31]

REFLECTANCE CONFOCAL MICROSCOPY: LESS (PENETRATION) IS SOMETIMES MORE (INFORMATION)

RCM is rapidly becoming a useful tool to widen the knowledge of the dermatologist regarding a specific lesion. Although the actual z penetrance limit of RCM is set around 200 μm, right under the superficial dermis, its xyz resolution is much higher than that of dermoscopy at this level, and its noninvasive nature (shared with dermoscopy) allows the consecutive examination of the lesion using both techniques, which is very useful to disambiguate equivocal lesions. This approach: dermatoscopy first, followed by RCM to disambiguate, enables us to obtain specific data when dermatoscopy does not reveal specific features or the findings are ambiguous. As detailed in later discussion, reports on RCM findings of different skin diseases, including pink lesions, have been increasing in number in recent years (reviewed recently in Ref.[32]), enabling the elaboration of several formal atlases of RCM findings.[33,34]

Box 1
Reflectance confocal microscopy features of benign nonmelanocytic pink tumors

Sebaceous hyperplasia

- Regular epidermal honeycomb pattern
- Dilated central follicular infundibulum
- Enlarged sebaceous ducts surrounded by nodules of cuboidal cells, each with a central dark round nucleus and abundant cytoplasm filled with reflective granules
- Crown vessels

Sebaceous adenoma/sebaceoma

- Nodules of cuboidal cells, each with a central dark round nucleus and abundant cytoplasm filled with reflective granules
- Peripheral rim of cells without abundant cytoplasm or reflective granules
- Sebaceoma shows fewer cuboidal cells and expansion of the peripheral cells

Trichoepithelioma

- Regular epidermal honeycomb pattern
- Dark tumor islands in the dermis
- Brightly reflective stroma arranged in parallel bundles encasing tumor islands
- Horn cysts within tumor islands

Seborrheic keratosis

- Regular epidermal honeycomb pattern
- Increased density of dermal papillae at DEJ
- Epidermal projections and keratinized invaginations (cerebriform epidermal architecture)
- Corneal cysts
- Dilated linear blood vessels in the papillary dermis

Clear cell acanthoma

- Sharp lateral circumscription by collarette of hyperreflective hyperkeratotic cells
- Parakeratosis
- Epidermal disarray
- Acanthosis with papillomatosis
- Dilated blood vessels expanding dermal papillae and extending into the spinous layer
- Inflammatory cell infiltrate

Dermatofibroma

- Regular epidermal honeycomb pattern
- Increased density of dermal papillary rings, most pronounced peripherally
- Thickened, bright collagen bundles, most pronounced centrally
- Orientation of collagen bundles from dermal papillary rings to central deeper dermal focus

Angioma

- Regular epidermal honeycomb pattern
- Dilated dark vascular lumina separated by thin reflective septa in the upper dermis
- Blood cells moving briskly through the vascular lumina

REFLECTANCE CONFOCAL MICROSCOPY: THE STEPWISE APPROACH TO SOLITARY PINK TUMORS

A stepwise approach is helpful when examining an ambiguous solitary (presumably tumoral) pink lesion on RCM. Initially, one must establish whether the lesion is melanocytic or nonmelanocytic in nature, and then whether specific features of malignancy are present. Thereafter, one can attempt to further achieve a specific diagnosis using the established criteria (**Box 1, Fig. 1**).

In order to establish that a melanocytic neoplasm is present, one looks closely for junctional nests, junctional thickenings, and/or widespread atypical nucleated cells at the dermal-epidermal junction (DEJ) and/or nests in the dermis. If one finds features suggestive of a melanocytic neoplasm, one then must assess the lesion for features of melanoma, such as (on non-facial lesions) widespread round Pagetoid cells, widespread atypical cells along the basal layer, greater than 10% of DEJ showing nonedge papillae, individual nucleated cells in the dermal papillae, and cerebriform nests. Differentiating melanoma from nevus or other benign macules is described in detail elsewhere in this issue. Step 2 is to look for widespread round Pagetoid cells. If

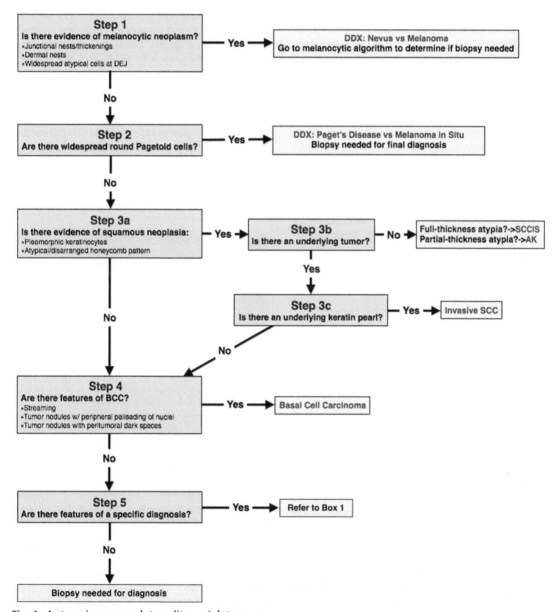

Fig. 1. A stepwise approach to solitary pink tumors.

these are identified, the lesion is probably either amelanotic superficial spreading melanoma or Paget disease, mammary or extramammary.

Once it is established that there is no evidence of a melanocytic tumor or Pagets disease, one must rule out squamous neoplasia and BCC. First, one looks for evidence of squamous neoplasia (pleomorphic keratinocytes and an atypical or disarranged epidermal honeycomb pattern). If present, one then must look for evidence of an underlying tumor because both invasive SCC and BCC can show overlying features of AK or SCCIS. If no underlying tumor is present and the changes of squamous neoplasia are partial thickness or patchy and mild, AK is likely. If the changes are full thickness, SCCIS is likely. If there is evidence of an underlying tumor and a keratin pearl is identified, invasive SCC should be suspected. If no keratin pearl is seen, one proceeds to the next step, which is to evaluate for features of BCC (streaming, tumor nodules with peripheral palisading of nuclei, and tumor nodules with peritumoral dark spaces).

Once melanocytic neoplasms, Paget disease, squamous neoplasms, and BCC have been excluded, one can then begin searching for constellations of features that suggest specific benign diagnoses (see **Box 1**). If no specific features are identified or if the lesion appears too deep for visualization using confocal, biopsy for histopathology is needed to allow for diagnosis to steer appropriate management. In the following paragraphs the RCM features of several benign and malignant pink tumors are described in detail.

REFLECTANCE CONFOCAL MICROSCOPY FINDINGS OF NONINFLAMMATORY BENIGN PINK LESIONS

Amelanotic nevi can be subtle on RCM, but close inspection reveals diagnostic clues indicating a melanocytic lesion, such as nests and junctional thickenings described in detail elsewhere in this issue. Importantly, in poorly melanized melanocytic neoplasms, the relative absence of melanin pigment means there is less contrast between the nucleus and the cytoplasm, making nuclear visualization more difficult. In the case of intradermal nevi, one may simply see tumor nodules in the dermis with no clear cellular or nuclear outlines. As such, one relies more heavily on the absence of specific features of other tumors with overlapping characteristics (such as peripheral palisading of nuclei or peritumoral dark spaces associated with tumor nodules in BCC in the case of some intradermal nevi) and architecture to exclude malignancy.

The unique appearance of sebocytes (**Fig. 2**) on RCM (cuboidal cells with a central dark round nucleus and abundant glistening cytoplasm) makes distinguishing well-differentiated sebaceous tumors from other pink tumors fairly straightforward using this technology.[33] One report of SH studied using RCM revealed arrangements of cuboid cells, each with reflective particles filling the cytoplasm and a central dark round nucleus, and enlarged sebaceous ducts.[35] Similar findings are reported in sebaceoma and sebaceous adenoma where nodules of the characteristic cells with reflective granular cytoplasms are surrounded by a rim of cells without abundant cytoplasm with reflective granules.[6]

Trichoepitheliomas, conventional and desmoplastic, often pose a diagnostic challenge clinically and histopathologically because both can show overlapping features with BCC, and the desmoplastic variant can also be confused with microcystic adnexal carcinoma. On RCM, diagnostic struggles are similar. Both variants of this tumor show dark tumor islands with varying numbers of horn cysts containing reflective keratin concentrically ramified by parallel bundles of reflective collagen. In desmoplastic trichoepithelioma, the tumor islands are often smaller and may be present as cords.[7] Clues that favor trichoepithelioma over BCC are the absence of parakeratosis,

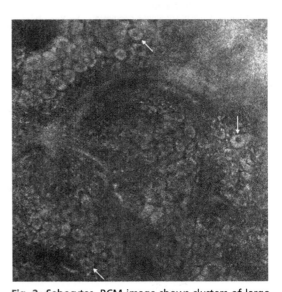

Fig. 2. Sebocytes. RCM image shows clusters of large oval-shaped cells (*arrows*) with defined borders, which are separated from one another by narrow dark intercellular spaces. Each cell harbors abundant cytoplasm containing numerous small reflective particles and a central round dark nucleus. The cells are arranged in clusters of lobules, giving a morulalike appearance. (*Courtesy of* Harold Rabinovitz, MD, Plantation, FL.)

pleomorphic keratinocytes, epidermal disarray, or streaming (localized areas with polarization of nuclei along the same axis) in the overlying epidermis and the absence of peritumoral dark spaces in the dermis. The stroma encasing tumor aggregates in trichoepithelioma is also fairly distinctive, but further studies are needed to determine the feasibility of using RCM to definitively exclude BCC when trichoepithelioma is suspected.

Benign nonpigmented epithelial tumors have also been described on RCM. Nonpigmented SK shows a regular epidermal honeycomb pattern and dense dermal papillae at the DEJ. The unique features of SK as seen using RCM include epidermal projections and keratinized invaginations as well as corneal cysts and dilated linear blood vessels in the papillary dermis. These observations correlate well with histologic examination of the lesions.[36] One study found that on RCM CCA displays clear edges composed of hyperkeratotic cells with parakeratosis, an inflammatory infiltrate, blood vessel dilation as well as acanthosis with papillomatosis causing epidermal disorganization.[37]

RCM offers a more detailed view of DF than that seen on dermoscopy. At the DEJ, nonpigmented DF shows dermal papillary rings, which are more densely packed at the periphery and more widely spaced centrally. Most prominently noted in the central portion of the lesion are thickened bright collagen bundles, which may be seen extending downward from the dermal papillary rings, giving the impression that they are tethering the rings to a common focus deeper in the dermis in the center of the lesion (Fig. 3). The overlying epidermis usually shows a normal honeycomb pattern and may be acanthotic.[33]

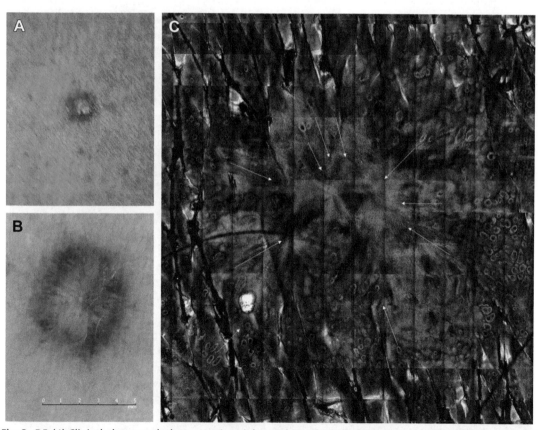

Fig. 3. DF. (A) Clinical photograph shows a satiny pink papule on the leg of a 51-year-old woman with a personal history of melanoma. Patient reported recent increase in size of lesion. (B) Dermoscopic image shows an erythematous papule with some light pigmentation at the periphery and central white streaks with a somewhat radial arrangement. (C) RCM mosaic at the level of the DEJ shows peripheral dense dermal papillary rings and central flattening of the DEJ with thickened collagen bundles. The collagen bundles and papillary rings are somewhat radially arranged toward a central focus with some papillary rings being oblong but arranged in the same axis as collagen bundles, giving the impression that the collagen bundles are tethering them to a central focus (arrows). No biopsy was performed because RCM confirmed clinical and dermoscopic impression of DF.

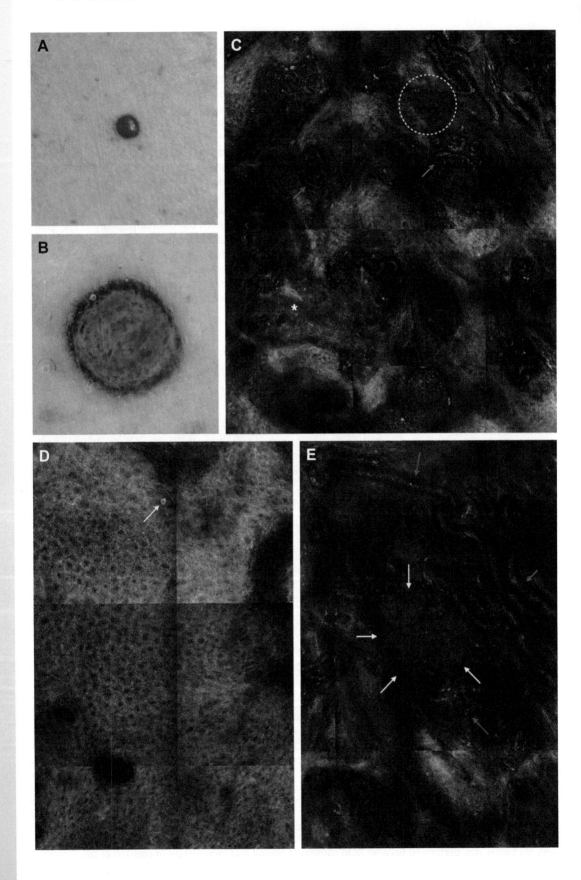

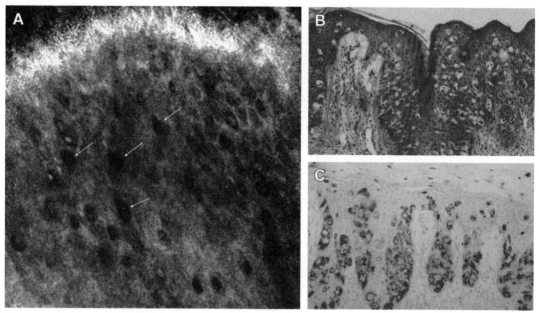

Fig. 5. Extramammary Paget disease. (*A*) RCM image from an erythematous patch on the penile shaft showing numerous roundish hyporeflective Pagetoid cells (*arrows*) in the upper epidermis. (*B*) Histopathology (hematoxylin-eosin) shows numerous atypical epithelioid Pagetoid cells at all levels of the epidermis. (*C*) Histopathology (carcinoembryonic antigen immunohistochemical stain) shows diffuse strong staining of all Pagetoid cells.

Noninvasive interpretation of benign vascular lesions is also aided by RCM. Examination of angiomas using RCM reveals dilated blood vessels perpendicular to the superficial dermis, which appear as dark variably sized lacunae with intervening brighter septa. These blood vessels contain 2 types of particles displaying real-time motion: larger, bright particles consistent with circulating leukocytes and smaller, darker particles consistent with erythrocytes.[33,38] PG is a difficult lesion to distinguish clinically and dermoscopically from Spitzoid nevi and amelanotic melanoma; hence, histology is almost invariably required. RCM suggests PG when, in addition to the absence of evidence of a melanocytic lesion, RCM reveals a well-delineated lesion with a bright collar and oval dark areas breaking the honeycombed pattern of the epidermis. Within these dark areas,

very thin vascular channels with blood flow are seen.[39]

REFLECTANCE CONFOCAL MICROSCOPY FINDINGS OF MALIGNANT PINK LESIONS

Several studies have addressed the sensitivity and accuracy of RCM for the visualization of melanoma. RCM is potentially useful for the diagnosis of hypomelanotic and amelanotic melanoma because it reveals clearly the architectural disarray of the skin structure due to the malignancy.[40] However, its lack of penetrance beyond the papillary dermis limits its usefulness for invasive lesions.

In studies of melanoma, RCM has yielded a 93% sensitivity, which means that 7 of 100 cases of melanoma could be misdiagnosed as benign.

Fig. 4. Nodular amelanotic malignant melanoma. (*A*) Clinical photograph shows on the abdomen of a middle-aged woman a satiny pink-maroon papule not dissimilar from the DF in **Fig. 3**. (*B*) Dermoscopic image shows an erythematous papule with white streaks and a peripheral ring of reticular pigmentation, which shows parallels to DF, but unlike DF, the white streaks are not radially arranged. (*C*) RCM mosaic at the DEJ shows complete disruption of the DEJ with no recognizable pattern (aspecific pattern), an irregular internally dishomogenous junctional thickening (*white asterisk*), a hint of the surface of a cerebriform nest (*circle*), and numerous large polymorphous vessels (*red arrows*). (*D*) RCM mosaic in the upper epidermis shows a broadened honeycomb pattern and a rare roundish Pagetoid cell (*yellow arrow*). (*E*) RCM mosaic in the upper dermis shows a poorly reflective cerebriform nest (*yellow arrows*) and numerous prominent polymorphous vessels (*red arrows*). (*Courtesy of* Caterina Longo, MD, PhD, Reggio Emilia, Italy.)

Conversely, a 76% specificity means that 76 of 100 benign lesions could be clearly diagnosed without resorting to biopsy specimen collection. Although far from ideal, these numbers are superior to those of dermoscopy in terms of specificity (sensitivity is similar for both techniques).[41–43]

Amelanotic and hypomelanotic melanoma account for almost 10% of melanoma diagnosis. Using RCM, the main features of amelanotic melanoma are similar to those of pigmented melanoma, that is, enlarged cytologically atypical cells in the basal layer, poorly defined dermal papillae at the DEJ, Pagetoid cells throughout the lesion, particularly in the superficial layers, cerebriform nests, and nucleated cells inside dermal papillae (Fig. 4).[44,45] Interestingly, Pagetoid cells of melanoma cannot be distinguished yet from intraepidermal Paget cells in Paget disease.[46,47] These cells, usually loaded with melanin in pigmented melanoma, are often devoid of the pigment in amelanotic melanoma. The hyporeflective Pagetoid cells seen in amelanotic melanoma and nonpigmented Paget disease appear as dark round to oval-shaped cells, sometimes referred to as dark holes in the epidermis, on RCM. These cells are observed in 85% of amelanotic melanoma, but seldom appear in pigmented melanoma. This feature is particularly relevant to distinguish amelanotic melanoma from other pink skin malignancies, because they are mostly absent in nonmelanocytic skin tumors, particularly BCC.[48] Used in combination with the features of pigmented melanoma described above, this feature enhances the use of RCM as a diagnostic tool for melanoma.

Mammary and extramammary Paget disease may be pigmented, but usually presents as a pink patch or plaque. On RCM, nonpigmented

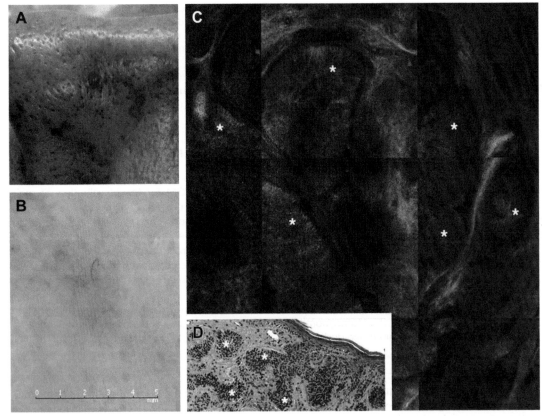

Fig. 6. Nodular BCC. (A) Clinical photograph shows a flesh-pink–colored papule on the lateral nose of a 45-year-old woman without extensive sun damage. (B) Dermoscopic image shows a flesh-colored lesion with arborizing fine telangiectasia, which is otherwise featureless (H&E stain). (C) RCM mosaic image in the dermis shows horizontal vessels with leukocyte trafficking (arrows) and tumor islands (asterisks) with peripheral palisading seen as fine white streaks perpendicular to the curved tumor border surrounded by a narrow dark space. (D) Corresponding histopathology shows islands of basaloid cells (asterisks) with peripheral palisading of nuclei and thin peritumoral clefts and/or subtle surrounding mucin deposition. Telangiectatic vessels are seen in the superficial dermis.

Paget disease shows numerous large (1.5–2 times the size of neighboring keratinocytes), round, hyporeflective cells sometimes surrounded by a dark halo or targetlike cells, each with a central small reflective area and a surrounding prominent dark halo, singly or in clusters at all levels of the epidermis (**Fig. 5**). Florid nesting of lesional cells is usually noted at the level of the DEJ, and, thus far, invasive Paget disease has been indistinguishable from in situ Paget disease on RCM. The surrounding epidermis usually shows a disarrayed honeycomb pattern and occasionally a broadened honeycomb pattern. Prominent vertically oriented blood vessels are also typical, but may simply be related to site.[47,49] It is important to keep in mind that hyporeflective Pagetoid cells seen in amelanotic melanoma are virtually indistinguishable from those seen in Paget disease.[48] However, as both lesions require biopsy for staging to determine proper management, final diagnosis can be deferred to histopathology without causing delay in treatment.[50]

BCC has been extensively characterized using RCM.[51,52] Within the lower epidermis, BCC may show localized areas demonstrating bright, elongated tumor cells with nuclear polarization along the same axis, also called "streaming."[51] Within the dermis, tumor nodules or islands, which may appear dark or bright, are surrounded by a layer of cells with minimal cytoplasm and oval nuclei lined up perpendicular to the outer edge of the "tumor island" (peripheral palisading of nuclei).[53] Sometimes, the palisading is appreciated as peripheral fine white streaks, similar to a picket fence. Mucin surrounding tumor islands, which often causes peritumoral clefting on histology, appears as peritumoral dark spaces on RCM (**Fig. 6**).[54] Epidermal actinic damage, frequently present overlying BCC, appears as keratinocyte disarray above the basal layer.[51] Similar to dermoscopy, RCM also reveals dilated branching horizontal vessels. In addition, real-time or video-capture RCM allows for observation of leukocyte trafficking, which is prominent in BCC.[55] Similar to histology, fibroepithelioma of Pinkus shows a distinct pattern on RCM viewed at the level of the DEJ: a fenestrated pattern outlined by islands of tumor cells.[56,57]

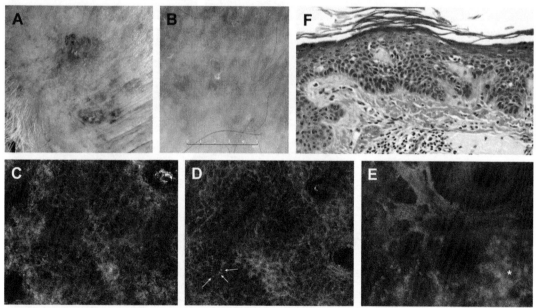

Fig. 7. AK. (*A*) Clinical photograph shows a pink plaque with patchy scaling on the forehead of an 82-year-old man who has nearby field cancerization on his scalp. (*B*) Dermoscopic image shows homogenous pink and milky white areas with small foci of scale. (*C*) RCM image at the level of stratum corneum/stratum granulosum shows mild keratinocytic pleomorphism and mild epidermal disarray. (*D*) RCM image at the level of the stratum spinosum shows more subtle keratinocytic pleomorphism and minimal keratinocytic disarray on the right side of the image as well as exocytosis of a few lymphocytes (*arrows*). (*E*) RCM image in the upper dermis shows solar elastosis (*asterisk*) and a focal inflammatory cell infiltrate. No tumor is noted beneath the epidermis. Keratin pearls are notably absent in all RCM images. (*F*) Histopathology (hematoxylin-eosin) shows solar elastotic skin with focal parakeratosis and broader subjacent mild partial-thickness keratinocytic atypia. A few lymphocytes are noted in the epidermis, and there is an aggregate of lymphocytes in the subjacent dermis.

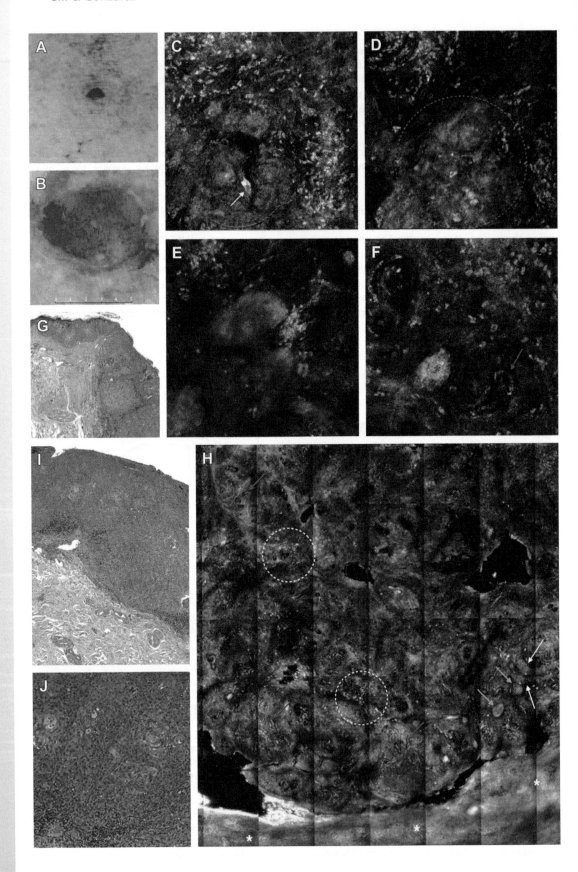

An algorithm has also been established to diagnose BCC using RCM.[58] Major criteria include (i) nuclear polarization (streaming), (ii) peripheral palisading of nuclei, (iii) leukocytic infiltrates, (iv) dilated or more numerous blood vessels oriented parallel to the observation plane, and (v) epidermal pleomorphism. Identification of 3 criteria yielded 94% and 78% sensitivity and specificity, respectively, whereas 4 criteria yielded 83% and 96% sensitivity and specificity, respectively.[58] Additional positive parameters have been identified that help in refining the diagnosis, including dendritic cells, basaloid nodules, telangiectasia, tortuous blood vessels, and peritumoral dark spaces (peritumoral clefting).[54,59,60] Conversely, other parameters can be used to discard BCC, including diffuse papillae, epidermal disorganization, and cerebriform nests.[61] Finally, it is worth noting that recent efforts have used RCM to discriminate among the different subtypes of BCC.[62,63]

Squamous neoplasia includes the spectrum of AK to SCCIS to invasive SCC. RCM can be used to distinguish AK from SCC.[64] As squamous neoplasia generally involves at least areas that are easily evaluated by RCM (epidermis and superficial dermis), its features are usually well visualized by RCM. AK displays highly reflective polygonal cells and dark corneocytes at the level of the stratum corneum as well as epidermal disarray and pleomorphism of the nucleated epidermis, which can be limited to the basal layer or extend into the spinous and granular layers, corresponding to parakeratosis and partial-thickness keratinocytic atypia on histology, respectively (Fig. 7).[65,66] A recent study has used RCM to diagnose and grade AK. Grade 1 AK displays zones of disarranged honeycomb pattern in the stratum spinosum mixed with regions of typical honeycomb pattern. Grade 2 AK displays atypical keratinocytes in both the stratum spinosum and the granulosum. Finally, grade 3 AK displays a severely disrupted atypical honeycomb pattern and widespread pleomorphic keratinocytes.[67] On RCM, SCCIS shows scaling of heterogeneous brightness and parakeratotic cells (dark center delineated by a bright contour) in the stratum corneum, roundish blood vessels that correspond to the dotted vasculature observed using dermoscopy, and both epidermal disarray and keratinocytic pleomorphism at all epidermal levels.[65] When there appears to be tumor within the dermis below the overlying epidermal changes of squamous neoplasia and a keratin pearl (well-defined, blurry, pale gray aggregate distinct from the surrounding tumor) is noted, invasive SCC is likely (Salvador González, Martina Ulrich, unpublished data, 2013) (Fig. 8). Invasive SCC occasionally arises from the base of the epidermis with only very focal epidermal involvement. In this situation, like superficial shave biopsy, it may be difficult to achieve an accurate diagnosis using a superficial modality, such as RCM, and deep biopsy for histopathological evaluation would be required.

SUMMARY

Although histology remains the gold standard for the diagnosis of skin cancers, dermoscopy and RCM have made strides toward their adoption as the first line of diagnostic tools. Dermoscopy lacks resolution but is able to hint at the presence of

Fig. 8. Invasive SCC. (A) Clinical photograph of a well-circumscribed pink-red papule that appeared suddenly on the chest of a 78-year-old man with extensive sun damage. (B) Dermoscopic image shows a well-demarcated homogenous pink papule with numerous serpiginous blood vessels. (C) RCM image at the level of the stratum corneum shows corneal disruption (oval), an atypical parakeratotic corneocyte (white arrow), and erosions covered with a neutrophilic crust (red asterisks). (D) RCM image in the upper dermis shows epidermal disarray and a bulging acanthotic aggregate of pleomorphic keratinocytes (dashed red circle). (E) RCM image around the level of DEJ shows complete disarray and a well-demarcated blurry hyporeflective aggregate, called a keratin pearl (red asterisk). In the lower half of the image, one sees a bulbous aggregate of pleomorphic keratinocytes, which are losing resolution. An inflammatory cell infiltrate is noted in the upper left corner. (F) RCM image in the upper dermis reveals a keratin pearl (red asterisk), amorphous masses of atypical cells, and admixed inflammatory cells. A prominent vascular loop is also noted (red arrow). (G) Histopathology (hematoxylin-eosin) low-magnification overview shows solar elastotic skin with SCCIS shouldering an eroded, inflamed invasive SCC. (H) RCM mosaic in the upper dermis shows a well-demarcated tumor papule and a rim of background solar elastotic dermis (white asterisks). Fingerlike projections of pleomorphic keratinocytes (white arrows) are seen in association with keratin pearls (aqua arrows). There are numerous round, curved, and serpiginous prominent blood vessels (red arrows) and inflammatory infiltrates (dashed yellow circles). (I) Histopathology (hematoxylin-eosin) low-magnification overview shows an eroded invasive SCC with squamous pearls and an inflammatory cell infiltrate. (J) Histopathology (hematoxylin-eosin) at higher magnification shows aggregates of atypical keratinocytes with variably developed keratin pearls and inflammation.

deeper structures. Confocal is more time-consuming, requires expensive equipment, and lacks penetrance, but it is able to achieve cellular resolution identifying structures in vivo that were formerly only possible to visualize on histopathology. As such, the combined use of dermoscopy and RCM provides an ample palette for the trained dermatologist to enhance the diagnosis. In addition to the lack of invasiveness, a major advantage is the "repeatability" of the imaging, which enables therapeutic follow-up of the lesion. A drawback is that both techniques, particularly RCM, require extensive specialist training. However, the publication of dermoscopy and RCM standards together with simpler, more accessible equipment will widen the number of users and consolidate these tools at the forefront of dermatology diagnosis.

REFERENCES

1. Giacomel J, Zalaudek I. Pink lesions. Dermatol Clin 2013;31(4):649–78, ix.
2. Argenziano G, Zalaudek I, Corona R, et al. Vascular structures in skin tumors: a dermoscopy study. Arch Dermatol 2004;140(12):1485–9.
3. Ferrara G, Gianotti R, Cavicchini S, et al. Spitz nevus, spitz tumor, and spitzoid melanoma: a comprehensive clinicopathologic overview. Dermatol Clin 2013;31(4):589–98, viii.
4. Zaballos P, Ara M, Puig S, et al. Dermoscopy of sebaceous hyperplasia. Arch Dermatol 2005; 141(6):808.
5. Bryden AM, Dawe RS, Fleming C. Dermatoscopic features of benign sebaceous proliferation. Clin Exp Dermatol 2004;29(6):676–7.
6. Moscarella E, Argenziano G, Longo C, et al. Clinical, dermoscopic and reflectance confocal microscopy features of sebaceous neoplasms in Muir-Torre syndrome. J Eur Acad Dermatol Venereol 2013;27(6): 699–705.
7. Ardigo M, Zieff J, Scope A, et al. Dermoscopic and reflectance confocal microscope findings of trichoepithelioma. Dermatology 2007;215(4):354–8.
8. Braun RP, Rabinovitz HS, Krischer J, et al. Dermoscopy of pigmented seborrheic keratosis: a morphological study. Arch Dermatol 2002;138(12):1556–60.
9. Blum A, Metzler G, Bauer J, et al. The dermatoscopic pattern of clear-cell acanthoma resembles psoriasis vulgaris. Dermatology 2001;203(1):50–2.
10. Lacarrubba F, de Pasquale R, Micali G. Videodermatoscopy improves the clinical diagnostic accuracy of multiple clear cell acanthoma. Eur J Dermatol 2003;13(6):596–8.
11. Blum A, Bauer J. Atypical dermatofibroma-like pattern of a melanoma on dermoscopy. Melanoma Res 2003;13(6):633–4.
12. Zaballos P, Llambrich A, Cuellar F, et al. Dermoscopic findings in pyogenic granuloma. Br J Dermatol 2006;154(6):1108–11.
13. Jaimes N, Halpern JA, Puig S, et al. Dermoscopy: an aid to the detection of amelanotic cutaneous melanoma metastases. Dermatol Surg 2012;38(9): 1437–44.
14. Rubegni P, Lamberti A, Mandato F, et al. Dermoscopic patterns of cutaneous melanoma metastases. Int J Dermatol 2014;53(4):404–12.
15. Chernoff KA, Marghoob AA, Lacouture ME, et al. Dermoscopic findings in cutaneous metastases. JAMA Dermatol 2014;150(4):429–33.
16. Costa J, Ortiz-Ibanez K, Salerni G, et al. Dermoscopic patterns of melanoma metastases: interobserver consistency and accuracy for metastasis recognition. Br J Dermatol 2013;169(1):91–9.
17. Rader RK, Payne KS, Guntupalli U, et al. The pink rim sign: location of pink as an indicator of melanoma in dermoscopic images. J Skin Cancer 2014; 2014:719740.
18. Crignis GS, Abreu L, Bucard AM, et al. Polarized dermoscopy of mammary Paget disease. An Bras Dermatol 2013;88(2):290–2.
19. Mun JH, Park SM, Kim GW, et al. Clinical and dermoscopic characteristics of extramammary Paget's disease: a study of 35 cases. Br J Dermatol 2016; 174(5):1104–7.
20. Liebman TN, Jaimes-Lopez N, Balagula Y, et al. Dermoscopic features of basal cell carcinomas: differences in appearance under non-polarized and polarized light. Dermatol Surg 2012;38(3):392–9.
21. Puig S, Cecilia N, Malvehy J. Dermoscopic criteria and basal cell carcinoma. G Ital Dermatol Venereol 2012;147(2):135–40.
22. Popadic M. Dermoscopic features in different morphologic types of basal cell carcinoma. Dermatol Surg 2014;40(7):725–32.
23. Liebman TN, Wang SQ. Detection of early basal cell carcinoma with dermoscopy in a patient with psoriasis. Dermatol Online J 2011;17(2):12.
24. Pyne JH, Fishburn P, Dicker A, et al. Infiltrating basal cell carcinoma: a stellate peri-tumor dermatoscopy pattern as a clue to diagnosis. Dermatol Pract Concept 2015;5(2):21–6.
25. Zalaudek I, Ferrara G, Broganelli P, et al. Dermoscopy patterns of fibroepithelioma of Pinkus. Arch Dermatol 2006;142(10):1318–22.
26. Rosendahl C, Cameron A, Argenziano G, et al. Dermoscopy of squamous cell carcinoma and keratoacanthoma. Arch Dermatol 2012;148(12):1386–92.
27. Peris K, Micantonio T, Piccolo D, et al. Dermoscopic features of actinic keratosis. J Dtsch Dermatol Ges 2007;5(11):970–6.
28. Zalaudek I, Giacomel J, Argenziano G, et al. Dermoscopy of facial nonpigmented actinic keratosis. Br J Dermatol 2006;155(5):951–6.

29. Zalaudek I, Argenziano G, Leinweber B, et al. Dermoscopy of Bowen's disease. Br J Dermatol 2004; 150(6):1112–6.

30. Zalaudek I, Di Stefani A, Argenziano G. The specific dermoscopic criteria of Bowen's disease. J Eur Acad Dermatol Venereol 2006;20(3):361–2.

31. Zalaudek I, Giacomel J, Schmid K, et al. Dermatoscopy of facial actinic keratosis, intraepidermal carcinoma, and invasive squamous cell carcinoma: a progression model. J Am Acad Dermatol 2012; 66(4):589–97.

32. Longo C, Moscarella E, Argenziano G, et al. Reflectance confocal microscopy in the diagnosis of solitary pink skin tumours: review of diagnostic clues. Br J Dermatol 2015;173(1):31–41.

33. Gonzalez S, Gill M, Halpern A. Reflectance confocal microscopy of cutaneous tumors: an atlas with clinical, dermoscopic and histological correlations. London: Informa Healthcare; 2008.

34. Hofmann-Wellenhof R, Pellacani G, Malvehy J, et al. Reflectance confocal microscopy for skin diseases. Heidelberg: Springer; 2012.

35. Propperova I, Langley RG. Reflectance-mode confocal microscopy for the diagnosis of sebaceous hyperplasia in vivo. Arch Dermatol 2007;143(1):134.

36. Ahlgrimm-Siess V, Cao T, Oliviero M, et al. Seborrheic keratosis: reflectance confocal microscopy features and correlation with dermoscopy. J Am Acad Dermatol 2013;69(1):120–6.

37. Ardigo M, Buffon RB, Scope A, et al. Comparing in vivo reflectance confocal microscopy, dermoscopy, and histology of clear-cell acanthoma. Dermatol Surg 2009;35(6):952–9.

38. Marks V, Tcheung WJ, Burton C 3rd, et al. Reflectance confocal microscopy features of angioma serpiginosum. Arch Dermatol 2011;147(7):878.

39. Moscarella E, Zalaudek I, Agozzino M, et al. Reflectance confocal microscopy for the evaluation of solitary red nodules. Dermatology 2012;224(4): 295–300.

40. Kaur R, Albano PP, Cole JG, et al. Real-time supervised detection of pink areas in dermoscopic images of melanoma: importance of color shades, texture and location. Skin Res Technol 2015;21(4): 466–73.

41. Pellacani G, Guitera P, Longo C, et al. The impact of in vivo reflectance confocal microscopy for the diagnostic accuracy of melanoma and equivocal melanocytic lesions. J Invest Dermatol 2007;127(12): 2759–65.

42. Stevenson AD, Mickan S, Mallett S, et al. Systematic review of diagnostic accuracy of reflectance confocal microscopy for melanoma diagnosis in patients with clinically equivocal skin lesions. Dermatol Pract Concept 2013;3(4):19–27.

43. Guitera P, Pellacani G, Crotty KA, et al. The impact of in vivo reflectance confocal microscopy on the diagnostic accuracy of lentigo maligna and equivocal pigmented and nonpigmented macules of the face. J Invest Dermatol 2010;130(8):2080–91.

44. Maier T, Sattler EC, Braun-Falco M, et al. Reflectance confocal microscopy in the diagnosis of partially and completely amelanotic melanoma: report on seven cases. J Eur Acad Dermatol Venereol 2013;27(1):e42–52.

45. Braga JC, Scope A, Klaz I, et al. The significance of reflectance confocal microscopy in the assessment of solitary pink skin lesions. J Am Acad Dermatol 2009;61(2):230–41.

46. Cinotti E, Perrot JL, Labeille B, et al, Groupe imagerie cutanée non invasive de la Société française de dermatologie. The contribution of reflectance confocal microscopy in the diagnosis of Paget's disease of the breast. Ann Dermatol Venereol 2013; 140(12):829–32 [in French].

47. Pan ZY, Liang J, Zhang QA, et al. In vivo reflectance confocal microscopy of extramammary Paget disease: diagnostic evaluation and surgical management. J Am Acad Dermatol 2012;66(2):e47–53.

48. Losi A, Longo C, Cesinaro AM, et al. Hyporeflective pagetoid cells: a new clue for amelanotic melanoma diagnosis by reflectance confocal microscopy. Br J Dermatol 2014;171(1):48–54.

49. Guitera P, Scolyer RA, Gill M, et al. Reflectance confocal microscopy for diagnosis of mammary and extramammary Paget's disease. J Eur Acad Dermatol Venereol 2013;27(1):e24–9.

50. Scope A, Longo C. Recognizing the benefits and pitfalls of reflectance confocal microscopy in melanoma diagnosis. Dermatol Pract Concept 2014; 4(3):67–71.

51. Gonzalez S, Tannous Z. Real-time, in vivo confocal reflectance microscopy of basal cell carcinoma. J Am Acad Dermatol 2002;47(6):869–74.

52. Witkowski AM, Ludzik J, DeCarvalho N, et al. Noninvasive diagnosis of pink basal cell carcinoma: how much can we rely on dermoscopy and reflectance confocal microscopy? Skin Res Technol 2016;22(2):230–7.

53. Segura S, Puig S, Carrera C, et al. Development of a two-step method for the diagnosis of melanoma by reflectance confocal microscopy. J Am Acad Dermatol 2009;61(2):216–29.

54. Ulrich M, Roewert-Huber J, Gonzalez S, et al. Peritumoral clefting in basal cell carcinoma: correlation of in vivo reflectance confocal microscopy and routine histology. J Cutan Pathol 2011;38(2):190–5.

55. Gonzalez S, Sackstein R, Anderson RR, et al. Real-time evidence of in vivo leukocyte trafficking in human skin by reflectance confocal microscopy. J Invest Dermatol 2001;117(2):384–6.

56. Perrot JL, Labeille B, Douchet C, et al, Groupe imagerie cutanée non invasive de Société française de dermatologie. Contribution of reflectance confocal

microscopy to the diagnosis of fibroepithelioma of Pinkus. Ann Dermatol Venereol 2014;141(10):643–5 [in French].

57. Longo C, Soyer HP, Pepe P, et al. In vivo confocal microscopic pattern of fibroepithelioma of Pinkus. Arch Dermatol 2012;148(4):556.

58. Nori S, Rius-Diaz F, Cuevas J, et al. Sensitivity and specificity of reflectance-mode confocal microscopy for in vivo diagnosis of basal cell carcinoma: a multicenter study. J Am Acad Dermatol 2004;51(6):923–30.

59. Segura S, Puig S, Carrera C, et al. Dendritic cells in pigmented basal cell carcinoma: a relevant finding by reflectance-mode confocal microscopy. Arch Dermatol 2007;143(7):883–6.

60. Ahlgrimm-Siess V, Horn M, Koller S, et al. Monitoring efficacy of cryotherapy for superficial basal cell carcinomas with in vivo reflectance confocal microscopy: a preliminary study. J Dermatol Sci 2009; 53(1):60–4.

61. Ahlgrimm-Siess V, Massone C, Scope A, et al. Reflectance confocal microscopy of facial lentigo maligna and lentigo maligna melanoma: a preliminary study. Br J Dermatol 2009;161(6):1307–16.

62. Longo C, Lallas A, Kyrgidis A, et al. Classifying distinct basal cell carcinoma subtype by means of dermatoscopy and reflectance confocal microscopy. J Am Acad Dermatol 2014;71(4):716–24.e1.

63. Peppelman M, Wolberink EA, Blokx WA, et al. In vivo diagnosis of basal cell carcinoma subtype by reflectance confocal microscopy. Dermatology 2013; 227(3):255–62.

64. Peppelman M, Nguyen KP, Hoogedoorn L, et al. Reflectance confocal microscopy: non-invasive distinction between actinic keratosis and squamous cell carcinoma. J Eur Acad Dermatol Venereol 2015; 29(7):1302–9.

65. Rishpon A, Kim N, Scope A, et al. Reflectance confocal microscopy criteria for squamous cell carcinomas and actinic keratoses. Arch Dermatol 2009;145(7):766–72.

66. Aghassi D, Anderson RR, Gonzalez S. Confocal laser microscopic imaging of actinic keratoses in vivo: a preliminary report. J Am Acad Dermatol 2000;43(1 Pt 1):42–8.

67. Zalaudek I, Piana S, Moscarella E, et al. Morphologic grading and treatment of facial actinic keratosis. Clin Dermatol 2014;32(1):80–7.

Shining into the White

The Spectrum of Epithelial Tumors from Actinic Keratosis to Squamous Cell Carcinoma

 CrossMark

Martin Ulrich, MD[a],*, Iris Zalaudek, MD[b], J. Welzel, MD[c]

KEYWORDS

- Actinic keratosis • Bowen disease • Squamous cell carcinoma • Reflectance confocal microscopy
- Dermoscopy • Skin imaging

KEY POINTS

- Reflectance confocal microscopy (RCM) allows the evaluation of the superficial parts of the skin at high resolution.
- In the past 15 years, the research of RCM has continuously been growing, and several independent groups have shown its applicability for non-hyperkeratotic actinic keratosis.
- Although the applicability of RCM has clearly been proven, RCM also has limitations in this field.
- RCM may be very useful in the diagnosis and monitoring of squamous neoplasia, but future studies are required to show its additional use in clinical practice.

INTRODUCTION

Invasive squamous cell carcinoma (SCC) represents the second most common skin cancer in humans, but their earliest form, namely actinic keratoses (AK), affects up to 60% of the elderly population.[1] AKs typically arise in the context of field cancerization, representing one step in the continuum from chronic photo damage with subclinical dysplasia to invasive SCC.[2,3] In this regard, AKs have been referred to as early in situ SCC with different grades describing the level of epidermal involvement[4] (Table 1).

Despite this classic pathway that describes the stepwise progression from AK to invasive SCC, recent data suggest an alternative pathway of AK grade 1 directly progressing to invasive SCC.[5]

The clinical grading of AKs is mainly based on the grade of hyperkeratosis,[6] which has not yet been shown to correlate with histologic grading of AK. In fact, although the clinical grade III refers to hyperkeratotic AKs, grade III in histopathology refers to fully developed intraepithelial carcinoma affecting the whole epidermis.

In most cases, the diagnosis of AK has been made clinically. However, the distinction between AK and other forms of nonmelanoma skin cancer, such as superficial basal cell carcinoma or benign lesions, may pose a diagnostic challenge. Furthermore, the distinction from different grades of AK, in situ SCC/Bowen disease, or even invasive SCC may be difficult, but is of major importance for treatment selection. Dermoscopy seems to aid the differentiation between the different stages in the continuum of keratinocyte skin cancer, because AK, in situ SCC/Bowen disease, and invasive SCC have been related to different patterns.[7,8]

[a] Private Dermatology Office/CMB Collegium Medicum Berlin, Luisenstrasse 54/55, Berlin 10117, Germany; [b] Non-Melanoma Skin Cancer Unit, Department of Dermatology and Venereology, Medical University of Graz, Graz, Austria; [c] Department of Dermatology, General Hospital Augsburg, Germany
* Corresponding author.
E-mail addresses: martinaulrich@gmx.net; m.ulrich@collegiummedicum.de

Dermatol Clin 34 (2016) 459–467
http://dx.doi.org/10.1016/j.det.2016.05.008
0733-8635/16/$ – see front matter © 2016 Elsevier Inc. All rights reserved.

Table 1
Histologic grading of actinic keratosis, modified according to Roewert-Huber and colleagues
AK grade 1 — Intraepidermal dysplasia of keratinocytes involving the lower third of the epidermis
AK grade 2 — Intraepidermal dysplasia of keratinocytes involving the lower two-thirds of the epidermis
AK grade 3 — Intraepidermal dysplasia of keratinocytes involving the complete epidermis. By some investigators, AK grade 3 are defined as SCC in situ, whereas others define AK in general as SCC in situ

The criteria of AK have already been described in the beginning of the era of reflectance confocal microscopy (RCM) by Aghassi and colleagues,[9] and further studies have analyzed the sensitivity and specificity of the AK criteria as well as the differentiation of AK from Bowen disease/SCC in situ and invasive SCC.[10–13]

Herein, the morphologic criteria of the complete spectrum of squamous neoplasia on RCM evaluation are described. Furthermore, the use of RCM for the monitoring of AK is discussed.

REFLECTANCE CONFOCAL MICROSCOPY CRITERIA OF SQUAMOUS NEOPLASIA
Actinic Keratosis and Actinic Cheilitis

On RCM, mosaics AK are characterized by central or multilocal disruption of the stratum corneum by overlying hyperkeratotic or parakeratotic scale (Fig. 1A). On higher magnification, RCM single images (0.5 mm × 0.5 mm) allow the identification of single detached keratinocytes and small bright round structures corresponding to parakeratosis. In hyperkeratotic lesions, the scale may be compact, and if covering the complete or majority of a lesion, it may significantly impair the evaluation. Rarely, inflammatory cells may be observed within the stratum corneum as a sign of impetiginization. At the level of the stratum granulosum and spinosum, an atypical honeycomb pattern may be observed. Atypical keratinocytes show pleomorphism by variations in their size and shape, thus resulting in an architectural disarray of the epidermis. In the papillary dermis, discrete increase in vasculature may be observed showing small, elongated vessels. Curled fibers may commonly be observed in the upper dermis, corresponding to solar elastosis. Furthermore, other changes of the collagen such as huddles may often be seen as a sign of photoaging.[14] Recently, it has been shown that according to the grading, a histopathology of different grades of AK may also be differentiated by RCM, thus allowing an improved severity assessment and better selection of treatment.[15] Actinic cheilitis shows similar criteria with atypical keratinocytes at the epidermal layers[16] (see Fig. 1).

REFLECTANCE CONFOCAL MICROSCOPY FEATURES OF ACTINIC KERATOSES

- Bright cells in the stratum corneum (parakeratosis)
- Atypical honeycombed pattern
- Upper dermis with curled fibers and slightly elongated vessels

SQUAMOUS CELL CARCINOMA IN SITU/BOWEN DISEASE

AK and SCC in situ/Bowen disease share some findings on RCM evaluation because both represent different stages of the same disease continuum and also molecular and histopathological characteristics. Although SCC in situ arising in AK and typical Bowen disease arising as single lesions on trunk and/or extremities may show slight differences on histology, they are summarized in this paragraph and are synonymously used. Parakeratosis, hyperkeratosis, and atypical honeycomb pattern may similarly be seen in AK and SCC in situ. However, marked atypia in the stratum granulosum is highly suggestive of SCC in situ as a sign for atypical proliferation of keratinocytes involving the complete epidermis. When applying RCM in clinical practice, the correct identification of the stratum granulosum may pose a significant challenge, especially for less-experienced observers. In that regard, atypical honeycomb pattern that appears directly underneath the stratum corneum is a good indicator for SCC in situ. Furthermore, SCC in situ is characterized by the presence of targetoid cells in the epidermis. Targetoid cells represent apoptotic epidermal keratinocytes, and corresponding to different stages of apoptosis, they may occur either as bright round cells with a dark rim or as a round structure with a dark center, a bright rim, and another dark rim in the periphery. The first type of targetoid cells is more common and represents apoptotic cells without nuclei, whereas the latter corresponds to apoptotic cells still containing a central nucleus.[13] Marked pleomorphism of

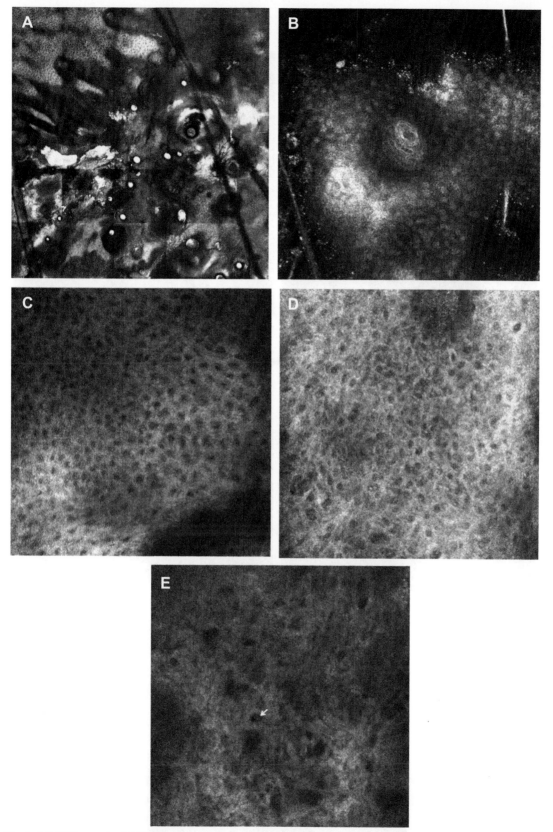

Fig. 1. (*A*) RCM mosaic of AK illustrating disruption of the stratum corneum with several areas of overlying scale and parakeratosis. (*B*) RCM single image showing small bright structures within the stratum corneum corresponding to parakeratosis. (*C*) RCM single image of the stratum granulosum. (*D*) RCM single image of the stratum spinosum. Please note the atypical honeycombed pattern. (*E*) RCM single image of the upper dermis illustrating solar elastosis with curled and clumped fibers and small dilated vessels (*arrow*).

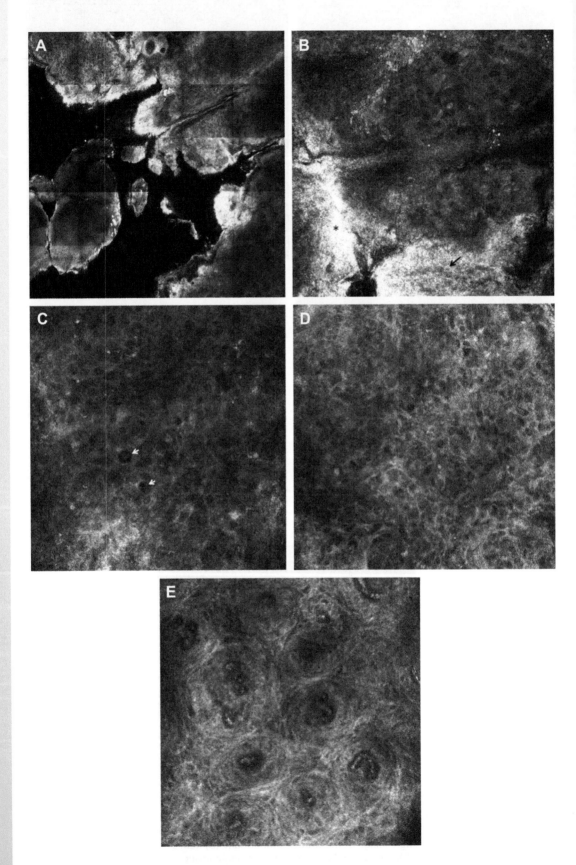

the keratinocytes is common, resulting in an atypical honeycomb pattern, or if severe, in complete disarray of the epidermis. Corresponding to the glomerular pattern of vessels seen in dermoscopy of SCC in situ, the vasculature also shows distinct features on RCM that also helps in the differentiation of SCC in situ from AK and invasive SCC. The vessels of SCC in situ appear in the papillary dermis and are often grouped together, surrounded by compact collagen. The morphology of the single vessels varies from round to S-shaped, depending on the level of examination. Solar elastosis may additionally be observed in the dermis (**Fig. 2**).

REFLECTANCE CONFOCAL MICROSCOPY FEATURES OF SQUAMOUS CELL CARCINOMA IN SITU/BOWEN DISEASE

- Disruption of the stratum corneum
- Atypical honeycombed pattern in all skin layers, also in the stratum granulosum
- Targetoid cells (apoptosis)
- Upper dermis with S-shaped vessels

INVASIVE SQUAMOUS CELL CARCINOMA

The detection of early SCC often represents a diagnostic challenge because clear clinical and dermoscopy criteria are lacking. On RCM evaluations, the detection of early invasion of SCC remains difficult because of several limitations. Hyperkeratosis that is often associated with invasive SCC impairs the evaluation of underlying structures, and because of the en face images, early invasion from the basal part of the epidermis into the upper dermis cannot reliably be determined. Tumor nests in the dermis represent the most important criterion for invasive SCC. These tumor nests show morphologic variations and may either be hyporefractile or hyperrefractile in well-differentiated SCC. When compared with AK and SCC in situ, invasive SCC also shows differences in tumor vasculature with enlarged and elongated vessels. Corresponding to dermoscopy, hairpin vessels may commonly be observed. Currently, only few studies have

analyzed the criteria of invasive SCC. Of these, one recent study reported the predictive parameters of AK in SCC.[17] In this study of 30 lesions (24 AKs and 6 invasive SCC), the presence of architectural disarray of the stratum granulosum in combination with dermal nestlike structures had a correct prediction of 88.5% of the SCC cases (**Fig. 3**).

REFLECTANCE CONFOCAL MICROSCOPY FEATURES OF SQUAMOUS CELL CARCINOMA

- Severe hyperkeratosis
- Atypical honeycombed pattern
- Upper dermis with dilated hairpin vessels and bright keratinizing tumor nests

REFLECTANCE CONFOCAL MICROSCOPY FOR TREATMENT MONITORING OF ACTINIC KERATOSIS

When evaluating the in vivo effects of a specific treatment and its efficacy to clear AK, sequential biopsies are often not feasible because they require multiple invasive interventional procedures. Moreover, biopsies are associated with scarring and inflammation, which itself leads to an artificial alteration of the tissue and limits the objective evaluation. The use of RCM allows the monitoring of treatment response over time without any alteration of the lesions and is therefore applicable for the evaluation of treatment effects, individual response, and efficacy. In addition to the changes in AK, RCM is also able to visualize the changes in clinically noninvolved, but biologically affected tissue, which has been referred to as subclinical AK lesion (SC-AK). Imiquimod is known for its ability to highlight and treat these SC-AKs, and the morphologic changes of apoptosis, induction of Langerhans cells, and inflammation have been described for AK as well as for SC-AK.[18] Further studies have included RCM for the monitoring of AK treatment response to low-dose 5-fluorouracil with salicylic acid and diclofenac in hyaluronic acid as well as to ingenol mebutate (**Fig. 4**).[19–23]

Fig. 2. (*A*) RCM mosaic of SCC in situ illustrating disruption of the stratum corneum with several areas of overlying scale as well as marked disarray of the epidermal architecture. (*B*) RCM single image of the stratum corneum illustrating single detached corneocytes and Parakeratosis. (*C*) RCM single image of the stratum granulosum illustrating marked pleomorphism of the keratinocyte resulting in an atypical honeycomb pattern and the presence of targetoid cells (*arrows*). (*D*) RCM single image of the spinous layer showing complete disarray of the epidermal architecture and the presence of multiple targetoid (apoptotic) cells. (*E*) RCM single image of the upper dermis with typical round to S-shaped vessels being grouped together and surrounded by compact collagen.

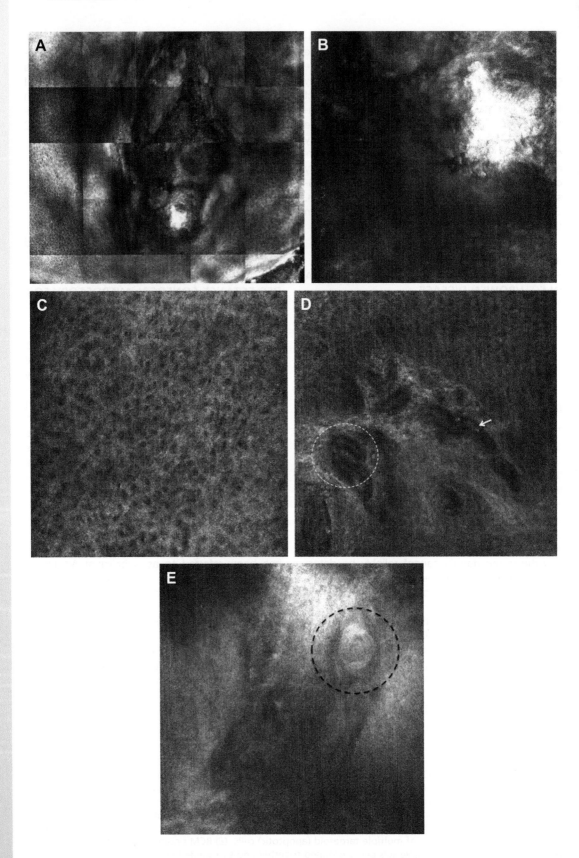

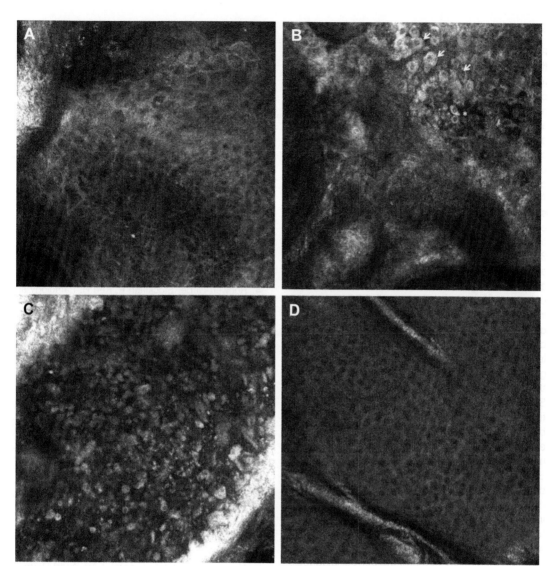

Fig. 4. Illustration of the treatment response of AK to ingenol mebutate. (*A*) AK before treatment. A representative image at the level of the granular/spinous layer with the presence of atypical keratinocytes is shown. (*B*) RCM showing acute changes 1 day after first application of ingenol mebutate gel 0.05% on the upper extremities. Apoptosis of keratinocytes with swelling of the cells (*arrows*), visible dark nucleus, and acantholysis (*asterisk*) is seen. (*C*) The changes during treatment with ingenol mebutate gel 0.05% of the same site at day 3 (1 day after second application) with multiple apoptotic cells and numerous small bright cells within the vesicles that correspond to neutrophils. (*D*) Clearance of AK after treatment with ingenol mebutate gel as seen on day 57. A representative image at the level of the granular/spinous layer is shown. A regular honeycomb pattern of the epidermis is observed.

Fig. 3. (*A*) RCM mosaic of an invasive SCC illustrating central hyperkeratosis. (*B*) RCM single image of the stratum corneum illustrating severe compact hyperkeratosis. (*C*) RCM single image of the stratum granulosum illustrating pleomorphism of the keratinocyte resulting in an atypical honeycomb pattern. (*D*) RCM single image illustrating dilated (*arrow*) and hairpin vessels (*circle*). (*E*) RCM single image of the dermis illustrating tumor nests central keratinization (*circle*).

SUMMARY

RCM allows the evaluation of the superficial parts of the skin at high resolution. Therefore, its applicability for the diagnosis of AK has already been the subject of early, preliminary studies. In the past 15 years, the research of RCM has continuously been growing, and several independent groups have shown its applicability for non-hyperkeratotic AK. Ulrich and colleagues[11] performed a study of 46 AKs and reported the presence of architectural disarray and cellular pleomorphism as the best predictor for AK. The sensitivity and specificity values in this study ranged from 80% to 98.6%. A further study by Horn and colleagues[10] analyzed 30 actinic keratoses and a sensitivity of 93.34% and specificity of 88.34% with a positive predictive value of 88.94%; a negative predictive value of 93.15% could be achieved by 2 clinical dermatologists. Rishpon and colleagues[24] analyzed 7 AKs, 25 SCCs in situ, 3 invasive SCCs, and 3 keratoacanthomas and described the presence of an atypical honeycomb or a disarranged pattern of the spinous-granular layer, round nucleated cells at the spinous-granular layer, and round blood vessels traversing through the dermal papilla as key RCM features of SCC. Furthermore, dyskeratotic cells, marked keratinocyte atypia, and a distinct vascular pattern have been suggested as key features of Bowen disease.[13] More recently, Peppelman and colleagues[17] have reported criteria for differentiation of AK and SCC. In their study, the combination of architectural disarray in the stratum granulosum, architectural disarray in the spinous layer, and nestlike structures in the dermis showed significant odds ratios. The forward multivariate logistic regression analysis showed that the combination of these features increased the ability to make the correct diagnosis of AK and SCC noninvasively. In this regard, the ability of RCM for the complete spectrum from SC-AK to AK, Bowen disease, and invasive SCC has been shown.

Moreover, RCM has also been applied in different studies for monitoring of biological treatment effects as well as for clearance of AK through different topicals.

Although the applicability of RCM has clearly been proven, RCM also has limitations in this field. Most importantly, hyperkeratosis impairs the evaluation significantly and can make the correct diagnosis or the differentiation of AK and SCC impossible. The en face evaluation of RCM also limits the detection of early invasion. Furthermore, RCM is strongly user-dependent as are all diagnostic techniques relying on subjective analysis, including also dermatopathology.

In conclusion, RCM may be very useful in the diagnosis and monitoring of squamous neoplasia, but future studies are required to show its additional use in clinical practice.

REFERENCES

1. Drake LA, Ceilley RI, Cornelison RL, et al. Guidelines of care for actinic keratoses. Committee on Guidelines of Care. J Am Acad Dermatol 1995;32(1):95–8.
2. Slaughter DP, Southwick HW, Smejkal W. Field cancerization in oral stratified squamous epithelium; clinical implications of multicentric origin. Cancer 1953;6(5):963–8.
3. Braakhuis BJ, Tabor MP, Kummer JA, et al. A genetic explanation of Slaughter's concept of field cancerization: evidence and clinical implications. Cancer Res 2003;63:1727–30.
4. Roewert-Huber Stockfleth E, Kerl H. Pathology and pathobiology of actinic (solar) keratosis—an update. Br J Dermatol 2007;157(Suppl 2):18–20.
5. Fernández-Figueras MT, Carrato C, Sáenz X, et al. Actinic keratosis with atypical basal cells (AK I) is the most common lesion associated with invasive squamous cell carcinoma of the skin. J Eur Acad Dermatol Venereol 2015;29(5):991–7.
6. Olsen EA, Abernethy ML, Kulp-Shorten C, et al. A double-blind, vehicle-controlled study evaluating masoprocol cream in the treatment of actinic keratoses on the head and neck. J Am Acad Dermatol 1991;24(5 Pt 1):738–43.
7. Zalaudek I, Piana S, Moscarella E, et al. Morphologic grading and treatment of facial actinic keratosis. Clin Dermatol 2014;32(1):80–7.
8. Zalaudek I, Kreusch J, Giacomel J, et al. How to diagnose nonpigmented skin tumors: a review of vascular structures seen with dermoscopy: part II. Nonmelanocytic skin tumors. J Am Acad Dermatol 2010;63(3):377–86.
9. Aghassi D, Anderson RR, Gonzalez S. Confocal laser microscopic imaging of actinic keratoses in vivo: a preliminary report. J Am Acad Dermatol 2000;43(1 Pt 1):42–8.
10. Horn M, Gerger A, Ahlgrimm-Siess V, et al. Discrimination of actinic keratoses from normal skin with reflectance mode confocal microscopy. Dermatol Surg 2008;34(5):620–5.
11. Ulrich M, Maltusch A, Rius-Diaz F, et al. Clinical applicability of in vivo reflectance confocal microscopy for the diagnosis of actinic keratoses. J Dermatol Surg 2008;34(5):610–9.
12. Ulrich M, Maltusch A, Röwert J, et al. Actinic keratoses: non-invasive diagnosis for field cancerisation. Br J Dermatol 2007;156(3):13–7.
13. Ulrich M, Kanitakis J, González S, et al. Evaluation of Bowen disease by in vivo reflectance confocal microscopy. Br J Dermatol 2012;166(2):451–3.

14. Pellacani G, Ulrich M, Casari A, et al. Grading kerati-nocyte atypia in actinic keratosis: a correlation of reflectance confocal microscopy and histopathology. J Eur Acad Dermatol Venereol 2015;29(11):2216–21.

15. Longo C, Casari A, Beretti F, et al. Skin aging: in vivo microscopic assessment of epidermal and dermal changes by means of confocal microscopy. J Am Acad Dermatol 2013;68(3):e73–82.

16. Ulrich M, González S, Lange-Asschenfeldt B, et al. Non-invasive diagnosis and monitoring of actinic cheilitis with reflectance confocal microscopy. J Eur Acad Dermatol Venereol 2011;25(3):276–84.

17. Peppelman M, Nguyen KP, Hoogedoorn L, et al. Reflectance confocal microscopy: non-invasive distinction between actinic keratosis and squamous cell carcinoma. J Eur Acad Dermatol Venereol 2015; 29(7):1302–9.

18. Ulrich M, Krueger-Corcoran D, Roewert-Huber J, et al. Reflectance confocal microscopy for noninvasive monitoring of therapy and detection of subclinical actinic keratoses. Dermatology 2010;220(1):15–24.

19. Label of Picato®: Available at: http://www.ema. europa.eu/docs/en_GB/document_library/EPAR_Pro duct_Information/human/002275/WC500135327.pdf. Accessed August 22, 2016.

20. Maier T, Cekovic D, Ruzicka T, et al. Treatment monitoring of topical ingenol mebutate in actinic keratoses with the combination of optical coher-ence tomography and reflectance confocal micro-scopy: a case series. Br J Dermatol 2015;172(3): 816–8.

21. Ulrich M, Alarcon I, Malvehy J, et al. In vivo reflectance confocal microscopy characterization of field-directed 5-fluorouracil 0.5%/salicylic acid 10% in actinic keratosis. Dermatology 2015;230(3): 193–8.

22. Malvehy J, Roldán-Marín R, Iglesias-García P, et al. Monitoring treatment of field cancerisation with 3% diclofenac sodium 2.5% hyaluronic acid by reflectance confocal microscopy: a histo-logic correlation. Acta Derm Venereol 2015;95(1): 45–50.

23. Ulrich M, Pellacani G, Ferrandiz C, et al. Evidence for field cancerisation treatment of actinic keratoses with topical diclofenac in hyaluronic acid. Eur J Der-matol 2014;24(2):158–67.

24. Rishpon A, Kim N, Scope A, et al. Reflectance confocal microscopy criteria for squamous cell car-cinomas and actinic keratoses. Arch Dermatol 2009;145(7):766–72.

Application of Handheld Confocal Microscopy for Skin Cancer Diagnosis
Advantages and Limitations Compared with the Wide-Probe Confocal

Syril Keena T. Que, MD[a],*, Jane M. Grant-Kels, MD[a],
Harold S. Rabinovitz, MD[b], Margaret Oliviero, FNP-C[b],
Alon Scope, MD[c]

KEYWORDS

- Handheld reflectance confocal microscopy • Wide-probe reflectance confocal microscopy
- Melanoma • Nonmelanoma skin cancer • Face • Eyes • Mucosa

KEY POINTS

- Handheld reflectance confocal microscopy (HH-RCM) can be useful for diagnosing lesions on the curved surfaces of the face, eyes and mucosa.
- The HH-RCM's small probe can be glided across the skin, allowing access to narrow surfaces, compared with the wide-probe RCM, which requires affixation to broad, flat skin surfaces.
- The main disadvantage of the HH-RCM is its smaller field of view, which limits the extent of optical sampling of lesions.
- Another advantage of the wide-probe RCM is its built-in navigation system, guided by a dermoscopic image, which the HH-RCM lacks.
- Studies have also investigated use of the handheld RCM in presurgical assessment of tumor margins and for monitoring the efficacy of nonsurgical skin cancer therapies.

INTRODUCTION

The clinical diagnosis of tumors on the curved surfaces of the face, around the eyes, and on the mucosal surfaces can be difficult, while biopsies and excisions can have functional and aesthetic consequences at these sites. A lower diagnostic accuracy and higher biopsy threshold at these sites could lead to delayed diagnosis of skin cancers that may be more difficult to manage.

Noninvasive imaging technologies have improved upon the accuracy of early diagnosis of skin cancers. However, acquisition of high-quality images with dermoscopy and with wide-probe reflectance confocal microscopy (WP-RCM, VivaScope 1500, CaliberID, Rochester, New York) have been hampered with technical difficulties in these curved, narrow, or relatively inaccessible surfaces. To this end, the newly introduced handheld reflectance confocal microscope

Conflicts of Interest: H.S. Rabinovitz and M. Oliviero are both clinical investigators and speakers for Caliber.
[a] Department of Dermatology, University of Connecticut Health Center, 263 Farmington Avenue, MC 6231, Farmington, CT 06030-6231, USA; [b] Department of Dermatology, University of Miami School of Medicine, 1295 NW 14th St., University of Miami South Bldg., Suites K-M, Miami, FL 33125, USA; [c] Department of Dermatology, Sheba Medical Center, Tel Hashomer, Ramat Gan 5262000, Affiliated with the Sackler School of Medicine, Tel Aviv University, Ramat Gan 52621, Israel
* Corresponding author.
E-mail address: keenaq@gmail.com

Dermatol Clin 34 (2016) 469–475
http://dx.doi.org/10.1016/j.det.2016.05.009
0733-8635/16/$ – see front matter © 2016 Elsevier Inc. All rights reserved.

(HH-RCM, Vivascope 3000, CaliberID) has a small probe, which allows rapid access to narrow surfaces. The use of the HH-RCM can potentially reduce the number of biopsies performed for benign lesions, while allowing earlier diagnosis of skin cancers, both melanoma and nonmelanoma skin cancers (NMSCs), on the face, eyes, and mucosal surfaces. Other potential applications are the use of HH-RCM for guiding management of skin cancers, such as RCM-guided excisions or laser ablation, and for monitoring response to nonsurgical treatments. This article discusses the technical parameters of the HH-RCM, as well as its advantages and limitations compared with the WP-RCM, and surveys the handful of studies focusing on HH-RCM.

COMPARISON OF IMAGES ACQUISITION BY HANDHELD REFLECTANCE CONFOCAL MICROSCOPE AND WIDE-PROBE REFLECTANCE CONFOCAL MICROSCOPY

The differences between WP-RCM and HH-RCM are summarized (Table 1).

The traditional WP-RCM (Fig. 1A) uses an 830 nm laser to acquire images that are characterized by a lateral (horizontal) resolution of less than 1.25 μm and an axial (vertical) resolution of less than 5.0 μm at the center field of view, and a maximal imaging depth of about 250 μm. The WP-RCM images are acquired as single 500×500 μm^2 optical sections, which can be stitched together via computer software to create a mosaic image along the X-Y axis with a field of view of up to 8×8 mm^2. An automated stack of images, acquired along the Z-axis, from the stratum corneum to the superficial dermis, can be obtained at the same location in the lesion. Video streaming of RCM images can also be recorded.

The HH-RCM (Fig. 1B) became commercially available in the United States in 2011. The handheld device also uses an 830 nm laser light source, and its images are characterized by lateral and axial resolution and maximal imaging depth that are comparable to that of the WP-RCM. The HH-RCM has 3 image acquisition modes: single optical sections, image stacks, and video recording. The main differences in acquisition from the WP-RCM are (1) HH-RCM acquires single optical sections that are 750×750 μm^2 (compared to 500×500 μm^2 for WP-RCM), and (2) the HH-RCM cannot acquire mosaic images (see Fig. 1, Table 1).

ADVANTAGES AND LIMITATIONS OF WIDE-PROBE REFLECTANCE CONFOCAL MICROSCOPE

The WP-RCM has demonstrated high specificity and increased sensitivity in the diagnosis of melanoma[1,2] and nonmelanoma skin cancers,[3]

Table 1
A comparison of the handheld reflectance confocal microscopy and wide-probe reflectance confocal microscopy

	HH-RCM	WP-RCM
Individual RCM optical section field of view	1 mm × 1 mm	0.5 mm × 0.5 mm
Maximal field of view	1 mm × 1 mm	8 mm × 8 mm
Average imaging time	1–4 min	5–10 min
Automated capture functions	Stack of individual images	• Axial stack of individual images • Horizontal mosaic of captured images
Advantages	• Access to contoured surfaces • Rapid examination of multiple areas of interest	• Wide field of view = assessment of lesion for overall pattern and symmetry • Built-in navigation guided by dermoscopy • Tissue fixation = systematic navigation and orientation
Limitations	• Small field of view • Difficult to achieve orientation within a lesion	• Requires fixation with adhesive, which takes longer and requires flat skin surface • Limited access to contoured surfaces

Adapted from Fraga-Braghiroli NA, Stephens A, Grossman D, et al. Use of handheld reflectance confocal microscopy for in vivo diagnosis of solitary facial papules: a case series. J Eur Acad Dermatol Venereol 2014;28(7):940; with permission.

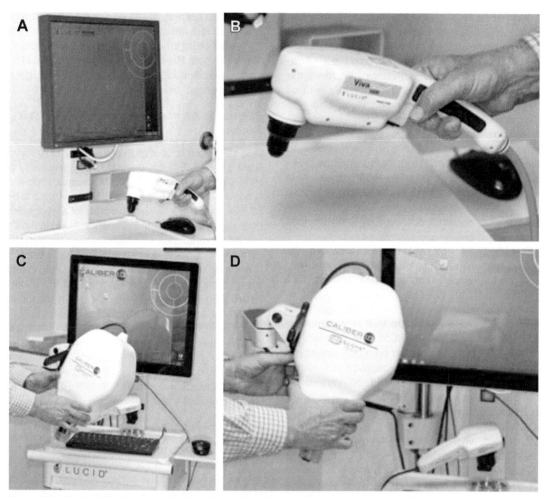

Fig. 1. (*A*) HH-RCM (*B*) Close-up of HH-RCM probe (*C*) WP-RCM (*D*) Close-up of WP-RCM. The differences between the WP-RCM and HH-RCM are summarized in **Table** 1. (*Courtesy of* CaliberID, Andover, MA; with permission.)

compared with clinical and dermoscopic examination. Advantages of the WP-RCM include the wide field of view (enables the clinician to evaluate the entire tumor for the overall pattern, size of the lesion, and symmetry of structures and brightness) the presence of built-in navigation guided by dermoscopy, and the systematic navigation and orientation provided by tissue fixation.

However, the WP-RCM requires affixation to flat skin surface of about 2 cm in diameter to obtain high-quality images. If adhesion to the skin is not firm and steady, air bubbles may block the path of RCM laser light and obscure tissue imaging, and skin folding and motion artifacts may reduce image quality and seamlessness. The authors often encounter such imaging technical difficulties when attempting to image lesions on the curved and narrow surfaces of the face (eg, the nose or ear lobe). In other locations, such as around the eyes or at mucosal surfaces, imaging with

WP-RCM is inaccessible. This has been a limitation to the use of RCM, since a majority of NMSCs occurs on face.

Additionally, setting up the bulky imaging apparatus and acquiring the images with the WP-RCM are also time consuming, particularly on the face, taking at least 15 minutes. This may pose a barrier for adoption of RCM in the busy dermatologic practices.

ADVANTAGES AND LIMITATIONS OF HANDHELD REFLECTANCE CONFOCAL MICROSCOPE

The HH-RCM has advantages. It is well suited for curved and narrow surfaces because of its small probe, whose tip measures 5 mm in diameter. The HH-RCM allows for imaging of lesions in less accessible sites, such as the medial canthus of the eye or oral or genital mucosa.

The HH-RCM also acquires images faster than the WP-RCM, is lighter in weight, and is relatively easy to handle after some initial practice. Although WP-RCM requires skin preparation by the application of a disposable adhesive window, the HH-RCM can be applied to skin directly with oil immersion fluid, making imaging faster and less cumbersome. As such, it also allows for rapid examination of multiple lesions of concern on the patient. Finally, most of the previously published diagnostic algorithms, delineated for the WP-RCM, can be applied to HH-RCM, since most criteria can be evaluated on optical sections and do not require mosaic image acquisition. The RCM optical sections obtained by both devices are similar in quality and appearance.

The HH-RCM also has inherent limitations. Its optical sections are 1×1 mm^2 in areas that only allow partial optical sampling of skin lesions. This is in contrast to the WP-RCM, in which adjacent individual optical sections can be pieced together to form large mosaic images up to 8×8 mm^2. The limited field of view of HH-RCM may diminish the ability to distinguish between benign melanocytic nevi and melanomas. In the evaluation of melanocytic lesions, the lesion should be viewed as a whole in order to adequately assess the symmetry, circumscription, overall pattern, and RCM features.

That said, when the differential diagnosis is between unrelated pathologic entities, identifying the cellular morphology of the lesion may suffice for diagnosis. For example, HH-RCM can allow distinction between basal cell carcinoma (BCC) from intradermal nevi; similarly, if dendritic pagetoid melanocytes are noted in an HH-RCM stack from the face, the likely diagnosis of a lentigo maligna can be established over a solar lentigo, pigmented actinic keratosis, or lichen planus-like keratosis.

Another disadvantage of the current HH-RCM is that navigation is only guided by the clinical eye, and not by the dermoscopic image of the lesion, nor by the RCM software. In contrast, the WP-RCM has a built-in navigation system, which can be guided by the dermoscopic image; this simplifies orientation and identification of suspicious foci within a lesion.

APPLICATIONS OF HANDHELD REFLECTANCE CONFOCAL MICROSCOPE

The HH-RCM can be used to diagnose melanoma[4,5] and NMSC,[6–9] can preoperatively or intra-operatively map out tumor margins,[10] and can help monitor the efficacy of nonsurgical treatments for skin cancers.[11,12] It can also be used to identify the correct site to perform Mohs surgery, when site identification is uncertain.

The HH-RCM studies are summarized (**Table 2**). Although most HH-RCM studies involved facial lesions, use on mucosal lesions in the mouth, genitals, or perianal skin has also been reported.

Diagnostic Accuracy for Nonmelanoma Skin Cancers

One study carried out at the University Hospital of Saint-Etienne, France, evaluated the sensitivity of HH-RCM for the diagnosis of 344 histopathologically confirmed BCCs.[7] The sensitivity was found to be 87.5%, with the learning curve for BCC diagnosis improving over time with experience. No statistically significant difference was found in the sensitivity for different histopathologic subtypes or body sites.

Another study evaluating 54 lesions compared the accuracy measures for diagnosis of BCC using HH-RCM versus WP-RCM. The study reported sensitivity of 100% versus 93%, respectively, a specificity of 78% for both probes, a positive predictive value of 96% versus 95%, and a negative predictive value of 100% versus 70%, respectively.[6] The authors attributed the higher sensitivity negative predictive value of WP-RCM to its broader field of view.

Periorbital Neoplasms

The HH-RCM has been used by ophthalmologists to visualize conjunctival tumors.[13] In 1 prospective, observational case series, 53 conjunctival lesions on 46 patients were examined. Twenty-three lesions were excised (3 nevi, 10 melanomas, 5 SCCs, 2 lymphomas, 3 pinguecula/pterygium), while the other 20 lesions that did not show malignant features on RCM remained under follow-up. In all cases examined, the RCM diagnosis was in agreement with the histopathologic diagnosis, and lesions that were followed did not show any clinical progression. The HH-RCM has also been useful for examining lesions on the eyelid margin[9] or on other periorbital skin. In 1 study, 47 eyelid margin lesions were examined, 35 of which were excised and 12 of which were followed clinically for at least 1 year. The HH-RCM was 100% sensitive and 69.2% specific for malignancy, and none of the lesions deemed benign by HH-RCM features showed any clinical progression.

Future studies will likely compare the diagnostic accuracy of HH-RCM with the current ophthalmologic standard of care.

Mucosal Tumors

The oral mucosa is a difficult biopsy site for dermatologists, and an area prone to bleeding and

Table 2
Studies involving handheld Vivascope 3000

	Number of Patients/ Lesions	Lesion Type	Head and Neck Lesions	Extrafacial Body Sites	Mucosal Lesions	Guiding Surgery	Skin Lesion Type/Purpose of Examination
Menge et al,[4] 2016	17 patients 63 lesions	39 lentigo maligna; 24 benign lesions	x				Lentigo maligna
Cinotti et al,[5] 2012	10 lesions	8 melanoses; 2 melanomas			x		Vulvar melanoma ad melanosis
Castro et al,[6] 2015	54 lesions	45 BCC	x	x			BCC
Cinotti et al,[7] 2015	344 lesions	315 BCC	x	x	x		BCC
Fraga-Braghiroli et al,[8] 2014	6 patients 6 lesions	2 BCC; 1 SCC; 1 melanocytic nevus; 1 sebaceous hyperplasia; 1 desmoplastic trichoepithelioma	x				Solitary facial papules: BCC, SCC, sebaceous hyperplasia, desmoplastic trichoep, compound nevus
Cinnotti et al,[9] 2014	47 lesions	5 melanomas; 9 melanocytic nevi; 14 BCC; 3 SCC	x				Eyelid margin tumors
Chen et al,[10] 2014	2 lesions	2 BCC	x	x		x	Confocal-guided laser ablation of BCCs
Kai et al,[11] 2016	40 lesions	40 lentigo maligna	x				Lentigo maligna after imiquimod treatment
Cinotti et al,[12] 2014	1 lesion	1 SCC in situ			x		SCC on the glans penis after photodynamic therapy
Cinotti et al,[13] 2015	46 patients 53 lesions	3 nevi; 10 melanomoas; 5 SCC; 2 lymphomas; 3 pinguencula/pterygium; 30 other benign	x				Conjunctival tumors
Erfan et al,[14] 2012	56 lesions	46 benign melanotic macules; 10 melanomas			x		Labial melanotic macule
Contaldo et al,[15] 2013	6 patients 24 mucosal areas	24 areas of normal oral mucosa			x		Healthy oral mucosa
Ferrari et al,[16] 2014	1 patient 1 lesion	1 benign vulvar mucosal melanotic macule			x		Vulvar mucosal melanotic macules
Debarbieux et al,[17] 2014	56 lesions	46 benign melanotic macules; 10 melanomas			x		Labial or genital pigmented macules, including melanomas
Cinotti et al,[18] 2014	1 lesion	1 benign melanotic macules on anus			x		Anal melanosis

patient discomfort. Suspicious lesions of the lips and oral mucosa are oftentimes referred to oral surgeons for management. The HH-RCM provides a way for dermatologists to rapidly image the oral mucosa[14,15] and offers in-office evaluation of oral growths without surgical procedures. Contaldo and colleagues[15] examined 100 healthy mucosal sites, including 38 lips, 24 cheeks, 10 gingivae, and 28 tongues, using the HH-RCM and correlated the findings with conventional histopathology. Results showed reproducible RCM features across participants and in different mucosal sites. To date, no studies have investigated the appearance of oral malignancies with the HH-RCM, and no studies have documented the diagnostic accuracy of this device for malignant tumors; however, this early study of healthy oral mucosa shows that the use of HH-RCM in the dermatology setting may be of practical value.

The HH-RCM can also be used to distinguish between vulvar melanosis[16,17] and vulvar melanoma,[5] which can be challenging. In 1 study by Cinotti and colleagues,[5] the authors used the standard RCM criteria to diagnose pigmented lesions of the vulva. In all 10 cases examined, RCM diagnosis corresponded well with histopathology. Vulvar melanosis showed on RCM as dark spaces rimmed by bright monomorphous basal cells (edged papillae), with dendritic bright cells in the basal layer of the epithelium. Vulvar melanomas, on the other hand, exhibited atypical cells throughout the epithelium and loss of normal architecture, allowing them to be distinguished from benign lesions.

Diagnosis of lesions on the anal mucosa[18] is similarly challenging and less accessible for biopsy by the dermatologist. One case report describes patient with human immunodeficiency virus (HIV) who presented with acquired pigmentation of the anal mucosa. The HH-RCM showed features suggestive of hypomelanosis: a honeycomb pattern of the epidermis, with hyperrefractive elongated dermal papillary rings, homogeneous round cells, and no atypical cells. Histopathologic examination confirmed this diagnosis. In future cases, the HH-RCM could be used to diagnose anal melanosis and to rule out a melanoma.

Monitoring of Nonsurgical Skin Cancer Therapies

Another potential application for HH-RCM is the monitoring of treatment efficacy after nonsurgical therapies, such as topical chemotherapy, photodynamic therapy, cryosurgery, or radiation therapy. These therapies often lack histopathologic confirmation of diagnosis and of clearance of the neoplasm after therapy. Rather, diagnosis and monitoring rely on clinical and dermoscopic judgments, which can be limited for nonpigmented neoplasms. This can be problematic, as rates of NMSC clearance are lower for non-surgical therapies. Nonetheless, in many cases, the patient may decline a diagnostic or post-treatment biopsy. For example, a mutilating surgery for SCC in situ of the penis[12] can be avoided by treating the skin cancer with topical chemotherapy or photodynamic therapy. After treatment, tumor clearance can be assessed using the HH-RCM.

The HH-RCM has also been used to monitor for recurrence after topical chemotherapy with imiquimod. Kai and colleagues[11] treated 40 patients with lentigo maligna with imiquimod. They biopsied select areas to assess for clearance of tumor. HH-RCM was used to monitor for lentigo maligna recurrence for 5 years after imiquimod treatment. Patients who were clear on histology immediately after treatment had a 0% recurrence rate 5 years later based HH-RCM imaging. Of note, there was no histopathologic confirmation of tumor clearance at 5 years follow-up.

Surgical Adjunct

A study by Chen and colleagues[10] demonstrates that HH-RCM may also be useful for the assessment of tumor margins prior to surgery or intraoperatively. In this study, the authors used both WP- and HH-RCM to guide Er:YAG laser ablation of 2 cases of superficial and early nodular BCC. The RCM was used to define the lateral border and thickness of the tumor, which on a note of caution, cannot be relied upon completely, because the RCM has a limited depth of detection (of about 250 μm). Intraoperatively, the RCM was also used to detect residual BCC after initial laser ablation. Both RCM imaging and histopathologic sections confirmed final clearance of tumor. The authors note that motion artifact was not a significant limitation, even though HH-RCM is held directly to the skin without fixation (see **Table 2**).

SUMMARY AND FUTURE DIRECTIONS

In summary, studies have demonstrated the potential utility of HH-RCM for the diagnosis of melanoma and NMSC on curved surfaces and its possible applications in defining tumor margins and monitoring for clearance of skin cancers after nonsurgical therapy. HH-RCM is smaller, faster, and easier to use than WP-RCM. Current limitations of HH-RCM include its inability to form larger mosaic images, resulting in a small field of view that prevents visualization of the entire tumor.

This limitation may reduce the applicability of HH-RCM in differentiation of melanoma from nevi. The smaller window also lowers the sensitivity for the detection of NMSC. Therefore, HH-RCM and WP-RCM are complementary technologies that fulfill different clinical needs and are not mutually exclusive.

Studies of HH-RCM have been mostly preliminary and have focused mostly on the face, and to a lesser extent, on external mucosa. Future studies might include a comparison of HH- and WP-RCM diagnosis of the same lesions. Studies may also test HH-RCM utility for lesions on the trunk and extremities to evaluate the overall applicability of this device. It would also be interesting to see if a fluorescence-based HH confocal may be useful for diagnosis and delineation of neoplasms, particularly on mucosal surfaces in which dyes can be easily absorbed.

REFERENCES

1. Guitera P, Pellacani G, Longo C, et al. In vivo reflectance confocal microscopy enhances secondary evaluation of melanocytic lesions. J Invest Dermatol 2009;129(1):131–8.
2. Guitera P, Pellacani G, Crotty KA, et al. The impact of in vivo reflectance confocal microscopy on the diagnostic accuracy of lentigo maligna and equivocal pigmented and nonpigmented macules of the face. J Invest Dermatol 2010;130(8):2080–91.
3. Kadouch DJ, Schram ME, Leeflang MM, et al. In vivo confocal microscopy of basal cell carcinoma: a systematic review of diagnostic accuracy. J Eur Acad Dermatol Venereol 2015;29(10):1890–7.
4. Menge TD, Hibler BP, Cordova MA, et al. Concordance of handheld reflectance confocal microscopy (RCM) with histopathology in the diagnosis of lentigo maligna (LM): A prospective study. J Am Acad Dermatol 2016;74(6):1114–20.
5. Cinotti E, Perrot JL, Labeille B, et al. Reflectance confocal microscopy for the diagnosis of vulvar melanoma and melanosis: preliminary results. Dermatol Surg 2012;38(12):1962–7.
6. Castro RP, Stephens A, Fraga-Braghiroli NA, et al. Accuracy of in vivo confocal microscopy for diagnosis of basal cell carcinoma: a comparative study between handheld and wide-probe confocal imaging. J Eur Acad Dermatol Venereol 2015;29(6):1164–9.
7. Cinotti E, Jaffelin C, Charriere V, et al. Sensitivity of handheld reflectance confocal microscopy for the diagnosis of basal cell carcinoma: a series of 344 histologically proven lesions. J Am Acad Dermatol 2015;73(2):319–20.
8. Fraga-Braghiroli NA, Stephens A, Grossman D, et al. Use of handheld reflectance confocal microscopy for in vivo diagnosis of solitary facial papules: a case series. J Eur Acad Dermatol Venereol 2014;28(7):933–42.
9. Cinotti E, Perrot JL, Campolmi N, et al. The role of in vivo confocal microscopy in the diagnosis of eyelid margin tumors: 47 cases. J Am Acad Dermatol 2014;71(5):912–8.e2.
10. Chen CS, Sierra H, Cordova M, et al. Confocal microscopy-guided laser ablation for superficial and early nodular basal cell carcinoma: a promising surgical alternative for superficial skin cancers. JAMA Dermatol 2014;150(9):994–8.
11. Kai AC, Richards T, Coleman A, et al. Five-year recurrence rate of lentigo maligna after treatment with imiquimod. Br J Dermatol 2016;174(1):165–8.
12. Cinotti E, Perrot JL, Labeille B, et al. Laser photodynamic treatment for in situ squamous cell carcinoma of the glans monitored by reflectance confocal microscopy. Australas J Dermatol 2014;55(1):72–4.
13. Cinotti E, Perrot JL, Labeille B, et al. Handheld reflectance confocal microscopy for the diagnosis of conjunctival tumors. Am J Ophthalmol 2015;159(2):324–33.e1.
14. Erfan N, Hofman V, Desruelles F, et al. Labial melanotic macule: a potential pitfall on reflectance confocal microscopy. Dermatology 2012;224(3):209–11.
15. Contaldo M, Agozzino M, Moscarella E, et al. In vivo characterization of healthy oral mucosa by reflectance confocal microscopy: a translational research for optical biopsy. Ultrastruct Pathol 2013;37(2):151–8.
16. Ferrari A, Agozzino M, Ardigò M, et al. Dermoscopic and confocal microscopy patterns of vulvar mucosal melanotic macules. J Am Acad Dermatol 2014;70(4):e81–2.
17. Debarbieux S, Perrot JL, Erfan N, et al. Reflectance confocal microscopy of mucosal pigmented macules: a review of 56 cases including 10 macular melanomas. Br J Dermatol 2014;170(6):1276–84.
18. Cinotti E, Chol C, Perrot JL, et al. Anal melanosis diagnosed by reflectance confocal microscopy. Australas J Dermatol 2014;55(4):286–8.

This limitation may reduce the applicability of HH-RCM for differentiation of melanoma from nevi. The smaller window also lowers the sensitivity for the detection of NMSC. Therefore, HH-RCM and WP-RCM are complementary technologies that fulfill different clinical needs and are not mutually exclusive.

Studies of HH-RCM have been mostly preliminary and have focused mostly on the face, and to a lesser extent, on external mucosa. Future studies might include a comparison of HH- and WP-RCM diagnosis of the same lesions. Studies may also test HH-RCM utility for lesions on the trunk and extremities to evaluate the overall applicability of this device. It would also be interesting to see if a team-reviewer-based HH protocol may be useful for discussion and delimitation of new lesions, particularly on mucosal surfaces in which these can be readily assessed.

TAKE-HOME...

Confocal Microscopy for Special Sites and Special Uses

Elisa Cinotti, MD, PhD*, Bruno Labeille, MD,
Frédéric Cambazard, PhD, Jean-Luc Perrot, MD

KEYWORDS

- Reflectance confocal microscopy • Special sites • Mucosa • Nail • Tumor • Infection • Parasites
- Microcirculation

KEY POINTS

- The in vivo hand-held reflectance confocal microscopy camera allows one to explore skin appendages and oral, genital, and ocular mucosa.
- In vivo and ex vivo confocal microscopy is not only valuable to identify skin cancers but also for the diagnosis of skin infections and inflammatory diseases.
- In vivo reflectance confocal microscopy can be used to guide presurgical mapping of skin tumors.
- Confocal microscopy can provide videos that are particularly useful to study the cutaneous microcirculation.

 Video content accompanies this article at http://www.derm.theclinics.com.

INTRODUCTION

In vivo reflectance confocal microscopy (RCM) was initially developed in dermatology for the evaluation of skin neoplasms. Recently, a hand-held (HH) camera (VivaScope 3000, Caliber, Rochester, NY; distributed in Europe by Mavig GmbH, Munich, Germany) has been developed expanding the applications of RCM. HH-RCM has three main advantages compared with the traditional wide probe (TWP) VivaScope 1500: (1) it is handy because it uses an optical fiber wiring the optical source to the detector, (2) it does not need fixation on the skin through a metal ring, and (3) it has a smaller tip (5 mm in diameter in the first version of the HH device, 1.5 cm in the second version of the HH device, and 2 cm in the TWP), enabling access to body sites with curved surfaces inaccessible to the TWP.[1]

All these advantages have enabled the use of RCM for the study of the whole body skin, of the mucosa, and of the skin appendages. The HH-RCM has increased the use of RCM in clinical practice because of faster image acquisition (1–3 minutes per lesion vs 10–20 minutes).[1] Moreover, it has allowed the use of RCM for a rapid diagnosis of cutaneous inflammatory and infectious diseases and of epithelial cancers that do not require the architectural information provided by the mosaic image reconstruction of the TWP.[2,3]

HH-RCM can be compared with modern dermoscopy, which started with the evaluation of tumors and now has been demonstrated to be a useful noninvasive diagnostic tool for a wide range of skin diseases.

A new field of confocal microscopy has also been opened by the development of an ex vivo device dedicated to the skin (VivaScope 2500,

Funding Sources: None.
Conflict of Interest: None.
Dermatology Department, University Hospital of Saint-Etienne, Cedex 2, Saint-Etienne, 42055, France
* Corresponding author.
E-mail address: elisacinotti@gmail.com

Dermatol Clin 34 (2016) 477–485
http://dx.doi.org/10.1016/j.det.2016.05.010
0733-8635/16/© 2016 Elsevier Inc. All rights reserved.

Caliber; distributed in Europe by Mavig GmbH). This new device has been conceived for the evaluation of cutaneous tumor margins in real-time, directly on freshly excised tissue in a perioperative setting. However, further applications are possible, such as the diagnosis of infectious diseases.

SPECIAL SITES

Mucosa, nails, and hairs can be examined by RCM. All these body sites are sensitive areas where noninvasive imaging techniques are of high interest to spare biopsies and excisions. RCM has a limit in the laser penetration depth and for this reason acral skin has not been initially investigated. However, in our experience RCM could also be useful in this area.

Genital and Oral Mucosa

Mucosa is particularly suitable for RCM because of its thin or absent cornified layer, which allows a deeper penetration of the laser and a resolution in the upper layers higher than in the skin. Thus, RCM permits a better-detailed visualization of the cellular morphology.[1]

RCM is a promising tool for the differential diagnosis of pigmented lesions in the genital and oral mucosa[4–6] and in particular to differentiate early melanoma from the more frequent melanosis.[4,5] Melanoses correspond to the benign hyperpigmentation of basal keratinocytes and are characterized under RCM by the presence of chorion papillae rimmed by hyperreflective monomorphous cells corresponding to hyperpigmented basal keratinocytes[4–6] (**Fig. 1**). Mucosal melanoma is characterized by four major features: (1) high density of basal hyperreflective dendritic cells, (2) presence of pagetoid bright large cells in the epithelium (mainly roundish or fusiform with plump body), (3) loss of normal architecture of chorion papillae, and (4) sheet-like proliferation of atypical cells in the chorion.[4,5]

RCM is also helpful for the differential diagnosis between in situ squamous cell carcinoma (SCC) and Zoon plasma cell balanitis, a benign idiopathic inflammatory disease.[7] RCM criteria for mucosal SCC are similar to those used in the skin: atypical honeycomb pattern and disarranged epidermal pattern. Moreover RCM can be used to monitor laser photodynamic treatment of in situ SCC of the glans over time in a total noninvasive modality.[8]

Ocular Mucosa

Our group first applied the RCM devices dedicated to dermatology to the study of the ocular mucosa.[9] HH-RCM can explore the whole cornea and conjunctiva surface, including the ciliary margin, the lacrimal punctum, the internal and external canthi, and both surfaces of the eyelids comprising the meibomian glands.[1] These regions have not previously been explored by RCM, because of the limited mobility of devices available for ophthalmology (Confoscan 4 slit-scanning confocal microscope, Nidek, Gamagori, Japan; and Heidelberg Retina Tomograph in association

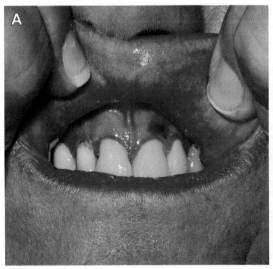
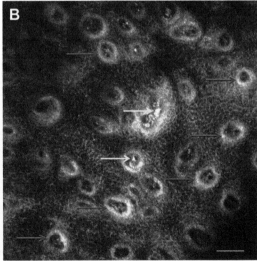

Fig. 1. Clinical (A) and in vivo RCM (B) aspect of a gingival melanosis. RCM shows roundish chorion papillae rimmed by hyperreflective cells (B, red arrows) at the epithelium-chorion junction. Some melanophages are visible inside the papillae (B, yellow arrows). Scale bar: 100 μm.

with the Rostock Cornea Module, Heidelberg Engineering GmbH, Heidelberg, Germany). RCM dedicated to the skin can diagnose lentigo (**Fig. 2**), primary acquired melanosis, nevi, basal cell carcinoma (BCC), SCC, melanoma, and lymphoma of eyelid margin and conjunctiva[9–12] with criteria similar to the cutaneous counterparts. However, compared with the skin (1) dilated vessels are common in normal conjunctiva and are less specific for malignancy; (2) inflammatory cells are common in the stroma of the normal conjunctiva; (3) dendritic cells can be found in the normal epithelium of the conjunctiva, especially in case of primary acquired melanosis; (4) nevi of the conjunctiva often have a cystic aspect; and (5) melanoma of the conjunctiva are invasive, whereas in situ melanoma are named primary acquired melanosis with atypia in ophthalmology.[1] RCM can also be used to diagnose ocular infections[1] and storage diseases with ocular involvement, such as cystinosis[12] and Fabry disease.[13] RCM can show the signs of postradiation blepharitis (**Fig. 3**) and can indicate foreign body material, such as pine processionary caterpillar hair in the cornea[14] and suture thread remaining in the eyelid after surgery and causing inflammation (**Fig. 4**).

Nail

The nail plate transparency allows a deep penetration of RCM that can image up to the nail bed in case of thin nails (<500 μm).[15] RCM can diagnose onychomycosis and could be used in the future as a noninvasive procedure for the investigation of different inflammatory nail diseases, such as psoriasis and lichen planus.[15] It is unable to directly explore the nail matrix located deep under the eponychium. However, it also helps in case of melanonichia to distinguish subungueal melanoma from lentigo and nevi because the matrix can be observed by reclining the eponychium.[15] In our

experience RCM is also useful to confirm the diagnosis of periungueal and subungueal pyogenic granuloma, by showing a lobulated proliferation of capillary-sized vessels with possible secondary ulceration, hemorrhage, and inflammatory infiltrate (**Fig. 5**).

Palms and Soles

Under RCM normal acral skin has a specific aspect: epidermal ridges appear as broad parallel bands with a regular honeycomb pattern, and furrows as parallel dark areas disrupting the honeycomb pattern (**Fig. 6**).[16] The openings of sweat ducts appear as hyperreflective circles plugged in lines inside the honeycomb pattern (see **Fig. 6**). When the image plan is not exactly parallel to the skin surface, the longitudinal section of acrosyringia can be seen as hyperreflective elongated coiled structures.

Although the presence of a thick corneum layer makes more difficult the examination of this region, RCM can help to diagnose acral lentiginous melanoma by showing inhomogeneous pagetoid cells with a particular tropism for acrosyringia.[16] However, acral lentiginous melanoma diagnosis cannot be excluded in the absence of RCM signs because early acral lentiginous melanoma can present only subtle atypia, such as slight proliferation of atypical melanocytes at the dermal-epidermal junction that may not be identified under RCM.[16] The superficial part of the stratum corneum can also be scraped off with a scalpel to have a deeper RCM examination in this special area.

SPECIAL USES
Infections and Infestations

RCM has a lateral resolution of up to 1.25 μm. This means that structures larger than 1.25 μm could

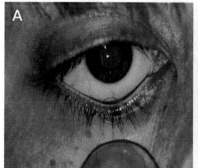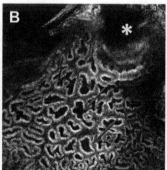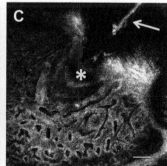

Fig. 2. Clinical (*A, red circle*) and in vivo RCM (*B, C*) aspect of an eyelid margin lentigo. RCM shows polycyclic and elongated dermal papillae rimmed by hyperreflective cells (*B, C, red arrows*) at the epidermal-dermal junction. An orifice of an eyelash (*B, C, yellow asterisk*) and the eyelash shaft (*C, yellow arrow*) are visible. Scale bar: 100 μm.

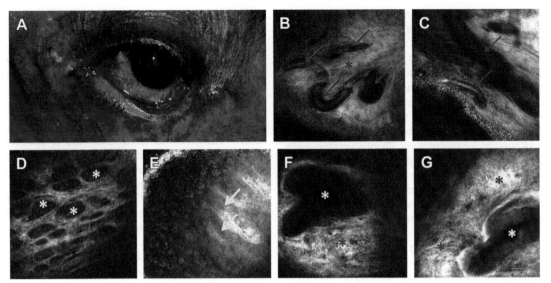

Fig. 3. Clinical (*A*) and in vivo RCM (*B–G*) aspect of postradiation blepharitis. RCM shows teleangectatic vessels (*B, C, red arrows*), fibrosis (*B, F, G, red asterisks*), alteration of meibomian glands in a transversal (*D*) and sagittal (*E*) view (*D, yellow asterisks; E, yellow arrows*), and distortion of the lacrimal punctum (*F, G, white asterisk*). Scale bar: 100 μm.

theoretically be identified. Parasites, such as *Sarcoptes scabiei* (**Fig. 7**), *Demodex folliculorum*, *Pyemotes ventricosus*, *Ixodes*, *Dermanyssus gallinae*, *Pediculus humanus*, pinworms, and *Pulex irritans* (**Fig. 8**), have been observed under RCM.[2,17–19] Some parasites are already visible to the naked eye but RCM can identify their different body parts helping the precise identification of the species (see **Fig. 8**). RCM can also quantify parasites, define their exact localization, and assess their viability after treatment.[20,21]

Some bacteria could also be theoretically identified, whereas virus cannot be observed because they are too small. However, viral cytopathic effects on keratinocytes can be observed in case of molluscipoxvirus, coxsackievirus, human papillomavirus, and herpes simplex and varicella-zoster herpes virus infection.[17]

RCM can also be used to identify filaments, pseudofilaments, and conidia on skin, and mucosa, and in skin appendages in case of mycosis. Filaments and pseudofilaments appear as thin,

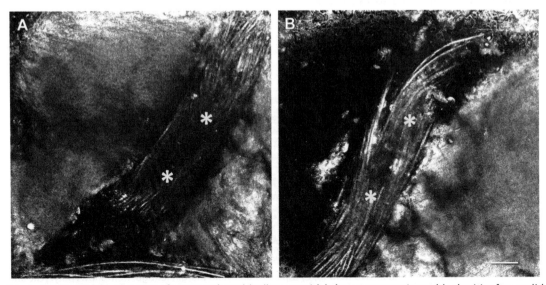

Fig. 4. In vivo RCM (*A, B*) aspect of a suture thread (*yellow asterisks*) that causes persistent blepharitis after eyelid surgery. Scale bar: 100 μm.

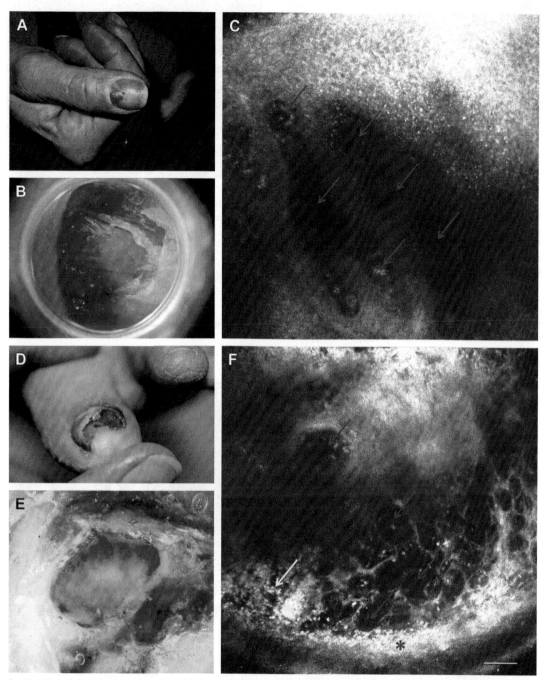

Fig. 5. Clinical (*A, D*), dermoscopical (*B, E*), and RCM (*C, F*) aspect of two cases of ungueal pyogenic granuloma. RCM shows a lobulated proliferation of capillary-sized vessels (*red arrows*), an inflammatory infiltrate (*yellow arrow*), and a well-defined hyperreflective collarette around the lesion (*red asterisk*). Scale bar: 100 μm.

hyperreflective, longitudinal structures with a serpentine shape,[15,22,23] whereas conidia are hyperreflective small roundish bodies.[23] RCM can confirm the diagnosis of mycosis during the clinical examination of patients avoiding them to wait for the microscopic and cultural examinations (**Fig. 9**).

Tumor Mapping

RCM can help surgery by indicating cutaneous tumor margins, especially in case of large BCC, lentigo maligna, and Paget disease. Our group developed a technique combining the staged excision of the "spaghetti type" and RCM[24,25] to

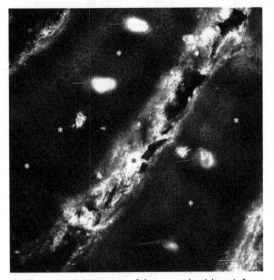

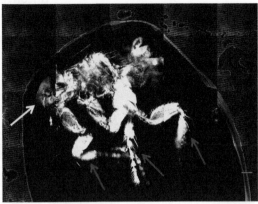

Fig. 8. In vivo RCM shows different body parts of a human flea (*Pulux irritans*) (mosaic image reconstruction acquired with VivaScope 1500; *yellow arrow* cephalic portion and *red arrows* legs). Scale bar: 100 μm.

Fig. 6. In vivo RCM aspect of the normal epidermis from the acral skin. Ridges appear as broad parallel bands with a regular honeycomb pattern (*yellow asterisks*) and furrows as parallel hyperreflective (in the superficial portion filled of keratin) and hyporeflective (in the deeper portion) areas disrupting the honeycomb pattern (*red asterisks*). Acrosyringia appear as hyperreflective circles plugged in lines in the center of the ridges (*red arrows*). Scale bar: 100 μm.

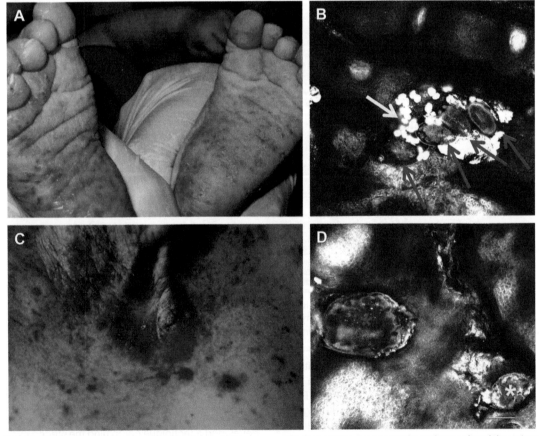

Fig. 7. Clinical (*A, C*) and in vivo RCM (*B, D*) aspect of two cases of scabies. RCM shows eggs (*B, red arrows*) and droppings (*B, yellow arrow*) and *Sarcoptes scabies* mites (*D, red asterisk* adult female and *yellow asterisk* larva). Scale bar: 100 μm.

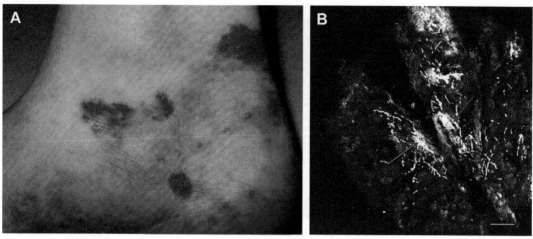

Fig. 9. Clinical (*A*) and in vivo RCM (*B*) aspect of a dermatophytosis. Dermatophytes are easily identified under RCM as thin, high-reflective, longitudinal structures with a linear shape (*red arrows*). Scale bar: 100 μm.

improve the definition of tumor margins. Subsequently, other groups invented new procedures, such as the combination of dermoscopy and RCM with a presurgical cut performed along the dermoscopical tumor margins before RCM examination.[26]

Understanding Clinical, Dermoscopic, and Histologic Features

Histology is the gold standard for examination of the architecture and cell components of the skin. However, histologic examination implies an invasive biopsy, requires a fixation that can alter the specimen, and is not always performed on the whole lesion. RCM has the advantage of being performed in vivo with possible direct correlation with the clinical and dermoscopic aspect. This is why RCM is of great interest in understanding the cellular substrate that is responsible for particular clinical and/dermoscopic features. For example, thanks to RCM, we could demonstrate that the gray color observed in mucosal melanoses is linked to the presence of melanophages.[27] Moreover, RCM showed that the clefts around the tumor islands of BCC are not artifacts induced by the tissue retraction following the fixation of the skin specimen but are present in vivo and correspond to mucin accumulation.[28] RCM could also add information to the histologic examination. For example, we observed that cells of Langerhans cell histiocytosis and epidermal Langerhans cells, which are considered different cell populations but are not possible to distinguish under histology, have different aspects under RCM.[29]

Videos

RCM produces real-time images that can be recorded as video with nine images per second. This modality is useful with HH-RCM to record the displacements of the operator, who "navigates" inside the skin. This is particularly interesting in case of large lesions and when the lesion architecture is important for the diagnosis.

Videos can also be useful to record in real-time blood cells circulating inside the lumina of dermal capillaries.[30] Blood cells appear as bright roundish spots inside roundish hyporeflective dermal capillaries. The capillaries appear in pairs, with the arterial and venous capillaries one next to the other. Our group quantified the capillary blood flow based on RCM videos in different vascular lesions.[31,32] Because microcirculation is a key element of tumor growth, quantification of blood flow could be helpful for the diagnosis of malignant tumors.

In case of parasitosis, videos also allow one to reconstruct the architecture of large parasites and to assess their viability through the identification of their movements, including intestinal peristalsis (Video 1) and defecation.

Ex Vivo Confocal Microscopy

Ex vivo confocal microscopy has been conceived for a fast alternative to frozen histopathology during Mohs micrographic surgery of cutaneous epithelial tumors. However, it is also useful for the diagnosis of melanocytic tumors and for tissues other than skin.[33,34] Moreover, it can be applied to the diagnosis of skin infections, such as herpes simplex[35] and mucormycosis.[36]

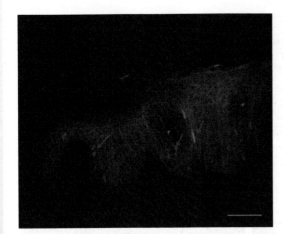

Fig. 10. Ex vivo fluorescence confocal microscopy of normal skin performed with a fluorescent antibody that target melanocytes allows to identify basal melanocytes (*red arrows*) that are usually not visible under reflectance confocal microscopy in nonpathologic conditions. Scale bar: 100 μm.

Because ex vivo confocal microscopy works with fluorescence and not only reflectance, in the future different fluorescent antibodies could be used to identify different cells and anatomic structures (**Fig. 10**), as used for immunohistochemistry in conventional histopathology.

SUPPLEMENTARY DATA

Supplementary data related to this article can be found at http://dx.doi.org/10.1016/j.det.2016.05.010.

REFERENCES

1. Cinotti E, Labeille B, Cambazard F, et al. Reflectance confocal microscopy for mucosal diseases. G Ital Dermatol Venereol 2015;150:585–93.
2. Cinotti E, Perrot JL, Labeille B, et al. Reflectance confocal microscopy for cutaneous infections and infestations. J Eur Acad Dermatol Venereol 2016; 30:754–63.
3. Cinotti E, Jaffelin C, Charriere V, et al. Sensitivity of handheld reflectance confocal microscopy for the diagnosis of basal cell carcinoma: a series of 344 histologically proven lesions. J Am Acad Dermatol 2015;73:319–20.
4. Debarbieux S, Perrot JL, Erfan N, et al. Reflectance confocal microscopy of mucosal pigmented macules: a review of 56 cases including 10 macular melanoma. Br J Dermatol 2014;170:1276–84.
5. Cinotti E, Perrot JL, Labeille B, et al. Reflectance confocal microscopy for the diagnosis of vulvar melanoma and melanosis: preliminary results. Dermatol Surg 2012;38:1962–7.
6. Cinotti E, Chol C, Perrot JL, et al. Anal melanosis diagnosed by reflectance confocal microscopy. Australas J Dermatol 2014;55:286–8.
7. Arzberger E, Komericki P, Ahlgrimm-Siess V, et al. Differentiation between balanitis and carcinoma in situ using reflectance confocal microscopy. JAMA Dermatol 2013;149:440–5.
8. Cinotti E, Perrot JL, Labeille B, et al. Laser photodynamic treatment for in situ squamous cell carcinoma of the glans monitored by reflectance confocal microscopy. Australas J Dermatol 2014;55:72–4.
9. Cinotti E, Perrot JL, Labeille B, et al. In vivo confocal microscopy for eyelids and ocular surface: a new horizon for dermatologists. G Ital Dermatol Venereol 2015;150:127–9.
10. Cinotti E, Perrot JL, Campolmi N, et al. The role of in vivo confocal microscopy in the diagnosis of eyelid margin tumors: 47 cases. J Am Acad Dermatol 2014;71:912–8.e2.
11. Cinotti E, Perrot J-L, Labeille B, et al. Handheld reflectance confocal microscopy for the diagnosis of conjunctival tumors. Am J Ophthalmol 2015;159: 324–33.e1.
12. Cinotti E, Perrot JL, Labeille B, et al. Optical diagnosis of a metabolic disease: cystinosis. J Biomed Opt 2013;18:046013.
13. Perrot J-L, Cinotti E, Labeille B, et al. In vivo confocal microscopy for the diagnosis of lysosomal storage diseases. Ann Dermatol Venereol 2014;141: 784–5.
14. Jullienne R, He Z, Manoli P, et al. In vivo confocal microscopy of pine processionary caterpillar hair-induced keratitis. Cornea 2015;34:350–2.
15. Cinotti E, Fouilloux B, Perrot JL, et al. Confocal microscopy for healthy and pathological nail. J Eur Acad Dermatol Venereol 2014;28:853–8.
16. Cinotti E, Debarbieux S, Perrot JL, et al. Reflectance confocal microscopy features of acral lentiginous melanoma: a comparative study with acral nevi. J Eur Acad Dermatol Venereol 2016;30: 1125–8.
17. Cinotti E, Labeille B, Cambazard F, et al. Reflectance confocal microscopy in infectious diseases. G Ital Dermatol Venereol 2015;150:575–83.
18. Cinotti E, Labeille B, Cambazard F, et al. Unusual reflectance confocal microscopy findings during the examination of a perianal nevus: pinworms. J Eur Acad Dermatol Venereol 2015. http://dx.doi.org/10.1111/jdv.13333.
19. Cinotti E, Labeille B, Bernigaud C, et al. Dermoscopy and confocal microscopy for in vivo detection and characterization of *Dermanyssus gallinae* mite. J Am Acad Dermatol 2015;73:e15–6.
20. Cinotti E, Perrot JL, Labeille B, et al. Reflectance confocal microscopy for quantification of *Sarcoptes scabiei* in Norwegian scabies. J Eur Acad Dermatol Venereol 2013;27:e176–8.

21. Cinotti E, Perrot J-L, Labeille B, et al. On the feasibility of confocal microscopy for the diagnosis of scabies. Ann Dermatol Venereol 2013;140:215–6.

22. Cinotti E, Perrot JL, Labeille B, et al. Tinea corporis diagnosed by reflectance confocal microscopy. Ann Dermatol Venereol 2014;141:150–2.

23. Cinotti E, Perrot JL, Labeille B, et al. Hair dermatophytosis diagnosed by reflectance confocal microscopy: six cases. J Eur Acad Dermatol Venereol 2015;29:2257–9.

24. Champin J, Perrot JL, Cinotti E, et al. In vivo reflectance confocal microscopy to optimize the spaghetti technique for defining surgical margins of lentigo maligna. Dermatol Surg 2014;40:247–56.

25. Terrier J-E, Tiffet O, Raynaud N, et al. In vivo reflectance confocal microscopy combined with the 'spaghetti' technique: a new procedure for defining surgical margins of genital Paget disease. Dermatol Surg 2015;41:862–4.

26. Venturini M, Gualdi G, Zanca A, et al. A new approach for pre-surgical margin assessment of basal cell carcinoma by reflectance confocal microscopy. Br J Dermatol 2016;174:380–5.

27. Cinotti E, Couzan C, Perrot JL, et al. In vivo confocal microscopic substrate of grey colour in melanosis. J Eur Acad Dermatol Venereol 2015;29:2458–62.

28. Ulrich M, Roewert-Huber J, González S, et al. Peritumoral clefting in basal cell carcinoma: correlation of in vivo reflectance confocal microscopy and routine histology. J Cutan Pathol 2011;38:190–5.

29. Cinotti E, Labeille B, Perrot JL, et al. Cells of Langerhans cell histiocytosis and epidermal Langerhans cells differ under reflectance confocal microscopy: first observation. Skin Res Technol 2014;20:385–7.

30. Cinotti E, Gergelé L, Perrot JL, et al. Quantification of capillary blood cell flow using reflectance confocal microscopy. Skin Res Technol 2014;20:373–8.

31. Perrot JL, Cinotti E, Labeille B, et al. Microscopie confocale et lésions vasculaires et analyse dynamique du débit vasculaire: un nouveau champ d'investigation de la microscopie confocale. Ann Dermatol Venereol 2014;141:S327–8.

32. Cinotti E, Perrot JL, Labeille B, et al. Reflectance confocal microscopy for the vascular flow analysis: a new field of exploration. Dermatol Pract Concept 2015;5:230.

33. Cinotti E, Haouas M, Grivet D, et al. In vivo and ex vivo confocal microscopy for the management of a melanoma of the eyelid margin. Dermatol Surg 2015;41:1437–40.

34. Forest F, Cinotti E, Yvorel V, et al. Ex vivo confocal microscopy imaging to identify tumor tissue on freshly removed brain sample. J Neurooncol 2015;124:157–64.

35. Cinotti E, Perrot JL, Labeille B, et al. First identification of the herpes simplex virus by skin-dedicated ex vivo fluorescence confocal microscopy during herpetic skin infections. Clin Exp Dermatol 2015;40:421–5.

36. Leclercq A, Cinotti E, Labeille B, et al. Ex vivo confocal microscopy: a new diagnostic technique for mucormycosis. Skin Res Technol 2016;22:203–7.

Reflectance Confocal Microscopy Algorithms for Inflammatory and Hair Diseases

Marco Ardigo, MD, PhD[a],*, Marina Agozzino, MD[a],
Chiara Franceschini, MD[b], Francesco Lacarrubba, MD, PhD[c]

KEYWORDS

- Reflectance confocal microscopy • Inflammatory diseases • Psoriasiform dermatitis
- Spongiotic dermatitis • Interface dermatitis • Confocal diagnostic algorithm • Diagnostic diagram

KEY POINTS

- Reflectance confocal microscopy (RCM) is a relatively novel noninvasive tool for microscopic evaluation of the skin recently applied on inflammatory skin conditions.
- RCM features useful for the differentiation between the 3 main inflammatory diseases groups, psoriasiform, spongiotic, and interface dermatitis, have been described.
- Algorithmic method of analysis for clinical fast application based on a multivariate analysis has been proposed.

INTRODUCTION

In vivo reflectance confocal microscopy (RCM) is an imaging technique that allows a real-time, microscopic view of the skin with cellular-level resolution close to conventional histopathological analysis. RCM provides "virtual" skin biopsies offering microscopic details of the different skin layers with an en face view.

RCM has been applied to the clinical setting for diagnosis and decision management of several inflammatory, neoplastic, and melanocytic skin diseases.[1–3] In dermatooncology, this technique is considered as a second-level examination positioned after dermoscopic examination in the clinical routine.

Recent prospective studies demonstrated that RCM improves diagnostic accuracy and spares numerous unnecessary surgical excisions.[4,5] Moreover, thanks to the possibility of detailed microscopic changes observation, RCM has been adopted for in vivo evaluation of therapeutic follow-up and diseases progression.[6,7]

More recently, starting from the description of the confocal microscopic patterns, RCM has been also applied on inflammatory skin conditions such as contact dermatitis,[8] psoriasis,[9] discoid lupus erythematosus,[10] lichen planus,[11] and seborrheic dermatitis[12] demonstrating high confocal–histology correlation. Consequently, the potential applicability of RCM to the diagnosis and differential diagnosis of inflammatory skin

Conflict of Interest: None.
Financial Disclosure: None.
[a] Clinical Dermatology Department, San Gallicano Dermatological Institute, Rome, Italy; [b] Department of Dermatology, University of Rome Tor Vergata, Rome, Italy; [c] Dermatology Clinic, University of Catania, Catania, Italy
* Corresponding author. Clinical Dermatology Department, San Gallicano Dermatological Institute, IRCCS, Via Chianesi 53, Rome 00144, Italy.
E-mail address: ardigo@ifo.it

Dermatol Clin 34 (2016) 487–496
http://dx.doi.org/10.1016/j.det.2016.05.011

derm.theclinics.com

diseases has been proposed, but the effective practical usefulness of RCM in the clinical practice still remained debated because a practical methodology for clinical routine is still lacking and, furthermore, a limited number of cases has been evaluated in different studies.

Similar to the approach used in histopathology, the identification of spongiosis, hyperkeratosis, and interface changes as seen on RCM permits to classify inflammatory skin diseases into 3 main groups: psoriasiform dermatitis, interface dermatitis, and spongiotic dermatitis. Later, additional disease-specific confocal features have been also demonstrated to be identifiable with RCM. The open issue was still related to the demonstration of an effective practical application of RCM in the real-life clinical setting for the diagnosis of distinct inflammatory skin diseases. To address this issue, more recently, a multicentric study designed and executed under the supervision of the International Confocal Group has been conducted with the aim of the identification of specific confocal features useful for the distinction between the 3 main groups of inflammatory skin diseases.[13] The study was conducted on a large number of cases affected by different superficial inflammatory skin diseases representing the different groups of entities. A multivariate model of prediction of individual case probability of diagnosis was built and applied to identify the significant confocal criteria describing each group of disease. The defined collection of confocal features have been translated into a diagnostic algorithm for practical application of RCM to the differentiation of the groups and later a tree diagram has been also proposed for a schematic and simplified analysis of confocal examinations.

SPONGIOTIC DERMATITIS

Spongiotic dermatitis are microscopically characterized by the presence of intercellular and/or intracellular edema at epidermal level associated with prevalence of inflammatory cells between keratinocytes and perivascular infiltration in the upper dermis. The prototype of this group of inflammatory skin diseases is irritant and allergic contact dermatitis. The presence of moderate to severe spongiosis and/or detection of vesicles are considered as the main findings characterizing those entities distinguishing spongiotic dermatitis from interface and psoriasiform dermatitis when present as the predominant microscopic features.

On RCM, spongiosis is detectable as dark areas involving the level of the epidermis in comparison with the darker surrounding epithelium appears with broadband intercellular spaces. Dark areas are associated with the presence of round-to-polygonal, mildly refractive cells corresponding on histopathology with inflammatory cells located between keratinocytes in the epidermis (Fig. 1). Notably, spongiosis, when mild to moderate, can be also detected in the other major groups of inflammatory skin diseases as sign of epidermal infiltration of inflammatory cells.

As mentioned, in spongiotic dermatitis semiquantitative estimation of the severity of the spongiosis that is generally detected at least moderate and more commonly severe until massive, has to be considered as more indicative for an acute spongiotic dermatitis. When the spongiosis is severe, it shows up as intraepidermal vesicle seen on RCM as round to polylobular, well-defined, deeply dark spaces delineated by keratinocytes pushed to the periphery of the area without an epithelial wall. The round intraepidermal area is filled by bright, round inflammatory cells in the context of a dark background corresponding with inflammatory cells (see Fig. 1). When fast developed (commonly detectable in irritant contact dermatitis), spongiosis appears as a large dark area with "intravesicular" septa clinically corresponding with fast developing blisters.

In spongiotic dermatitis, RCM of the superficial epidermal layers can reveal disrupted stratum corneum associated with detached corneocytes. Individual corneocytes may appear as floating, highly refractile polygonal cells that correspond to subtle desquamation, and reflecting the loss of cohesiveness of corneocytes in response to contact irritants agents.

The dermoepidermal junction (DEJ) is typically preserved with well visible and bright papillary rims. In the upper dermis, in real-time imaging, dilated vessels are generally detectable as round to canalicular structures filled by a prevalence of moving, mildly bright, not nucleated cellular structures (erythrocytes) and a minority of brighter cellular elements (leukocytes). Inflammatory cells are also detectable around dilated vessels.

Differentiation between irritant contact dermatitis and allergic contact dermatitis has been described to be possible through the evaluation of the changes involving the stratum corneum during time.[14] In detail, irritant contact dermatitis reaction typically shows a pronounced superficial disruption of the stratum corneum after the exposure to contact irritants (<24 hours); this dynamic evolution of the stratum corneum involvement is generally absent in allergic contact dermatitis. Dilated vessels and dermal inflammation can be visualized as secondary confocal features in both the subtype of spongiotic dermatitis. It has been shown that irritant and allergic contact dermatitis

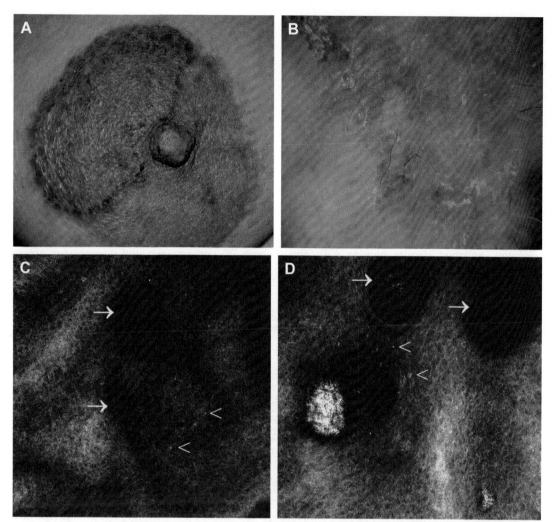

Fig. 1. Nipple eczema. (*A*) Clinical aspect. (*B*) Dermoscopy showing a pinkish–reddish background and yellowish crusts (original magnification, ×10). (*C*) Reflectance confocal microscopy (RCM; 1 × 1 mm) at the level of the epidermis showing spongiosis (*arrows*) and inflammatory cells (*arrowheads*). (*D*) RCM (1 × 1 mm) at the level of the epidermis showing bright inflammatory cells (*arrowheads*) and vesicles (*arrows*).

differ in term of kinetic evolution; irritant contact dermatitis reactions have a more rapid onset and shows a faster recovery compared with allergic contact dermatitis.[15] In addition, it was demonstrated that RCM allows in the detection of subclinical reaction to in experimental application of antigens when clinical features are absent or subtle, thereby verifying clinical readings of patch test (Ardigo, unpublished data, 2009).

PSORIASIFORM DERMATITIS

The prototypic entities of this group are plaque psoriasis (PP) and seborrheic dermatitis.[9,16] Reports on therapeutic follow-up of PP using RCM during topical[17] and systemic[6] treatment have

been also reported in literature, demonstrating the possibility of detailed monitoring of microscopic changes during treatment and actives efficacy noninvasive evaluation at a microscopic level.

Psoriasiform dermatitis, also named hyperkeratotic disease, is characterized by thickened stratum corneum and epidermis associated with papillomatosis (elongation of the rete ridges). The thickening of the stratum corneum can be evaluated using Viva Stack software analysis calculating the number of single steps needed to move above the stratum corneum (where the plastic window is seen as a bright round circle) and progressing deeper in 5-μm steps to the first cellulated epidermal layer; the stratum corneum is considered thickened when the total thickness is greater than 20 μm on the face or 40 μm on the other location. Moreover, at the level of the stratum corneum, the presence of high refractive round to polygonal structures corresponds to parakeratosis typical for PP at histology. The thickness of the epidermis can be also calculated using Stack acquisition starting from the first cellulated layer up to the first appearance of papillary dermis, progressing through stack images of 5-μm steps. The epidermis is "thickened" when the minimum keratinocytes layer thickness is greater than 60 μm on the face or 90 μm on the other body sites.

Other RCM criteria commonly detected and generally indicative for PP are the presence of uplocated, enlarged dermal papillae (DP) and nonrimmed DP at the spinous layer with thin interpapillary epidermal spaces (Fig. 2). In detail, the papillae are increased in number and density at the level of the spinous layer as well as at the DEJ compared with normal skin and according to the anatomic site. This is considered an indirect feature of papillomatosis viewed from the horizontal approach to the skin of RCM. The confocal features characterizing papillomatosis are generally seen diffusely involving the erythematous lesion in PP and only focal in seborrheic dermatitis.

Another interesting distinctive confocal feature is represented by the absence of DP rimming in PP, corresponding with the absence the DEJ pigmentation of keratinocytes, that is probably related to the tumor necrosis factor-α effects on both PP pathogenesis and melanocytes activity

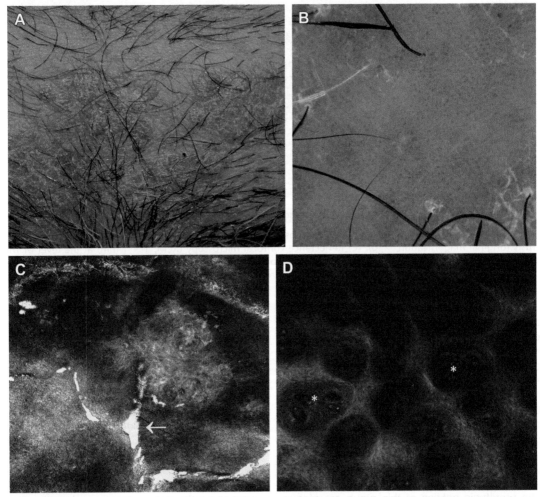

Fig. 2. Plaque psoriasis of the pubic region. (A) Clinical aspect. (B) Dermoscopy showing white scales and regularly distributed dotted vessels (original magnification, ×10). (C) Reflectance confocal microscopy (RCM; 1 × 1 mm) at the level of the stratum corneum showing hyperkeratosis (arrow). (D) RCM (1 × 1 mm) at the level of the papillary dermis showing nonrimmed, enlarged dermal papillae (asterisks) fulfilled by dilated blood vessels.

inhibition. In fact, tumor necrosis factor-α has been already demonstrated to be able to inhibit melanocyte activity since inducing melanocyte apoptosis on melanoma lines.[18]

At the level of the upper dermis, enlarged DP (>80 microns) are associated with the presence of prominent round or linear dark canalicular structures filling the DP, visible with vertical orientation in PP, corresponding with dilated vessels filling the enlarged DP detectable in optical histology. In contrast, in seborrheic dermatitis dilated vessels are horizontally oriented and located typically around the adnexal structures.

Mild to moderate spongiosis, identified by darker areas relative to the surrounding epithelium of the stratum spinosum with intercellular spaces between keratinocytes larger than normal, can be also detected in both psoriasis and seborrheic dermatitis as a secondary feature.

On RCM, seborrheic dermatitis and PP show the same confocal features, but different distribution and amount.[12] Seborrheic dermatitis shows a more evident inflammation involving the epidermis (spongiosis) as well as the upper dermis, with horizontal vessels in the upper dermis and the confocal features of papillomatosis distributed more focally than psoriasis where papillomatosis is distributed regularly along the profile of the lesion.

INTERFACE DERMATITIS

DEJ obscuration, corresponding on histology with DEJ inflammatory involvement, is detectable on RCM at the level of the interface between the epidermis and the upper dermis, is the hallmark of the interface dermatitis. This peculiar confocal feature is owing to the focal or diffuse distribution of inflammatory cells at the level of the basal layer of the epidermis and the papillary dermis with injury and necrosis of basal cell keratinocytes associated with vacuolar or lichenoid microscopic changes. Lichen planus and discoid lupus erythematosus are the prototypes of this group of skin inflammatory diseases. For the both entities, several experiences with the use of RCM have been already collected demonstrating the usefulness of this method for interface dermatitis identification.[10,11,19] On RCM, the interface involvement is visualized as the presence of multiple refractive cells, corresponding with inflammatory cells, with a total obliteration of the ringlike structures around DP that appeared nonedged and nonrimmed (Fig. 3). In detail, according to the horizontal approach of RCM to the skin tissue, the detectable major difference in the DEJ involvement is showed by focal interface changes in discoid lupus erythematous; in contrast, lichen planus is typified by the presence of sheets of inflammatory cells distributed along the front of the lesion and corresponding histologically with the lymphocytic lichenoid infiltrate. Thanks to the different distribution of the interface changes (focal vs diffuse), it seems to be possible to discriminate lichen planus from lupus erythematosus.

More recently, using RCM, the presence of "signetlike ring cells" corresponding with basal cell vacuolization in histology have been reported in literature as detectable in interface dermatitis and characterizing the interface changes typical of lupus erythematosus.[20]

Confocal features of interface changes (DEJ obscuration on RCM) are exclusive for interface dermatitis and not detectable in the other groups of inflammatory diseases, representing a key confocal criterion for the evaluation of inflammatory diseases.

In interface dermatitis, inflammatory cells can be also detected at the level of the epidermis and around/inside the adnexal epithelium, with the loss of the normal honeycomblike architecture of the epidermis as expression of mild to moderate spongiosis. Inflammatory cells can be also detected in the upper dermis around dilated vessels.

Melanophages can be detected in all subtypes of interface dermatitis as an indirect expression of the basal layer damage and the consequent diffusion of melanin in the upper dermis. Melanophages are visible on RCM as polygonal, plump, bright cellular elements, usually without a visible nucleus, located in the upper dermis; they are considered as more significantly detectable in lichen planus as in lupus erythematosus, especially in late stages of the disease.

Moreover, in discoid lupus erythematosus a more prominent thickening of the dermal fibers characterizes lupus erythematosus. Dermal sclerosis is detectable on RCM as coarse dermal fibers, variably bright, forming a grossly arranged net or amorphous bundles and represents another example of RCM features useful for clinical–microscopic differential diagnosis between 2 entities of the same group of interface dermatitis.

INFLAMMATORY SCALP DISEASES

Scarring alopecia represent an explicative example of the involvement of different skin sites with different anatomic structures owing to the same pathologic process. This group of inflammatory diseases involving the scalp and characterized by hair loss and cicatrical evolution have same pathophysiology of the interface dermatitis

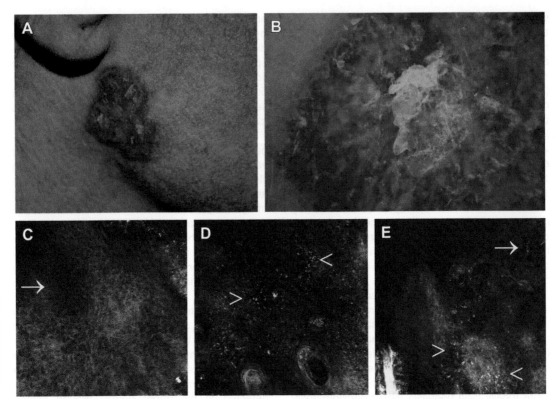

Fig. 3. Discoid lupus erythematous of the face. (*A*) Clinical aspect. (*B*) Dermoscopy showing intense, reddish background and white/yellowish scales (original magnification, ×10). (*C*) Reflectance confocal microscopy (RCM; 1 × 1 mm) showing epidermal disarray and spongiosis (*arrows*). (*D*) RCM (1 × 1 mm) at the level of the dermoepidermal junction showing an inflammatory cell infiltrate (*arrowheads*) obscuring the junction. (*E*) RCM (1 × 1 mm) showing bright inflammatory cells (*arrowheads*) and dilated blood vessels (*arrow*).

affecting the skin. Lichen planus pilaris and discoid lupus erythematosus are the most common causes of scarring alopecias. The microscopic evidence of interface dermatitis involving the DEJ and/or the adnexal epithelium characterizes them both. Upon RCM, the scalp tissue can be visualized starting from the cornified layer down to the papillary dermis with the possibility to examine the epidermis, the upper dermis, the hair shafts, the upper part of the adnexal infundibular epithelium, and the surrounding dermis. Consequently, information about adnexal structures distribution and density, hair shaft integrity and dimension, distribution and amount of inflammatory cells in different layers can be obtained. In this specific dermatology field, RCM can be considered as an intermediate step between dermoscopy and horizontal histology for the evaluation and therapeutic management of scalp inflammatory diseases.[21,22] Limited and promising experiences on this topic describe RCM as a noninvasive approach for the diagnosis and monitoring of patients affected by scarring alopecias.[23]

The main RCM criterion giving a real-time discrimination between scarring and nonscarring alopecias is represented by the detection of an active inflammation prevalently involving the adnexal epithelium and the interface with the upper dermis (the interface dermatitis) associated with different degree of dermal sclerosis typically located around adnexal structures (**Fig. 4**). In detail, the dermal sclerosis can be visualized as thickened and increased dermal fibers radially disposed around the hair follicle. Loss of the normal honeycombed pattern of the epidermis, inflammatory cells in the epidermis associated with spongiosis, dilated vessels, and inflammatory cells in the upper dermis can be also detached.

ALGORITHMIC METHOD FOR INFLAMMATORY SKIN DISEASE DIAGNOSIS

An initial comparison between the different entities has been done to obtain practical information on RCM examination of inflammatory diseases to be translated into the clinical routine. A large number

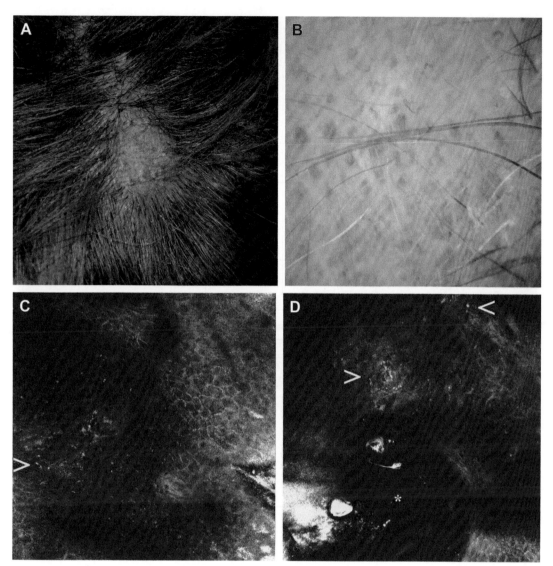

Fig. 4. Discoid lupus erythematous of the scalp. (*A*) Clinical aspect. (*B*) Typical dermoscopic image showing reduction of follicular openings, red roundish dots, and perifollicular hyperkeratosis (original magnification, ×10); (*C*) Reflectance confocal microscopy (RCM; 1 × 1 mm) showing epidermal disarray and bright inflammatory cells (*arrowheads*). (*D*) RCM (1 × 1 mm) close to a follicle (*asterisk*) showing obscuration of the dermoepidermal junction and bright inflammatory cells (*arrowheads*).

of cases comprehensive of different inflammatory skin diseases has been evaluated.[13] For each case, a total of 19 confocal features have been evaluated and good to very good concordance between observers has been demonstrated.

Stating from the 19 confocal criteria considered in the study that are generally identifiable in the evaluation of the most common inflammatory skin diseases part of the 3 main groups (**Fig. 5**), multivariate analysis of the results revealed that some are significant for diagnosis prediction. For interface dermatitis, the presence of DEJ obscuration in combination with melanophages in the

upper dermis and thickening of dermal fibers were highly descriptive; psoriasiform dermatitis was best described by thick epidermis, mild spongiosis, uplocated DP, and an absence of thickening of dermal fibers; and spongiotic dermatitis displayed moderate to severe spongiosis, presence of vesicles, irregular honeycombed epidermis, dilated vessels, and absence of uplocated DP and DEJ obscuration.

Individual scoring indexes for RCM descriptors and scoring range related to the different groups have been calculated according to the hazard ratios of multivariate analysis to define the optimal

SPONGIOTIC DERMATITIS	score 0–7	
Spongiosis, moderate to severe (a)	1	
Vescicles (b)	1	
Irregular honeycombed epidermis (c)	1	
Dilated vessels (d)	1	
No DEJ obscuration	2	
No up located DP	1	
	Optimal cut-off >4	

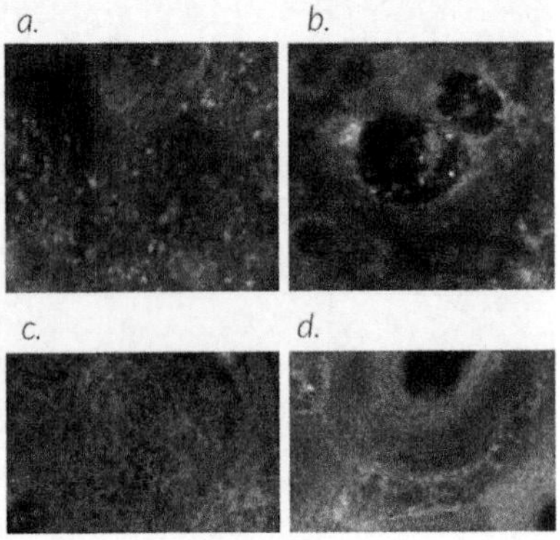

PSORIASIFORM DERMATITIS	score 0–5	
Thick epidermis (a)	1	
Spongiosis (b)	1	
Up located DP (c)	1	
No thickened dermal fibres	2	
	Optimal cut-off >3	

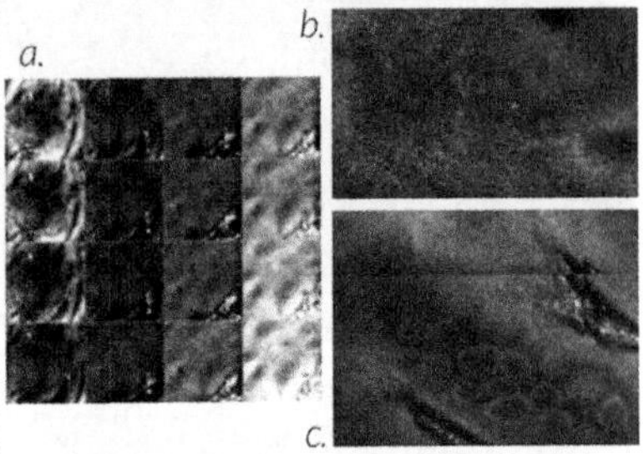

INTERFACE DERMATITIS	score 0–5	
DEJ obscuration (a)	2	
Thickened dermal fibres (b)	2	
Melanophages (c)	1	
	Optimal cut-off >1	

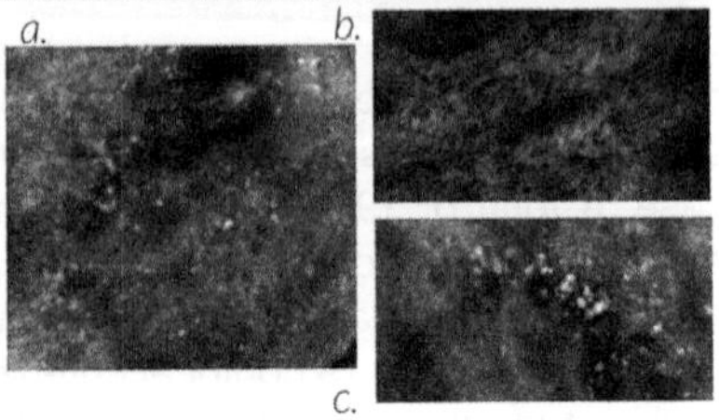

Fig. 5. Reflectance confocal microscopy descriptors for inflammatory diseases groups and relative scores for the definition of the optimal "cutoffs." DEJ, dermoepidermal junction.

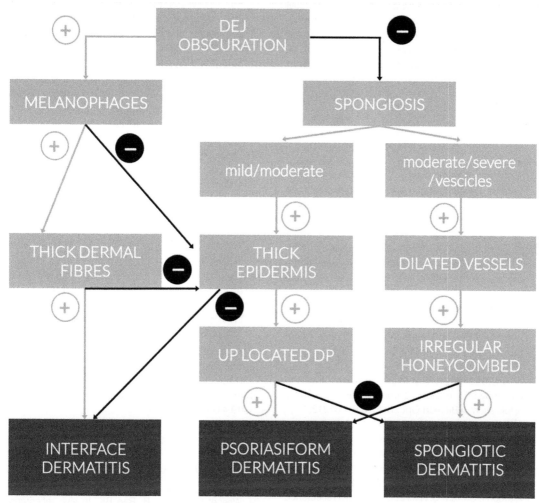

Fig. 6. Diagnostic tree starting from the identification of dermoepidermal junction (DEJ) obscuration. DP, dermal papillae.

cutoff for a high probability of diagnosis for each inflammatory groups (detected to be >81% accordingly to the receiver operating characteristic curve defined for each inflammatory skin disease group). Moreover, a simplified "tree diagram" for fast and practical application of RCM to the main superficial inflammatory skin diseases has been developed (**Fig. 6**). The tree diagram has been designed starting from the presence or absence of DEJ obscuration, because this microscopic features is exclusive for interface changes and not detectable in psoriasiform and spongiotic dermatitis. If DEJ obscuration is detected, the presence of thick dermal fibers associated with melanophages (secondary confocal descriptors comprising the pattern of interface dermatitis) highly confirm the diagnosis. If DEJ obscuration is absent, spongiosis and its

severity (mild to severe) have to be considered. According to the defined tree diagram, mild and moderate spongiosis associated with thick epidermis and uplocated DP is highly suggestive for psoriasiform dermatitis; conversely, the presence of severe spongiosis/vesicles, dilated vessels and irregular honeycombed pattern is predictive for spongiotic dermatitis.

SUMMARY

After the demonstration of the high correspondence of confocal features describing the most common inflammatory skin diseases with histology and their high reproducibility between different observers, the detection of statistical significance of the distribution of predominant features for each single group of inflammatory disease opens to the practical application of RCM to the clinical practice also in the field of inflammatory skin diseases. The next step is to apply the algorithmic analysis to other inflammatory skin diseases besides the 3 main groups and to conduct validation studies of the proposed algorithm.

REFERENCES

1. González S. Confocal reflectance microscopy in dermatology: promise and reality of non invasive diagnosis and monitoring. Actas Dermosifiliogr 2009;100(Suppl 2):59–69.

2. Guida S, Longo C, Casari A, et al. Update on the use of confocal microscopy in melanoma and non-melanoma skin cancer. G Ital Dermatol Venereol 2015;150(5):547–63.

3. Ulrich M, Lange-Asschenfeldt S, Gonzalez S. Clinical applicability of in vivo reflectance confocal microscopy in dermatology. G Ital Dermatol Venereol 2012;147:171–8.

4. Farnetani F, Scope A, Braun RP, et al. Skin cancer diagnosis with Reflectance Confocal Microscopy: reproducibility of feature recognition and accuracy of diagnosis. JAMA Dermatol 2015;151(10): 1075–80.

5. Ulrich M, Lange-Asschenfeldt S. In vivo confocal microscopy in dermatology: from research to clinical application. J Biomed Opt 2013;18(6):061212.

6. Ardigo M, Agozzino M, Longo C, et al. Reflectance confocal microscopy for plaque psoriasis therapeutic follow-up during an anti-TNF-α monoclonal antibody: an observational multicenter study. J Eur Acad Dermatol Venereol 2015;29(12):2363–8.

7. Alarcon I, Carrera C, Alos L, et al. In vivo reflectance confocal microscopy to monitor the response of lentigo maligna to imiquimod. J Am Acad Dermatol 2014;71(1):49–55.

8. Astner S, González S, Gonzalez E. Non invasive evaluation of allergic and irritant contact dermatitis by in vivo reflectance confocal microscopy. Dermatitis 2006;17:182–91.

9. Ardigo M, Cota C, Berardesca E, et al. Concordance between in vivo reflectance confocal microscopy and histology in the evaluation of plaque psoriasis. J Eur Acad Dermatol Venereol 2009;23:660–7.

10. Ardigò M, Maliszewski I, Cota C, et al. Preliminary evaluation of in vivo reflectance confocal microscopy features of Discoid lupus erythematosus. Br J Dermatol 2007;156:1196–203.

11. Moscarella E, González S, Agozzino M, et al. Pilot study on reflectance confocal microscopy imaging of lichen planus: a real-time, non-invasive aid for clinical diagnosis. J Eur Acad Dermatol Venereol 2012;26:1258–65.

12. Agozzino M, Berardesca E, Donadio C, et al. Reflectance confocal microscopy features of seborrheic dermatitis for plaque psoriasis differentiation. Dermatology 2014;229:215–21.

13. Ardigo M, Longo C, Gonzalez S. Multicenter study on inflammatory skin diseases from The International Confocal Working Group (ICWG): specific confocal microscopy features and an algorithmic method of diagnosis. Br J Dermatol 2016. http://dx.doi.org/10.1111/bjd.14516.

14. Windells K, Burnett N, Rius-Diaz F, et al. Reflectance confocal microscopy may differentiate acute allergic and irritant contact dermatitis in vivo. J Am Acad Dermatol 2004;50:220–8.

15. Guichard A, Fanian F, Girardin P, et al. Allergic patch test and contact dermatitis by in vivo reflectance confocal microscopy. Ann Dermatol Venereol 2014; 141(12):805–7.

16. Hoogedoorn L, Wolberink EA, van de Kerkhof PC, et al. Non invasive differentiation between stable and unstable chronic plaque psoriasis using in vivo reflectance confocal microscopy. J Am Acad Dermatol 2015;73(5):870–2.

17. Ardigo M, Agozzino M, Longo C, et al. Psoriasis plaque test with confocal microscopy: evaluation of different microscopic response pathways in NSAID and steroid treated lesions. Skin Res Technol 2013; 19:417–23.

18. Martinez-Esparza M, Jimenez-Cervantes C, Solano F, et al. Mechanisms of melanogenesis inhibition by tumor necrosis factor-alpha in B16/F10 mouse melanoma cells. Eur J Biochem 1998;255: 139–46.

19. Wassef C, Mateus R, Rao BK. In vivo reflectance confocal microscopy features of discoid lupus erythematosus. J Drugs Dermatol 2012;11(9):1111–3.

20. Amini-Adle M, Debarbieux S, Perier-Muzet M, et al. Signet ring-Like cells: a new reflectance confocal microscopy clue of interface dermatitis correlated to basal cell vacuolization in histopathology. Dermatology 2016;232(1):83–5.

21. Agozzino M, Tosti A, Barbieri L, et al. Confocal microscopic features of scarring alopecia: preliminary report. Br J Dermatol 2011;165:534–40.

22. Agozzino M, Donadio C, Franceschini C, et al. Therapeutic follow-up of Lichen Planopilaris using in vivo reflectance confocal microscopy: a case report. Skin Res Technol 2015;21(3):380–3.

23. Ardigò M, El shabrawi-Caelen L, Tosti A. In vivo reflectance confocal microscopy assessment of the therapeutic follow up of cutaneous T-cell lymphomas causing scalp alopecia. Dermatol Ther 2014;27(4):248–51.

In Vivo and Ex Vivo Confocal Microscopy for Dermatologic and Mohs Surgeons

Caterina Longo, MD, PhD[a],*, Moira Ragazzi, MD[b],
Milind Rajadhyaksha, PhD[c], Kishwer Nehal, MD[c], Antoni Bennassar, MD[d],
Giovanni Pellacani, MD[e], Josep Malvehy Guilera, MD, PhD[d]

KEYWORDS

- Confocal microscopy • In vivo • Ex vivo • Mohs surgery

KEY POINTS

- Confocal microscopy is an optimal device that offers a nearly histologic view of skin tissue.
- In vivo confocal microscopy helps to outline lateral basal cell carcinoma margins with accuracy, although it has been tested on a limited set of patients.
- Ex vivo confocal microscopy is a valid alternative to conventional frozen section pathology for BCC margin assessment.

INTRODUCTION

Micrographic Mohs surgery is a precise and complete excision of a skin cancer guided by the examination of margins with frozen histopathology during surgery. It was developed several years ago and is still applied in clinical dermatologic settings especially for some cancers, such as basal cell carcinoma (BCC) and squamous cell carcinoma (SCC). However, this technique has some drawbacks: the preparation of histopathology is labor intensive and time consuming, and multiple serial excisions are often necessary to achieve cancer-free margins, with frozen tissue preparation requiring 20 to 45 minutes for each stage. Furthermore, there are cost-related issues.

Confocal microscopy has been introduced in clinical settings in the last decades as a revolutionary tool capable of offering a quasi-histologic view of a given skin tumor in a few minutes.[1–4] Confocal microscopes works with two different modalities: in reflectance mode and in fluorescence mode. In reflectance confocal microscopy (RCM) contrast is achieved because of different refractive indices of cell structures and organelles, such as keratin and melanin; these serve as "endogenous chromophores" in the reflection-mode because of a higher refractive indices compared with water. This device is used in vivo at the patient's bedside.

Fluorescence confocal microscopy (FCM) uses as fluorescent agents several fluorophores among

The authors have no conflicts of interest to disclose.
Funding: Dr C. Longo and Prof G. Pellacani were partially funded by Research Project NET-2011-02347213, Italian Ministry of Health.
[a] Skin Cancer Unit, Arcispedale Santa Maria Nuova-IRCCS, viale Risorgimento 80, Reggio Emilia 42100, Italy;
[b] Pathology Unit, Arcispedale Santa Maria Nuova-IRCCS, viale Risorgimento 80, Reggio Emilia 42100, Italy;
[c] Dermatology Service, Memorial Sloan Kettering Cancer Center, 160 East 53rd Street, New York, NY 10022, USA; [d] Melanoma Unit, Dermatology Department, Hospital Clinic and Institut d'Investigacions Biomediques August Pi I Sunyer, Barcelona, Spain; [e] Dermatology Unit, UniMore, Modena, Italy
* Corresponding author.
E-mail address: longo.caterina@gmail.com

Dermatol Clin 34 (2016) 497–504
http://dx.doi.org/10.1016/j.det.2016.05.012
0733-8635/16/$ – see front matter © 2016 Elsevier Inc. All rights reserved.

which acridine orange is one of the most commonly used in the clinical setting. This tool works in the ex vivo setting on freshly excised specimens.[1–3]

Both modalities have been applied for Mohs surgery in skin cancer diagnosis and margin assessment. This article reviews the application of in vivo and ex vivo confocal microscopy in the Mohs surgery setting.

IN VIVO APPLICATIONS OF REFLECTANCE CONFOCAL MICROSCOPY

In vivo RCM has been applied at the patient's bedside for lateral margin detection in BCC and lentigo maligna (LM), because of its capability of exploring the skin at the cellular level, enabling the identification of tumor characteristics.

Basal Cell Carcinoma

Regarding BCC margin assessment, Venturini and colleagues[5,6] proposed a new feasible procedure for presurgical evaluation. Briefly, after the application of topical anesthesia, the lesion is analyzed by dermoscopy. Next, clear borders, approximately 2 mm from identifiable structures, are drawn with a dermographic pen, according to dermoscopic evaluation of the lesion. In the case of ill-defined tumor margins, a superficial cut with a lancet is made in correspondence with the presumed clear margin based on dermoscopy. Then, RCM is carried out by means of Vivascope 1500 (Mavig, Munchen, Germany), placing the cut at the center of the imaged area. A series of mosaics up to 4 × 4 mm in size at different depths are acquired to explore the area inside and outside the superficial cut and to determine if the margin is tumor-free (RCM-negative border corresponding to no BCC tumor features outside the cut or within 2 mm of the cut) or involved (RCM-positive border corresponding to BCC tumor features outside the cut or within 2 mm of the cut). In the case of an RCM-positive border, to perform radical excision, a clear border is redefined on RCM images and transposed onto the skin according to its direction and distance from the superficial cut.

In this study, RCM evaluation showed BCC foci beyond the presurgical mark in 3 of 10 (30%) lesions, demonstrated by polarization of elongated nuclei along the same axis of orientation, dark silhouettes, and increased dermal vasculature with tortuous and ectatic blood vessels. Thus, this method could represent a valid and relatively fast approach for lateral margin detection in BCC. However, because of the limited depth laser penetration, deep tumor margin cannot be assessed

and this is crucial for sclerosing BCC or deeply infiltrating tumors.

Another and different application of in vivo RCM involves the use of video mosaicking for rapid detection of residual tumor directly in the surgical wounds on patients.[7] A recent study used this approach on 25 patients, using aluminum chloride for nuclear contrast. Basically, imaging is performed in quadrants in the wound to simulate the Mohs surgeon's examination of pathology. Images and videos of the epidermal and dermal margins are acquired and bright nuclear morphology can be identified at the epidermal margin and detectable in residual nonmelanoma skin cancer tumors. Although this was a pilot feasibility study, intraoperative RCM imaging was found to be useful for the detection of residual tumor directly on patients during Mohs surgery. However, for routine clinical utility, a stronger tumor-to-dermis contrast may be necessary, and a smaller microscope head with an automated approach for imaging the entire wound in a rapid and controlled manner.

Lentigo Maligna

Delineating margins of LM preoperatively is often extremely challenging because of the pigmentation of the sun-damaged background and the intrinsic early changes of the tumor that is composed of single atypical melanocytic proliferation. Guitera and colleagues[8] in a subset of 29 patients have explored the use of in vivo RCM for LM mapping. A detailed procedure has been developed to ensure a presurgical definition of clear margins. When the lesion was visible clinically or on dermoscopy, the RCM field of view is centered in the middle of the lesion. Confocal images are obtained in four radial directions for margin determination until no evidence of LM is seen. The margins are explored in only four directions because of the time necessary to capture each mosaic. The histopathologic findings and diagnosis correlated with the RCM features in nearly all cases. In this study, there were four false-positive sites (diagnosed as an LM area by the LM score on RCM and not confirmed by pathologic findings) and five false-negative sites (diagnosed as LM by histopathologic study but not by the RCM assessment). Thus, this method is a reliable and easy method for presurgical margin assessment of LM.

Another interesting way to outline LM margin is the so-called "spaghetti" technique.[9] Marking is done at the visual limits of the LM, based on clinical and dermoscopy examination. The following evaluations are performed circumferentially, moving closer by 5 mm to the visual limits if the analysis is negative and moving away by

5 mm if malignant cells are identified. This spacing of 5 mm corresponds to the size of the tip of the Vivascope 3000 camera (Mavig). When applied to the skin, this tip creates a temporary footprint that serves as a transitional benchmark for the next exploration, with the tip applied adjacent to the mark left by the previous exploration. Then, a mark is made on the analyzed area using a dermographic pen as a dot in the center of the skin footprint of the camera after quickly mopping up the interface oil used for the RCM examination. These dots are interconnected by a line, drawn using a dermographic pen and then stained with a solution of fuchsin ink to avoid any possible deletion during preoperative disinfection of the skin. The outline of the lesion is marked. This method has been used only on 33 cases and thus limited conclusions can be drawn; however, the "spaghetti" technique allows accurate definition of the surgical margins of LM, with a low rate of multiple excisions.

Besides LM mapping, RCM has been successfully applied to accurately monitor the response of LM to nonsurgical treatment with topical imiquimod.[10] RCM identified 70% of all responders with no false-negative results, and when compared with histopathology, there was no significant difference in evaluating the response to imiquimod.

EX VIVO APPLICATIONS OF FLUORESCENCE CONFOCAL MICROSCOPY

Ex vivo FCM is used on freshly excised tumors in the operating room. Different fluorophores, such as fluorescein, Nile blue, patent blue, methylene blue, and acridine orange, can be used at different wavelengths. However, acridine orange is one of the most commonly used because of its capability to provide an excellent contrast. Confocal mosaics are acquired using an ex vivo fluorescence confocal microscope (Vivascope 2500, Mavig). The laser illumination wavelength is 488 nm. The depth is manually adjusted to image the surface. Imaging is with a 30×0.9 numerical aperture water immersion lens, which provides optical sectioning of approximately 1.5 μm and resolution of approximately 0.4 μm at the 488-nm wavelength. Acridine orange (0.6 mM, 10–20 seconds) is used as the contrast agent.

Basal Cell Carcinoma

FCM images provides an excellent correlation with conventional frozen sections while adding more information regarding fat tissue and other structures that can be altered by tissue processing in classic Mohs surgery.

A set of traditional histologic classic and new criteria has been developed to guide the reading and interpretation of the gray scale mosaics.[11–28] FCM criteria include the presence of the following:

1. *Fluorescence.* Presence of fluorescence was determined when bright images were seen on the screen. Fluorescence corresponds to nucleated cells stained with acridine orange. Areas of higher fluorescence consistently showed nuclear morphology compared with a darker appearing background of dermis (**Fig. 1**); fluorescence is typically seen as forming structures/aggregates.
2. *Tumor demarcation* (**Fig. 2**). Tumor shape corresponds to distinct histopathology subtypes.

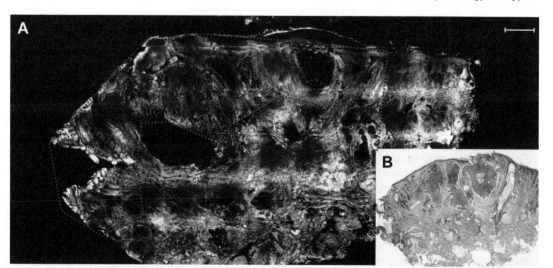

Fig. 1. (*A*) Tumor silhouette of BCC was highlighted by higher fluorescence signal (*dashed line*; scale bar, 750 μm). (*B*) Nodular BCC on frozen section revealing an excellent correlation with FCM image in *A* (hematoxylin-eosin, original magnification 2×).

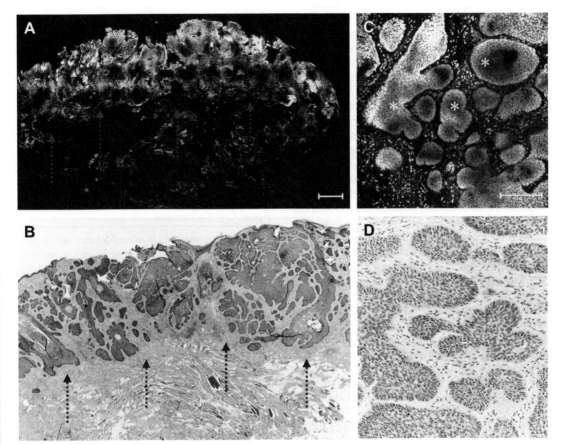

Fig. 2. (*A*) Low-resolution FCM image showing a BCC tumoral proliferation (*arrows*; scale bar, 750 μm). (*B*) Stained section depicted an excellent correlation with FCM image (*arrows*) in *A* (hematoxylin-eosin, original magnification 2×). (*C*) High-resolution FCM image showed the presence of basaloid islands (*asterisks*) with peripheral palisading and clefting that corresponded to the ones seen on histology (*D*) (hematoxylin-eosin, original magnification 10×).

3. *Nuclear crowding*. Nuclear crowding was determined when the nuclear density was higher than that of the surrounding epidermis and adnexal structures.
4. *Peripheral palisading*. Palisading is described, similar to that seen in frozen histology, by the prominent tendency of the outermost layer of basal cells to be arranged in a parallel-polarized way along the periphery of the BCC tumor. This is seen mainly in nodular subtypes of BCCs (Fig. 3).
5. *Clefting*. Hypofluorescent dark-appearing space surrounding basaloid islands partially outlines the islands in micronodular and infiltrative subtypes of BCCs; it is more evident in superficial and nodular tumors.
6. *Nuclear pleomorphism*. Nuclear pleomorphism is a deviation from the normal round or oval shapes of nuclei present in normal keratinocytes.
7. *Increased nucleus/cytoplasm ratio*. BCC nests are seen as crowded masses of elongated

heterogeneous nuclei with poor or absent cytoplasm.
8. *Stroma*. Tumoral stroma is the modified dermis surrounding the BCC nests. When viewed in FCM mosaics, the stroma is seen as more densely nucleated dermis, as fluorescent dots and filaments within a dark-appearing background.

Furthermore, distinct BCC subtypes reveal specific morphologic aspects. Superficial BCCs show a proliferation of atypical basaloid cells that form an axis parallel to the epidermal surface, are extensions from the dermal-epidermal junction, and demonstrate slitlike retraction of the palisaded basal cells from the subjacent stroma (cleft-like spaces). Nodular BCCs reveal small to large nodules with peripheral palisading and clefting, whereas the micronodular subtype shows monotonous small round and well-defined islands with roughly the same shape and contour. Infiltrative BCCs are the most challenging tumor

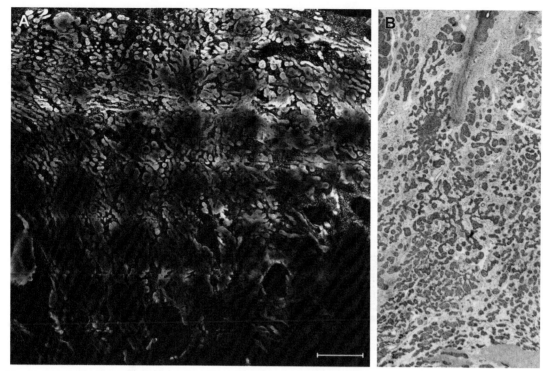

Fig. 3. (A) Highly fluorescent basaloid tumor islands sharply demarcated compared with background dermis (scale bar, 750 μm) and (B) their histologic correlates (hematoxylin-eosin, original magnification 2×).

because they appear as columns and cords of basaloid cells one to two cells thick with sharp angulation, enmeshed in a densely collagenized stroma; palisading and clefting are not always present.

Several studies have been conducted to assess the value of FCM for BCC margin assessment (Table 1). A study conducted by Bennassar and colleagues[28] on 80 BCCs using these FCM criteria demonstrated an overall sensitivity and specificity of detecting residual BCC of 88% and 99%, respectively. Moreover, the new technique reduced by almost two-thirds the time invested when compared with the conventional processing of frozen sections.[29] Several pitfalls may occur when evaluating FCM mosaics.[30] In particular, tiny and angulated cords and strands of fluorescent cells that are typically found in infiltrative BCCs can be more difficult to recognize. Furthermore, it is difficult to distinguish the infiltrative cords from the surrounding stroma, although the latter showed no tendency to cluster. Another possible pitfall is caused by the presence of several sebaceous glands that may be confused with BCC islands. However, the former showed no palisading, less fluorescence, and the presence of a centrally located nucleus compared with the tumors.

Squamous Cell Carcinoma

Few preliminary reports describe the feasibility of FCM for SCC diagnosis and margin assessment. Longo and colleagues[31] defined the FCM criteria to grade SCC tumors. This pilot study demonstrated that the presence of a well-defined tumor silhouette, numerous keratin pearls, keratin formation, and scarce nuclear pleomorphism on FCM images were correlated with the diagnosis of well-differentiated SCC (Fig. 4). Conversely, an ill-defined tumor silhouette, paucity or absence of keratin pearls, and marked nuclear pleomorphism was observed in poorly differentiated tumors. SCCs that were moderately differentiated revealed an intermediate pattern of growth with presence of keratin formation.

OTHER TUMORS

FCM has been used to assess the margins during micrographic mohs surgery (MMS) of eccrine syringomatous carcinoma.[32] On FCM the tumor appears highly fluorescent. Epidermis is spared of any neoplastic proliferation, whereas neoplastic cords of monomorphous fluorescent cells can be seen in the dermis. Those structures are similar to eccrine gland tubular structure.

Table 1
Comparison of FCM studies

Study	Mosaics Evaluated, N	Confocal Technique	Se	Sp	PPV	NPV	Scanning Time (min) for 12 × 12 mm	Staining Time (min)	Staining Technique
Patel et al,[3] 2007	—	FCM	—	—	—	—	9	0.5–5	Acetic acid
Rajadhyaksha et al,[1] 2001	—	RCM	—	—	—	—	3.5	0.5	Acetic acid
Gareau et al,[11] 2009	30	RCM	—	—	—	—	9	0.5–5	Acetic acid
Schüle et al,[12] 2009	284	FCM	0–89	29–89	—	—	—	2	Citric acid
Ziefle et al,[13] 2010	312	FCM	82	61	66.7	78	3	3.5	Acetic acid + toluidine blue
Al-Arashi et al,[16] 2007	37	FCM, RCM	—	—	—	—	—	2	Toluidine blue, methylene blue
Gareau et al,[17] 2008	50	FCM	—	—	—	—	9	0.5	Acridine orange
Gareau et al,[18] 2009 Karen et al,[19] 2009	48	FCM	96.6	89.2	93	94.7	9	0.3	Acridine orange
Larson et al,[23] 2013	17	FCM strip	94	94	—	—	<2	0.3	Acridine orange
Bennàssar et al,[29] 2014	150	FCM	88	99	98	97	3	0.3	Acridine orange
Longo et al,[30] 2014	35	FCM	94.9	96.8	—	—	3	0.3	Acridine orange

Abbreviations: NPV, negative predictive value; PPV, positive predictive value; Se, sensitivity; Sp, specificity.

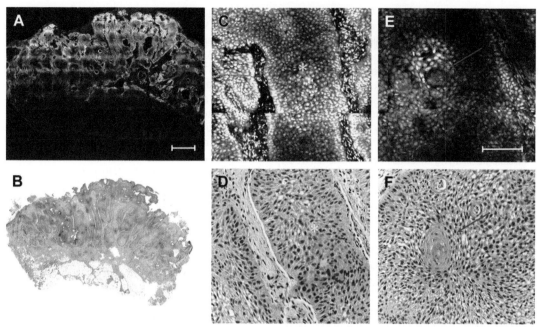

Fig. 4. (A) FCM mosaic reveals a well-defined cutaneous squamous cell carcinoma silhouette with sharp demarcation and highly fluorescent areas (scale bar, 750 µm). (B) Corresponding histopathologic images showing a well-differentiated tumor (hematoxylin-eosin, original magnification 2×). (C) Detail of the tumor showing keratynocitic tongue (*asterisk*) and (D) its histologic correlates (*asterisk*) (hematoxylin-eosin, original magnification 10×). (E) Keratin pearls (*arrow*; scale bar, µm) and corresponding histologic image (F) (hematoxylin-eosin, original magnification 10×).

SUMMARY

The need of defining skin cancer margins for a more accurate surgical excision has fueled the exploration of confocal microscopy in this special setting. In vivo and ex vivo confocal microscopy has been used with the great advantage of saving time and providing good diagnostic accuracy. For both techniques intense and dedicated training is required to learn how to use the device and even more relevant, how to interpret the images. For the near future we envision the routine application of confocal microscopy in the Mohs surgery setting.

REFERENCES

1. Rajadhyaksha M, Menaker G, Flotte T, et al. Confocal examination of nonmelanoma cancers in thick skin excisions to potentially guide Mohs micrographic surgery without frozen histopathology. J Invest Dermatol 2001;117:1137–43.

2. Chung VQ, Dwyer PJ, Nehal KS, et al. Use of ex vivo confocal scanning laser microscopy during Mohs surgery for nonmelanoma skin cancers. Dermatol Surg 2004;30:1470–8.

3. Patel YG, Nehal KS, Aranda I, et al. Confocal reflectance mosaicing of basal cell carcinomas in Mohs surgical skin excisions. J Biomed Opt 2007;12(3):034027.

4. Longo C, Zalaudek I, Argenziano G, et al. New directions in dermatopathology: in vivo confocal microscopy in clinical practice. Dermatol Clin 2012; 30(4):799–814.

5. Venturini M, Gualdi G, Zanca A, et al. A new approach for presurgical margin assessment by reflectance confocal microscopy of basal cell carcinoma. Br J Dermatol 2016;174(2):380–5.

6. Gualdi G, Venturini M, Zanca A, et al. Pre-surgical basal cell carcinoma margin definition: the SMART approach. J Eur Acad Dermatol Venereol 2016; 30(3):474–6.

7. Flores ES, Cordova M, Kose K, et al. Intraoperative imaging during Mohs surgery with reflectance confocal microscopy: initial clinical experience. J Biomed Opt 2015;20(6):61103.

8. Guitera P, Moloney FJ, Menzies SW, et al. Improving management and patient care in lentigo maligna by mapping with in vivo confocal microscopy. JAMA Dermatol 2013;149(6):692–8.

9. Champin J, Perrot JL, Cinotti E, et al. In vivo reflectance confocal microscopy to optimize the spaghetti technique for defining surgical margins of lentigo maligna. Dermatol Surg 2014;40(3):247–56.

10. Alarcon I, Carrera C, Alos L, et al. In vivo reflectance confocal microscopy to monitor the response of lentigo maligna to imiquimod. J Am Acad Dermatol 2014;71(1):49–55.

11. Gareau DS, Patel YG, Li Y, et al. Confocal mosaicing microscopy in skin excisions: a demonstration of rapid surgical pathology. J Microsc 2009;233(1): 149–59.

12. Schüle D, Breuninger H, Schippert W, et al. Confocal laser scanning microscopy in micrographic surgery (three-dimensional histology) of basal cell carcinomas. Br J Dermatol 2009;161(3):698–700.

13. Ziefle S, Schüle D, Breuninger H, et al. Confocal laser scanning microscopy vs 3-dimensional histologic imaging in basal cell carcinoma. Arch Dermatol 2010;146(8):843–7.

14. Kaeb S, Landthaler M, Hohenleutner U. Confocal laser scanning microscopy–evaluation of native tissue sections in micrographic surgery. Lasers Med Sci 2009;24(5):819–23.

15. Yaroslavsky AN, Barbosa J, Neel V, et al. Combining multispectral polarized light imaging and confocal microscopy for localization of nonmelanoma skin cancer. J Biomed Opt 2005;10(1):14011.

16. Al-Arashi MY, Salomatina E, Yaroslavsky AN. Multimodal confocal microscopy for diagnosing nonmelanoma skin cancers. Lasers Surg Med 2007;39(9): 696–705.

17. Gareau DS, Li Y, Huang B, et al. Confocal mosaicing microscopy in Mohs skin excisions: feasibility of rapid surgical pathology. J Biomed Opt 2008; 13(5):054001.

18. Gareau DS, Karen JK, Dusza SW, et al. Sensitivity and specificity for detecting basal cell carcinomas in Mohs excisions with confocal fluorescence mosaicing microscopy. J Biomed Opt 2009;14(3): 034012.

19. Karen JK, Gareau DS, Dusza SW, et al. Detection of basal cell carcinomas in Mohs excisions with fluorescence confocal mosaicing microscopy. Br J Dermatol 2009;160(6):1242–50.

20. Bennàssar A, Vilalta A, Carrera C, et al. Rapid diagnosis of two facial papules using ex vivo fluorescence confocal microscopy: toward a rapid bedside pathology. Dermatol Surg 2012;38(9): 1548–51.

21. Abeytunge S, Li Y, Larson B, et al. Rapid confocal imaging of large areas of excised tissue with strip mosaicing. J Biomed Opt 2011;16(5):050504.

22. Abeytunge S, Li Y, Larson B, et al. Confocal microscopy with strip mosaicing for rapid imaging over large areas of excised tissue. J Biomed Opt 2013; 18(6):61227.

23. Larson B, Abeytunge S, Seltzer E, et al. Detection of skin cancer margins in Mohs excisions with high-speed strip mosaicing confocal microscopy: a feasibility study. Br J Dermatol 2013;169:922–6.

24. Gareau DS. Feasibility of digitally stained multimodal confocal mosaics to simulate histopathology. J Biomed Opt 2009;14(3):034050.

25. Gareau DS, Jeon HS, Nehal KS, et al. Rapid screening of cancer margins in tissue with multimodal microscopy. J Surg Res 2012;178:533–8.

26. Gareau D, Bar A, Snaveley N, et al. Tri-modal confocal mosaics detect residual invasive squamous cell carcinoma in Mohs surgical excisions. J Biomed Opt 2012;17(6):066018.

27. Longo C, Ragazzi M, Castagnetti F, et al. Inserting ex vivo fluorescence confocal microscopy perioperatively in Mohs micrographic surgery expedites bedside assessment of excision margins in recurrent basal cell carcinoma. Dermatology 2013; 227(1):89–92.

28. Bennàssar A, Carrera C, Puig S, et al. Fast evaluation of 69 basal cell carcinomas with ex vivo fluorescence confocal microscopy: criteria description, histopathological correlation, and interobserver agreement. JAMA Dermatol 2013;149(7):839–47.

29. Bennàssar A, Vilata A, Puig S, et al. Ex vivo fluorescence confocal microscopy for fast evaluation of tumour margins during Mohs surgery. Br J Dermatol 2014;170(2):360–5.

30. Longo C, Rajadhyaksha M, Ragazzi M, et al. Evaluating ex vivo fluorescence confocal microscopy images of basal cell carcinomas in Mohs excised tissue. Br J Dermatol 2014;171(3):561–70.

31. Longo C, Ragazzi M, Gardini S, et al. Ex vivo fluorescence confocal microscopy in conjunction with Mohs micrographic surgery for cutaneous squamous cell carcinoma. J Am Acad Dermatol 2015; 73(2):321–2.

32. Longo C, Ragazzi M, Gardini S, et al. Ex vivo fluorescence confocal microscopy of eccrine syringomatous carcinoma: a report of 2 cases. JAMA Dermatol 2015;151(9):1034–6.

Telediagnosis with Confocal Microscopy
A Reality or a Dream?

Alexander Witkowski, MD, PhD[a],*, Joanna Łudzik, MD[b],
H. Peter Soyer, MD[c]

KEYWORDS

- Telemedicine • Teledermatology • Tele-confocal • Confocal microscopy • Dermoscopy

KEY POINTS

- Reflectance confocal microscopy (RCM) is a noninvasive tool allowing in vivo evaluation of cutaneous lesions at near histologic resolution.
- RCM has been shown to have high accuracy in diagnosing both pigmented and nonpigmented lesions and is increasing in popularity among the dermatology community.
- There is a need to evaluate diagnostic accuracy and safety of teleconfocal in real-world settings.
- Proper training programs and reading standards should be implemented and developed to ensure safe diagnostic sensitivity and avoid misdiagnosis of malignant lesions in telemedicine settings.

INTRODUCTION

The improvement of technology and modernization of medicine has completely changed the arena that doctors enter in everyday clinical practice. With the introduction of Internet-based communication, touch-screen mobile phones, and large data storage that can be streamed instantaneously, the demand to access information by both patients and their doctors has risen exponentially in the past decade.[1–3] The term *telemedicine* dates back to 1974 when Mark and colleagues[4] highlighted the potential for improving the traditional practice of exclusive face-to-face doctor-patient contact in a dedicated facility to other settings where a doctor could review patient information collected previously by a third party, such as another doctor, nurse, or technician, that could be reviewed at a later time.[5,6] Throughout the years telemedicine practice improved and made around-the-clock access to both general medical data and imaging, which allowed for improvement of patient care, scope of practice, and cost-benefit.[7–9] Telemedicine has enabled the rapid spread of interest in dermoscopy allowing a consultative expert opinion that was once done primitively by USB pendrive or e-mail and currently through secured Internet-based server software programs.[10–13] Mobile applications can be downloaded free of charge that provide either computer-based algorithm screening of melanocytic nevi photographed with a camera phone or human interpretation for a service fee.[14–17] With the ability for both doctors and patients to obtain nearly instant gratification, the question is if this connectivity can be transferred effectively and safely to more advanced tools in dermatology beyond those encompassing clinical imaging and dermoscopy.

Disclosure Statement: None of the authors have any commercial or financial conflicts of interest as well as any funding sources for this article.

[a] Department of Dermatology, University of Modena and Reggio Emilia, Via del Pozzo 71, 41100 Modena, Italy; [b] Department of Bioinformatics and Telemedicine, Jagiellonian University Medical College, ul. Sw. Łazarza 16, 31-530 Krakow, Poland; [c] Dermatology Research Centre, Translational Research Institute, School of Medicine, The University of Queensland, 37 Kent Street Woolloongabba QLD 4102, Australia
* Corresponding author.
E-mail address: alexander.witkowski@unimore.it

Dermatol Clin 34 (2016) 505–512
http://dx.doi.org/10.1016/j.det.2016.05.013
0733-8635/16/$ – see front matter © 2016 Published by Elsevier Inc

Reflectance confocal microscopy (RCM) is a noninvasive screening technique permitting in vivo view of cellular morphology at patients' bedside with relatively rapid acquisition of high-resolution images that can be used for real-time evaluation or subsequent review at a later time.[18] RCM has proven to be a reliable tool for improving diagnostic accuracy at patients' bedside and over the past decade has seen a substantial increase in interest among the dermatology community worldwide.[19,20] Thanks to streamlined confocal terminology and evaluation of RCM application to both pigmented and nonpigmented lesions in a large variety of studies, we can see a steady diffusion of RCM into clinical practice. Instead of replacing traditional biopsy with histopathology evaluation, RCM augments and bridges the clinico-dermoscopic presentation to the gold standard of pathology both improving earlier diagnosis and potential for significant reduction in unnecessary excisions.[21–24] The evaluation of RCM images requires specialized training that is not readily available despite the numerous publications in this field. The application of telemedicine with RCM (teleconfocal) may help overcome the deficit of experts through electronic learning (e-learning) training platforms as well as connect patients to experts at a distance.[25]

PRINCIPLES OF TELEMEDICINE

The principle of telemedicine use in dermatology is the use of telecommunication technology to send skin disorder–related medical data over a distance for the purpose of administration, research, disease prevention, patient management, and education. Teleconfocal provides access to particular dermatologic specialist knowledge that would be otherwise unavailable at a particular location by transferring the information via a store-and-forward (SAF) technique.[26–28] SAF teledermatology allows a referring physician or third party, such as a nurse or technical assistant, to acquire digital still images with accompanying patient data. In the case of teleconfocal, the collection of data includes patient information and a full set of images, including digital dermoscopy, 3 to 4 mosaic maps at the epidermis, dermal-epidermal junction (DEJ), and dermis as well as, a minimum of 4 VivaStacks® (Mavig, Munich, Germany) 2 in the center and 2 at the periphery of the lesion, with the option to add an RCM movie. These data are subsequently sent to a data storage unit (server) to be assessed by the reader, or reviewer, at a later time. As storage, retrieval, and privacy of information are crucial, the available confocal server (Vivanet) uses a secure server that secures information with Digital Imaging and Communications in Medicine–(DICOM) and Health Insurance Portability and Accountability Act–(HIPPA) compliant security in the United States, preventing intrusion and ensuring consistency in the presentation and sharing of information seamlessly between medical professionals.[29,30] During the initial implementation of the Vivanet, special single-purpose computer desktops with dual high-resolution monitors were connected by a virtual private network that allowed a secure 2-way interface between information being accessed and the user serving as a safety gate through which select information was passed. The limitation of this system relied on the large data size transfer (ranging from 300 mb to 1 Gb) and the high up-front expense of using a dedicated hardware desktop system to perform off-site telemedicine reads.[31]

CLOUD-BASED TELEMEDICINE

Recently the RCM manufacturer has updated the reading system through the use of a cloud-based server that relies on secure high-speed third-party servers, similar to well-known services, such as Dropbox, WeTransfer, and Gmail.[32] The latest version of the RCM hardware units are programmed to instantaneously upload the full set of images from the microscope to a distant cloud server through high-speed Internet connection (100 mbps recommended) (**Fig. 1**). This new cloud-based Vivanet is more advantageous because it requires minimal (or no) investment in hardware but still allows access to powerful processing and storage technologies resulting in a much more cost-effective solution. With the Vivanet cloud, the reader can access the required imaging and information via any computer, tablet, or mobile phone that is connected to high-speed Internet cable or WI-FI. Thanks to incorporation of similar software used in services, such as Google Maps, the large imaging files can be streamed in real time permitting fast scanning of mosaic maps and zoom-in and zoom-out functionality similar to what can be performed on the actual microscope units. From the authors' own experience, it is recommended to perform teleconfocal evaluation using a large high-resolution computer monitor; but in instances when a desktop is not available, similar effectiveness can be completed with a high-resolution laptop or large tablet. The DICOM- and HIPAA-compliant Vivanet cloud user interface is accessed securely through a URL (https://vivanet.caliberid.com) where the user is asked to input their dedicated username and password (**Fig. 2**). Once the user accesses the home screen, there is a patient list that shows

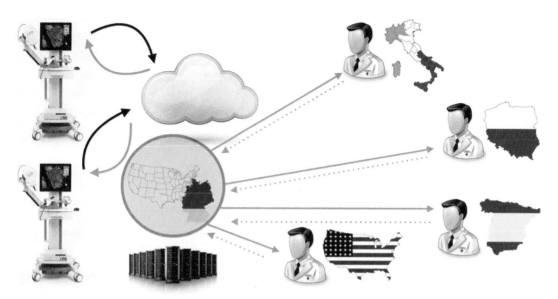

Fig. 1. The cloud-based teleconfocal system showing the connection between upload and current reading locations around the world.

completed and uncompleted evaluations (**Fig. 3**). After a patient case is selected, the user has access to the full imaging set via thumbnails (digital dermoscopy and RCM images) that can be clicked and expanded for more in-depth evaluation (**Fig. 4**). Finally, after completely viewing each image, the user is prompted to perform an evaluation helped by check boxes that highlight features found at the epidermis, DEJ, and dermis and overall diagnosis and treatment recommendations. Additionally, comments can be added if necessary. The final report is then stored on the cloud

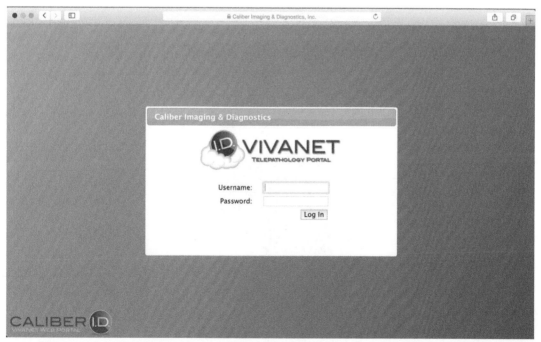

Fig. 2. Vivanet URL log-in window for the manufacturer's cloud-based telemedicine portal. (*Courtesy of* Caliber Imaging & Diagnostics, Inc, Andover, MA; with permission.)

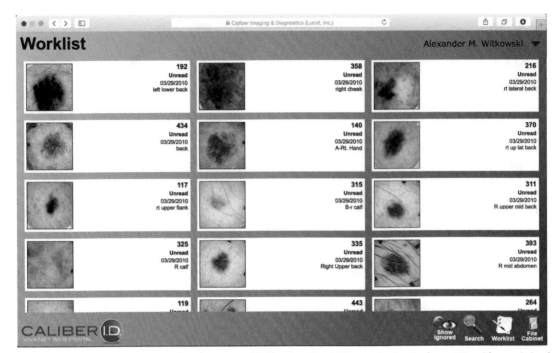

Fig. 3. Vivanet home page user interface. (*Courtesy of* Caliber Imaging & Diagnostics, Inc, Andover, MA; with permission.)

server and accessible by the upload site. Beta testing is underway to link full-body mapping (sequential digital dermoscopy or video dermoscopy) images with the patient file permitting a complete availability of patient information.

ELECTRONIC LEARNING AND TRAINING

In order to gain expertise in RCM, a novice must view and evaluate several lesions, which require a considerable amount of time dedicated to image

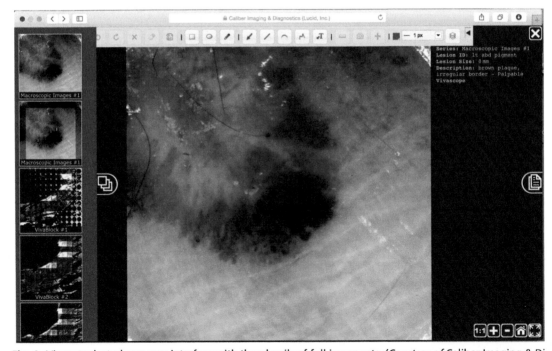

Fig. 4. Vivanet selected case user interface with thumbnails of full image sets. (*Courtesy of* Caliber Imaging & Diagnostics, Inc, Andover, MA; with permission.)

review and practice in a clinical setting. In order to make this process easier, a dedicated Web-based e-learning platform was developed (http://www.skinconfocalmicroscopy.org; http://www.confocaltraining.com) and launched in 2007 with the aim to provide access to teaching and test the reproducibility of RCM descriptors.[33] The platform teaches the user about the different features found at the 3 pertinent levels of evaluation (epidermis, DEJ, and dermis) and explains their correlations with dermoscopy and histopathology (Fig. 5). In the initial phase of its use, the efficacy of e-learning was demonstrated for melanoma (MM) diagnosis for physicians/dermatologists not previously skilled in the use of RCM and it was possible to evaluate the e-learning curve that resulted in an improvement of diagnostic accuracy over a long duration of time. But the question still remains: can RCM be used practically in a real telemedicine setting?

TELECONFOCAL PRACTICALITY AND SAFETY

Although it is now generally accepted that tele-dermoscopy is both safe and practical, few studies have been performed evaluating RCM application in a telemedicine setting.[34–38] Rao and colleagues[39] evaluated the RCM diagnostic accuracy in a support tele-consultation setting with retrospectively evaluating 340 lesions with 2 readers, one on-site and another at a distance. In the study, one reader was considered to be highly experienced in RCM evaluation (more than 10 years), whereas the other was less experienced. Diagnosis was based on the combination of dermoscopic and RCM images that resulted in an overall sensitivity greater than 90% and specificity of 60% with a combined sensitivity of 98% and 44% specificity. In this study, 3 MMs were misclassified as nevi; however, 2 were recommended for excision and one for follow-up. One basal cell carcinoma (BCC) was considered a melanocytic nevus; 3 of 40 squamous cell carcinomas (SCCs) were classified as benign lesions, and both readers considered histopathology-proven benign lesions to be malignant by RCM in 10.6% of cases. The investigators mentioned consideration of dual opinions because they found that all malignant lesions except for one SCC would have been excised based on at least one of the 2 readers' suggestions. This finding highlighted the potential for misdiagnosis by inexperienced single readers in telemedicine settings and the need for additional evaluation of reading technique and training requirements.

DOUBLE READER EVALUATION: A VALID CONSIDERATION

RCM reader experience may vary greatly and have quite a significant influence on the overall outcome of diagnostic accuracy and safe

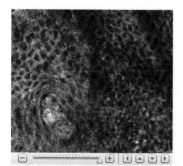

Fig. 5. Confocal training web site interface.

treatment recommendation. Therefore, the authors evaluated (submitted for publication) the diagnostic accuracy of RCM readers trained following a dedicated teaching program in order to determine whether the application of double reading can further improve the diagnostic accuracy of SAF telemedicine evaluation of RCM images, enhance MM detection, and reduce the risk of mismanagement and consequent liability. The authors performed a retrospective blind analysis of 1000 consecutive skin lesions that were evaluated by RCM for diagnostic decision during a 9-month period at the Dermatology Department at the University of Modena and Reggio Emilia. The images (clinical-dermoscopy-RCM image sets) were evaluated by 10 readers who received the same training program for 6 months plus 6 months of clinical exposure to bedside dermoscopy-RCM clinical decision-making. Each case was randomized in order that each case was blinded and evaluated by 2 different readers. Each reader was asked to provide their management decision, degree of confidence, and suspected diagnosis for 200 randomized cases. Based on histologic diagnosis, there were 176 malignant cases that included 83 MMs, 87 BCCs, and 6 SCCs.

The overall sensitivity for single-reader evaluation was 95% (ranging between 86%–100%) and specificity was 76% (ranging between 67%–84%). Excision was recommended with high confidence in 85% of malignancies and low confidence in 11% of malignancies with 9 MMs, 6 BCCs, and 2 SCCs (based on each 2000 total evaluations) misdiagnosed. Overall sensitivity for double-reader evaluation was 98% and specificity was 65%, respectively. Only 1 of 82 MMs (corresponding to an in situ MM) was misdiagnosed (concordant decision not to excise). When both readers concordantly chose to manage the lesion with no excision and high confidence, no malignant lesions were misclassified.

Of note, all readers followed a specific training program, including the individual study of clinical, dermoscopy, and RCM textbooks for skin cancer diagnosis as well as daily exposure for a 3- to 6-month period to dermoscopy and RCM outpatient clinics, with a minimum of 2000 clinical cases observed and discussed with a tutor. The authors' initial results show the potential limitation of novice single-reader evaluation at a distance, as the diagnostic sensitivity was not sufficient enough to keep the percentage of missed MMs at a safe level. This finding was attributable to a variety of factors, including lack of sufficient training, confidence variability, application of different evaluation criteria, fatigue, or stress of completion of a high volume of cases in a timely manner, all of which can be translated to real-life settings. Compared with previously reported methods and technology used for skin cancer screening, such as multispectroscopy, multiphoton, and optical coherence tomography, RCM resulted in a superior combined sensitivity in line with recent literature.[40–43] Additionally the previously mentioned technologies have limited applications in telemedicine settings and narrow application outside of pigmented skin lesions. The authors have not evaluated the cost-effectiveness of double-reader evaluation and its potential impact on cost sustainability of the technology implementation; this variable should be addressed.

SUMMARY

In retrospective evaluation settings, there is a tendency to achieve a higher performance because liability is absent. More variable results may occur in real-world settings. Although there is a very high sensitivity with RCM ruling in malignant lesions, particularly MM, there is a low specificity ruling them out in equivocal lesions. The implementation and availability of dedicated follow-up total-body clinical photography or sequential digital dermoscopy can help to avoid life-threatening mistakes by picking up subtle differences in cutaneous lesions over time. The mainstay of any new tool application in the telemedicine arena should encompass both high diagnostic accuracy and safety for patients. Training and evaluation guidelines should be implemented to guarantee proper and safe diffusion of the technology. Additional prospective studies can evaluate the potential for cost-effectiveness using this tool in telemedicine settings.

REFERENCES

1. Wang CW, Huang CT, Hung CM. VirtualMicroscopy: ultra-fast interactive microscopy of gigapixel/tera-pixel images over Internet. Sci Rep 2015;5:14069.
2. Varma S. Mobile teledermatology for skin tumour screening. Br J Dermatol 2011;164(5):939–40.
3. Taberner R. e-Dermatology: social networks and other web based tools. Actas Dermosifiliogr 2016; 107(2):98–106.
4. Mark RG. Telemedicine system: the missing link between homes and hospitals? Mod Nurs Home 1974; 32(2):39–42.
5. Park B, Bashshur R. Some implications of telemedicine. J Commun 1975;25(3):161–6.
6. Chouinard J. Satellite contributions to telemedicine: Canadian CME experiences. Can Med Assoc J 1983;128(7):850–5.

7. Gardner E, Tokarski C, Wagner M. Telemedicine goes the distance. Mod Healthc 1990;20(32):24–32.

8. Berek B, Canna M. Telemedicine on the move: health care heads down the information superhighway. Hosp Technol Ser 1994;13(6):1–65.

9. de la Torre-Díez I, López-Coronado M, Vaca C, et al. Cost-utility and cost-effectiveness studies of telemedicine, electronic, and mobile health systems in the literature: a systematic review. Telemed J E Health 2015;21(2):81–5.

10. Piccolo D, Smolle J, Argenziano G, et al. Teledermoscopy–results of a multicentre study on 43 pigmented skin lesions. J Telemed Telecare 2000;6(3):132–7.

11. Soyer HP. Dermoscopy and recently developed imaging techniques. Introduction. Semin Cutan Med Surg 2009;28(3):141.

12. Massone C, Brunasso AM, Campbell TM, et al. Mobile teledermoscopy–melanoma diagnosis by one click? Semin Cutan Med Surg 2009;28(3):203–5.

13. Arzberger E, Curiel-Lewandrowski C, Blum A, et al. Teledermoscopy in high-risk melanoma patients: a comparative study of face-to-face and teledermatology visits. Acta Derm Venereol 2016. http://dx.doi.org/10.2340/00015555-2344.

14. Manahan MN, Soyer HP, Loescher LJ, et al. A pilot trial of mobile, patient-performed teledermoscopy. Br J Dermatol 2015;172(4):1072–80.

15. Kroemer S, Frühauf J, Campbell TM, et al. Mobile teledermatology for skin tumour screening: diagnostic accuracy of clinical and dermoscopic image tele-evaluation using cellular phones. Br J Dermatol 2011;164(5):973–9.

16. Cook SE, Palmer LC, Shuler FD. Smartphone mobile applications to enhance diagnosis of skin cancer: a guide for the rural practitioner. W V Med J 2015;111(5):22–8.

17. Rudin RS, Auerbach D, Zaydman M, et al. Paying for telemedicine. Am J Manag Care 2014;20(12):983–5.

18. Rajadhyaksha M, Gonzalez S, Zavislan JM, et al. In vivo confocal scanning laser microscopy of human skin II: advances in instrumentation and comparison with histology. J Invest Dermatol 1999;113:293–303.

19. Coco V, Farnetani F, Cesinaro AM, et al. False-negative cases on confocal microscopy examination: a retrospective evaluation and critical reappraisal. Dermatology 2016;232(2):189–97.

20. Farnetani F, Scope A, Braun RP, et al. Skin cancer diagnosis with reflectance confocal microscopy: reproducibility of feature recognition and accuracy of diagnosis. JAMA Dermatol 2015;151(10):1075–80.

21. Longo C, Moscarella E, Argenziano G, et al. Reflectance confocal microscopy in the diagnosis of solitary pink skin tumours: review of diagnostic clues. Br J Dermatol 2015;173(1):31–41.

22. Longo C, Lallas A, Kyrgidis A, et al. Classifying distinct basal cell carcinoma subtype by means of dermatoscopy and reflectance confocal microscopy. J Am Acad Dermatol 2014;71(4):716–24.

23. Pellacani G, Pepe P, Casari A, et al. Reflectance confocal microscopy as a second-level examination in skin oncology improves diagnostic accuracy and saves unnecessary excisions: a longitudinal prospective study. Br J Dermatol 2014;171(5):1044–51.

24. Moscarella E, Rabinovitz H, Zalaudek I, et al. Dermoscopy and reflectance confocal microscopy of pigmented actinic keratoses: a morphological study. J Eur Acad Dermatol Venereol 2015;29(2):307–14.

25. Available at: http://www.confocaltraining.com/; Access date: August 25, 2016

26. Nelson CA, Takeshita J, Wanat KA, et al. Impact of store-and-forward (SAF) teledermatology on outpatient dermatologic care: a prospective study in an underserved urban primary care setting. J Am Acad Dermatol 2016;74(3):484–90.

27. Coates SJ, Kvedar J, Granstein RD. Teledermatology: from historical perspective to emerging techniques of the modern era: part II: emerging technologies in teledermatology, limitations and future directions. J Am Acad Dermatol 2015;72(4):577–86 [quiz: 587–8].

28. Coates SJ, Kvedar J, Granstein RD. Teledermatology: from historical perspective to emerging techniques of the modern era: part I: history, rationale, and current practice. J Am Acad Dermatol 2015;72(4):563–74 [quiz: 575–6].

29. Singh R, Chubb L, Pantanowitz L, et al. Standardization in digital pathology: supplement 145 of the DICOM standards. J Pathol Inform 2011;2:23.

30. Rubin CB, Kovarik CL. The nuts and bolts of teledermatology: preventing fragmented care. J Am Acad Dermatol 2015;73(5):886–8.

31. Massone C, Maak D, Hofmann-Wellenhof R, et al. Teledermatology for skin cancer prevention: an experience on 690 Austrian patients. J Eur Acad Dermatol Venereol 2014;28(8):1103–8.

32. Luan A, Momeni A, Lee GK, et al. Cloud-based applications for organizing and reviewing plastic surgery content. Eplasty 2015;15:e48.

33. Pellacani G, Vinceti M, Bassoli S, et al. Reflectance confocal microscopy and features of melanocytic lesions: an Internet-based study of the reproducibility of terminology. Arch Dermatol 2009;145(10):1137–43.

34. Leitch C, Jones R, Holme SA. Smartphone teledermoscopy referrals: comment on the paper by Börve et al. Acta Derm Venereol 2015;95(7):869, 871.

35. Börve A, Terstappen K, Sandberg C, et al. Mobile teledermoscopy-there's an app for that! Dermatol Pract Concept 2013;3(2):41–8.

36. Tan E, Oakley A, Soyer HP, et al. Interobserver variability of teledermoscopy: an international study. Br J Dermatol 2010;163(6):1276–81.

37. Warshaw EM, Gravely AA, Nelson DB. Accuracy of teledermatology/teledermoscopy and clinic-based dermatology for specific categories of skin neoplasms. J Am Acad Dermatol 2010; 63(2):348–52.

38. Massone C, Brunasso AM, Hofmann-Wellenhof R, et al. Teledermoscopy: education, discussion forums, teleconsulting and mobile teledermoscopy. G Ital Dermatol Venereol 2010;145(1): 127–32.

39. Rao BK, Mateus R, Wassef C, et al. In vivo confocal microscopy in clinical practice: comparison of bedside diagnostic accuracy of a trained physician and distant diagnosis of an expert reader. J Am Acad Dermatol 2013;69(6):e295–300.

40. Monheit G, Cognetta AB, Ferris L, et al. The performance of MelaFind: a prospective multicenter study. Arch Dermatol 2011;147(2):188–94.

41. Dimitrow E, Ziemer M, Koehler MJ, et al. Sensitivity and specificity of multiphoton laser tomography for in vivo and ex vivo diagnosis of malignant melanoma. J Invest Dermatol 2009;129(7):1752–8.

42. Gambichler T, Schmid-Wendtner MH, Plura I, et al. A multicenter pilot study investigating high-definition optical coherence tomography in the differentiation of cutaneous melanoma and melanocytic naevi. J Eur Acad Dermatol Venereol 2015; 29(3):537–41.

43. Hofmann-Wellenhof R, Pellacani G. Reflectance confocal microscopy for skin diseases. In: Wurm EMT, editor. Tele-reflectance confocal microscopy. Berlin: Springer; 2012. p. 469–74.

Well-aging
Early Detection of Skin Aging Signs

Caterina Longo, MD, PhD

KEYWORDS

- Reflectance confocal microscopy • Well-aging • Skin aging • Detection

KEY POINTS

- Skin aging is a complex and multifactorial biological process that involves a multistep pathway in which chronologic and photo aging are closely entangled.
- Reflectance confocal microscopy (RCM) can perform early detection of specific skin aging signs.
- Epidermal and papillary dermal changes can be morphologically assessed and readily monitored over time and over treatment with nearly histologic resolution and in a noninvasive manner.
- With RCM, aged skin typically displays an irregular honeycombed pattern with variable mottled pigmentation and the presence of flattened rete-ridges that coexists with polycyclic papillary contours. The papillary dermis shows a variable degree of changes of collagen with coarse collagen and huddled collagen. Finally, the presence of curled elastotic fibers, referred to as *solar elastosis*, is observable in elderly skin.

INTRODUCTION

"Age has no reality except in the physical world" Gabriel García Márquez (*Love in the Time of Cholera*). With this said, it is clear that aging is an ineluctable process that affects humans beings. Unlike the aging signs of internal organs, the skin demonstrates the first obvious signs of the passage of time with the consequent impact on a patient's social life.

Skin aging can be formally conceptualized into intrinsic and extrinsic aging, the latter not being easily disentangled from the former. The importance of aging lies in the enormous consumer demand for agents or treatments that can prevent or reverse its stigmata, its strong association with skin tumors, and the clues it provides regarding the nature of aging itself. In light of this, it is mandatory to detect early skin aging signs when the process can be readily reversed or, at least, minimized.

As a direct consequence, a precise and real-time quantification of aging is of outmost importance for in vivo staging of the dynamic process. Several bioengineering methods have been proposed to extensively and noninvasively assess skin aging in its early phase of development.

The current review focuses on the use of reflectance confocal microscopy (RCM) for the early detection of skin aging and for treatment monitoring.

Reflectance Confocal Microscopy

Minsky[1] developed RCM in 1957; since then, it has gained clinical and research popularity in the last decades, faster than any other devices. The reasons rely on the fact that RCM is a totally noninvasive technique that permits us to get optical en face sectioning of the skin with good contrast and high resolution, providing cytologic and architectural details.[2] Furthermore, the examination of a given skin lesion can be repeated over time, rendering this method extremely useful for treatment monitoring or dynamic evaluation of biological phenomena (ie, growing melanocytic nevi).[3]

Technical notes

Briefly, a confocal microscope consists of a point source of light, condenser, objective lenses, and a

The author has no conflict of interest to disclose.
Funding: none.
Skin Cancer Unit, Arcispedale Santa Maria Nuova-IRCCS, Viale Risorgimento 80, Reggio Emilia 42100, Italy
E-mail address: longo.caterina@gmail.com

Dermatol Clin 34 (2016) 513–518
http://dx.doi.org/10.1016/j.det.2016.05.014
0733-8635/16/$ – see front matter © 2016 Elsevier Inc. All rights reserved.

derm.theclinics.com

point detector.[1,2] The pinhole collects light emanating only from the in-focus plane. The mechanism of bright contrast in RCM is backscattering. In gray-scale confocal images, structures that appear reflective have components with high refractive index compared with their surroundings and are similar in size to the wavelength of light. Backscattering is primarily governed by the structures' refractive index compared with surrounding medium. Highly reflective skin components include melanin, collagen, keratin, and other elements, such as cytoplasmic organelles. The confocal scanning produces high-resolution black and white horizontal images (0.5 × 0.5 mm) with a lateral resolution of 1.0 μm and axial resolution of 3 to 5 μm. A sequence of full-resolution individual images at a given depth is acquired and combined together to create a mosaic ranging in size from 2 × 2 mm to 8 × 8 mm. A VivaCube (Mavig, Munich, Germany) composed of 3 to 4 mosaics with a 25-μm step is usually acquired for facial skin. Furthermore, a vertical VivaStack (Mavig, Munich, Germany) can be imaged. It consists of single high-resolution images acquired from the top skin surface up to 200 μm to obtain a sort of optic biopsy. The VivaStack modality is useful for the assessment of the epidermal thickness. Recently, a handheld RCM has been introduced on the market. This version is a smaller and flexible device that is quite useful in difficult-to-access areas (skin folds, ears). Unlike the wide-probe version, it has on-instrument control for laser power, imaging depth, and capture; but it does not allow scanning a large field of view.

Morphologic Aspects of Skin over the Age

Skin aging affects both epidermis and dermis; the process involves keratinocytes (KCs), melanocytes, and all cells that are present in the skin. In light of the nearly histologic resolution of RCM, it is readily feasible to detect morphologically the changes occurring over time. To start with, it is mandatory to know the overall picture of normal and young skin and then to progressively go through the changes observable in elderly skin.

Healthy Young Skin

In healthy young skin, the epidermis appears as a multilayer tissue with paradigmatic confocal findings depending on the skin level.[2,4] The stratum corneum appears as a highly refractive surface surrounded by darker skin furrows. Corneocytes are large, ranging from 10 to 30 μm, polygonal, and enucleated. Skin furrows appear as dark folds between islands of KCs that are typically arranged in a rhomboidal pattern formed by intersecting skin furrows (**Fig. 1**). Of note, the shape and arrangement of the skin folds strongly depends on the body site (being almost absent on the forehead and well represented on the abdomen) and the individual's age.

Going deeper, the stratum granulosum is composed of polygonal KCs presenting a grainy cytoplasm because of the presence of organelles. The KCs cohesively assemble, forming a honeycombed pattern because of its similarity with the honeycomb of bees (see **Fig. 1**). The contour of

Young skin

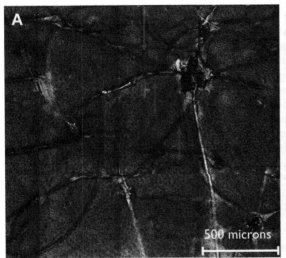
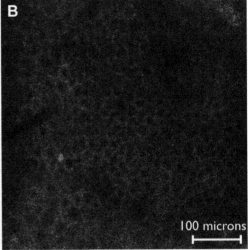

500 microns

100 microns

Fig. 1. (*A*) Epidermis in young subjects reveals a rhomboidal pattern of skin furrows (*arrows*). (*B*) Regular honeycombed pattern with KCs that are polygonal and with bright cell contours.

the cell is usually brighter than the cytoplasm and perfectly outlined. This pattern is commonly observed in light skin types. In contradistinction, dark skin types show pigmented KCs that are usually bright cells, small in size and always polygonal, separated by a darker contour (cobblestone pattern), resembling the negative of the honeycombed pattern.[3] On the face, a peculiar pattern is caused by the presence of numerous hair follicles that appear as dark round areas with a central roundish area from which arises the hair shaft. At the stratum spinosum level, the size of KCs tends to decrease but the cells still have a polygonal shape. The honeycombed pattern is easily observable. Below the spinous layer, there is a single layer of basal cells at the dermoepidermal junction (DEJ) that are uniform in size and shape but are smaller and more refractive than spinous KCs because of the melanin caps forming bright disks on top of the nuclei. It is intuitively obvious that the brightness of KCs depends strongly on the skin photo-type: the darker the skin photo-type, the brighter are the basal KCs. Conversely, skin photo-type I-II is characterized by basal KCs with low refractivity that constitutes barely visible dermal papillae. At the dermoepidermal level, in the presence of regular rete-ridges, basal cells form round or oval rings of bright cells (KCs) surrounding dark dermal papillae. On the face, rings are not usually observed. In young subjects, the dermis shows the presence of thin reflective reticulated fibers that form a weblike structure (Fig. 2).

Aged Skin

Regarding the epidermis, characteristic changes have been found in aged skin; the main findings have been reported for facial skin.[4–8] There is a decreased epidermal thickness with aging. Of note, a slight increase in epidermal thickness was found in middle-aged subjects whereby the presence of polycyclic papillary contours was simultaneously present. It is well known that polycyclic papillary contours correspond histopathologically to the presence of solar-lentigo features with bulbous and fused epidermal cristae. Thus, it could be speculated that the skin might became hyperplastic in response to solar insult and, later, severely atrophic with progressive thinning.

The overall epidermal surface analysis reveals a predominantly linear furrow pattern with the rhomboidal pattern becoming progressively larger and then completely linear without intersecting lines.

Unlike young skin, KCs in the elderly shows a wider variation in terms of shape, cellular outlines, and architecture. Those morphologies mirror a distinct epidermal pattern named irregular honeycombed pattern (Fig. 3); the changes occurring at different ages account for a variable degree of deviation from the regular honeycombed pattern until the complete disarray of the epidermis that occurs in presence of an actinic keratosis.[9–11]

When examining the changes occurring on melanocytes with age, it has to be clarified that in normal conditions melanocytes cannot be distinguished from KCs; they are detectable in tumors

Young skin

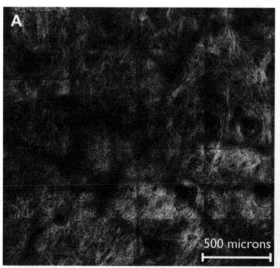 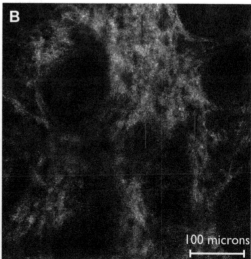

Fig. 2. (A) At dermal level a regular weblike arrangement of collagen fibers is seen throughout the skin area. (B) At higher magnification, RCM shows the presence of refractive and reticulated collagen fibers (arrows).

Aged skin

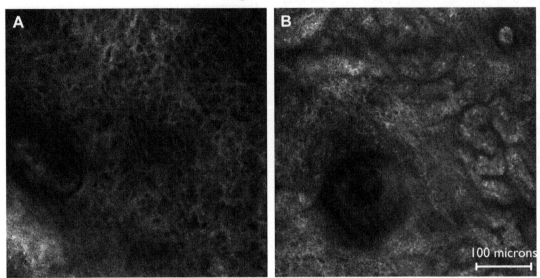

Fig. 3. (*A*) In aged skin, KCs shows variation in shape and refractive and they are assembled into an irregular honeycombed pattern. (*B*) At DEJ level, polycyclic contour are often detected even in absence of clinically visible solar lentigo.

(ie, melanocytic nevi and melanoma) or in inflammatory skin conditions (ie, melasma). With this said, the indirect effect on pigmentation can be observed with RCM, even in the preclinical stage.

More specifically, the presence of mottled pigmentation, defined as small clusters of bright KCs amid a honeycombed pattern, can be variably observed in different age groups. The late sign of aging or photoaging, clinically visible as age spots, is seen on confocal microscopy as changes of a solar lentigo.

At the dermal level, RCM provides an overview of the collagen and elastic tissue that might present different degrees of degeneration over time. In young subjects, the dermis shows the presence of thin reticulated fibers that are progressively replaced by thick coarse fibers or even amorphous huddles in the elderly (**Fig. 4**). Furthermore, when

Aged skin

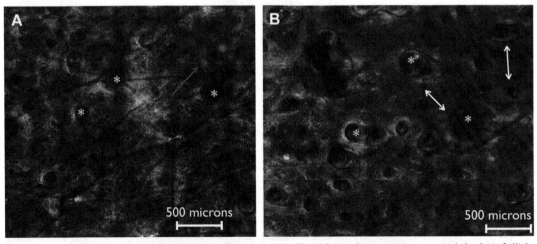

Fig. 4. (*A*) Aged skin is typified by coarse collagen with thick fibers (*arrow*) intersecting around the hair follicles (*asterisks*). (*B*) In severely sun-damaged skin or more than 80 years old, collagen fibers are no longer visible, and they are replaced by huddles of dark hyporefractive collaged (*double sided arrows*). (*Asterix* hair follicles).

severe solar elastosis is present, RCM highlights the presence of curled wavy fibers corresponding to elastotic changes.

Combining the previously identified confocal features, 3 different semiquantitative scores were calculated[7]: epidermal disarray score (irregular honeycombed pattern + epidermal thickness + furrow pattern); epidermal hyperplasia score (mottled pigmentation + extent of polycyclic papillary + epidermal thickness); collagen score (curled fibers, 2 for huddles of collagen, 1 for coarse collagen structures, and 0 for thin reticulated collagen). The epidermal disarray score showed a stable trend up to 65 years and a dramatic increase in the elderly more than 65 years old. The hyperplasia score was characterized by an ascending trend from younger subjects to middle age. The total collagen score showed a progressive trend with age with a different proportion of distinct collagen type.[7]

Besides facial skin, Wurm and colleagues[8] analyzed the dorsal and volar nonlesional skin of the lower forearm of 75 individuals with skin Fitzpatrick photo-types I to III in 2 age groups (20–30 years and 50–60 years) by means of RCM. From each participant and body site, 21 RCM features were assessed; statistically significant differences between the two age groups and different forearm sites were identified. Changes that were correlated with chronologic aging and that were aggravated on the UV-exposed dorsal forearm were as follows: loss of small skin furrows resulting in wider and less intersecting furrows; irregularity of the epidermal honeycomb pattern; irregularly distributed (mottled) pigmented keratinocytes/melanocytes; irregularity of the papillary rings and/or effacement of the rete ridges; and loss of thin collagen fibers and presence of collagen huddles.

Application of reflectance confocal microscopy for treatment monitoring

Sauermann and colleagues[12] evaluated the efficacy of a cream containing vitamin C applied twice a day for 4 months on the volar forearm in a study population of 33 women aged 45 to 67 years by using RCM.[12] Topical vitamin C resulted in a significant increase in the density of dermal papillae and in a reduction of granular layer cell size, indicating relevant effects in correcting the structural changes associated with the aging process.

Several studies investigated the morphologic changes due to laser treatment by RCM.[13–19] Recently, skin changes following ablative fractional carbon dioxide laser sessions by using RCM were analyzed in 10 patients.[13] Confocal microscopic images were acquired at baseline, 3 weeks, 6 weeks, and 12 weeks after the laser session. At week 3, the epidermis showed a complete disappearance of the mottled pigmentation with RCM along with the presence of few Langerhans cells. Newly formed collagen recognized as long, bright, and straight fibers replaced the coarse collagen observed at baseline before treatment (collagen remodeling). These fibers were arranged parallel to the surface epidermis and observed throughout the RCM mosaic. The collagen remodeling was still present after 3 months and confirms the long-term effect of the treatment.

SUMMARY

To sum up, RCM offers a dynamic view of the morphologic changes occurring at the epidermal and dermal level highlighting the different arrangement and cytology of KCs and melanocytes over time. New software will probably help the clinicians to precisely quantify those changes.

REFERENCES

1. Minsky M. Memoir on inventing the confocal scanning microscopy. Scanning 1988;10:128–38.
2. Rajadhyaksha M, Gonzalez S, Avislan JM, et al. In vivo confocal laser scanning microscopy of human skin II: advances in instrumentation and comparison with histology. J Invest Dermatol 1999;113:293–303.
3. Longo C, Zalaudek I, Argenziano G, et al. New directions in dermatopathology: in vivo confocal microscopy in clinical practice. Dermatol Clin 2012;30(4):799–814.
4. Sauermann K, Clemann S, Jaspers S, et al. Age-related changes in human skin investigated with histometric measurements by confocal laser scanning microscopy in vivo. Skin Res Technol 2002;8:52–6.
5. Neerken S, Lucassen GW, Bisschop MA, et al. Characterization of age-related effects in human skin: a comparative study that applies confocal laser scanning microscopy and optical coherence tomography. J Biomed Opt 2004;9:274–81.
6. Longo C, Casari A, Beretti F, et al. Skin aging: in vivo microscopic assessment of epidermal and dermal changes by means of confocal microscopy. J Am Acad Dermatol 2013;68(3):e73–82.
7. Longo C, Casari A, De Pace B, et al. Proposal for an in vivo histopathologic scoring system for skin aging by means of confocal microscopy. Skin Res Technol 2013;19(1):e167–73.
8. Wurm EM, Longo C, Curchin C, et al. In vivo assessment of chronological ageing and photoageing in forearm skin using reflectance confocal microscopy. Br J Dermatol 2012;167(2):270–9.

9. Pellacani G, Ulrich M, Casari A, et al. Grading keratinocyte atypia in actinic keratosis: a correlation of reflectance confocal microscopy and histopathology. J Eur Acad Dermatol Venereol 2015;29(11): 2216–21.

10. Moscarella E, Rabinovitz H, Zalaudek I, et al. Dermoscopy and reflectance confocal microscopy of pigmented actinic keratoses: a morphological study. J Eur Acad Dermatol Venereol 2015;29(2):307–14.

11. Wurm EM, Curchin CE, Lambie D, et al. Confocal features of equivocal facial lesions on severely sun-damaged skin: four case studies with dermatoscopic, confocal, and histopathologic correlation. J Am Acad Dermatol 2012;66(3):463–73.

12. Sauermann K, Jaspers S, Koop U, et al. Topically applied vitamin C increases the density of dermal papillae in aged human skin. Dermatology 2004;4: 13–8.

13. Longo C, Galimberti M, De Pace B, et al. Laser skin rejuvenation: epidermal changes and collagen remodeling evaluated by in vivo confocal microscopy. Lasers Med Sci 2013;28(3):769–76.

14. Mondon P, Hillion M, Peschard O, et al. Evaluation of dermal extracellular matrix and epidermal-dermal junction modifications using matrix-assisted laser desorption/ionization mass spectrometric imaging, in vivo reflectance confocal microscopy, echography, and histology: effect of age and peptide applications. J Cosmet Dermatol 2015;14(2):152–60.

15. Kawasaki K, Yamanishi K, Yamada H. Age-related morphometric changes of inner structures of the skin assessed by in vivo reflectance confocal microscopy. Int J Dermatol 2015;54(3):295–301.

16. Haytoglu NS, Gurel MS, Erdemir A, et al. Assessment of skin photoaging with reflectance confocal microscopy. Skin Res Technol 2014;20(3):363–72.

17. Lévêque JL, Fanian F, Humbert P. Influence of skin extension upon the epidermal morphometry, an in vivo study. Skin Res Technol 2014;20(1):58–61.

18. Raphael AP, Kelf TA, Wurm EM, et al. Computational characterization of reflectance confocal microscopy features reveals potential for automated photoageing assessment. Exp Dermatol 2013;22(7):458–63.

19. Shin MK, Kim MJ, Baek JH, et al. Analysis of the temporal change in biophysical parameters after fractional laser treatments using reflectance confocal microscopy. Skin Res Technol 2013;19(1): e515–20.

The Role of Reflectance Confocal Microscopy in Clinical Trials for Tumor Monitoring

 CrossMark

Josep Malvehy Guilera, MD, PhD[a,b,*], Alicia Barreiro Capurro, MD[a,b], Cristina Carrera Alvárez, MD, PhD[a,b], Susana Puig Sardá, MD, PhD[a,b]

KEYWORDS

- Reflectance confocal microscopy • Clinical trial • Tumor monitoring • Skin cancer

KEY POINTS

- RCM alone or in combination with dermoscopy or OCT has been shown to significantly improve accuracy in detection of tumor margins and recurrences in skin cancer.
- This tool can be useful in clinical trials and in clinical practice with this indication in melanocytic and nonmelanocytic tumors using either a handheld device or the standard RCM device to produce vivablocks.
- The main advantage of the first technical option is the reduced time of examination to a few minutes.
- It is probable that in the future faster scanners with higher resolution will be available in the market with the possibility of anatomic mapping of the tumor.

INTRODUCTION

Reflectance confocal microscopy (RCM) allows the evaluation with superb accuracy of some skin tumors before, during, and after treatment.[1] The clinician and the researcher may use RCM for the detection of tumor margins, recurrences, or the investigation of tissue changes during medical treatments.[2] Likewise in clinical trials RCM has been shown to provide useful information for evaluation of efficacy of topical or systemic medication. In this sense noninvasive evaluation of response to treatments substitutes the traditional approach of skin biopsy with the great advantage that the tissue changes can be evaluated in vivo. With the recent introduction of handheld RCM a fast examination of the tumor can be done in minutes. This solves the problem of time-consuming RCM examination using fixed RCM microscope examination. The handheld RCM modality allows a fast examination of tumor margins in melanoma or in patients with multiple tumors.

RCM evaluation is of major relevance in skin cancer assessment when ablative treatments are used or in the case of topical treatments, in particular indications in nonmelanoma skin cancer or in lentigo maligna.

In patients treated with surgery RCM plays a unique role to precisely map margins of the tumor in the skin surface and for the detection of subclinical recurrences. This has been used in melanoma in special situations, such as amelanotic melanoma or in lentigo maligna melanoma (LMM) on the face.

[a] Melanoma Unit, Department of Dermatology Hospital Clínic de Barcelona, IDIBAPS, Barcelona University, Carrer Villarroel 170, Barcelona 08036, Spain; [b] Centre of Biomedical Research on Rare Diseases (CIBERER), ISCIII, Barcelona 08036, Spain
* Corresponding author.
E-mail address: JMALVEHY@clinic.ub.es

Dermatol Clin 34 (2016) 519–526
http://dx.doi.org/10.1016/j.det.2016.06.001
0733-8635/16/© 2016 Published by Elsevier Inc

This article reviews evidence in the use of RCM in the research of different skin cancer tumor treatments.

REFLECTANCE CONFOCAL MICROSCOPY IN STUDIES OF SKIN CANCER TREATMENT
Reflectance Confocal Microscopy in Actinic Keratosis

Evaluation of efficacy of treatment of actinic keratosis (AK) and field cancerization in clinical trials traditionally has been done with naked examination and biopsies of lesions. For clinical evaluation, clinical pictures for documentation of the tumor can also be used. However, the clinical naked eye examination cannot assess with accuracy tissue changes or the presence of subclinical lesions, whereas biopsies have the inconvenience of local scar, pain, and the lack of dynamic information in vivo. Response of AKs to topical treatment modalities has been assessed by RCM in several clinical studies used alone or in combination with dermoscopy or different optical coherence tomography (OCT) modalities. The main advantage of RCM is that clinical and subclinical AKs can be monitored and dynamic changes in the tumor can be evaluated in vivo in real time (**Fig. 1**). This cannot be done with the biopsy of the tumor before, during,

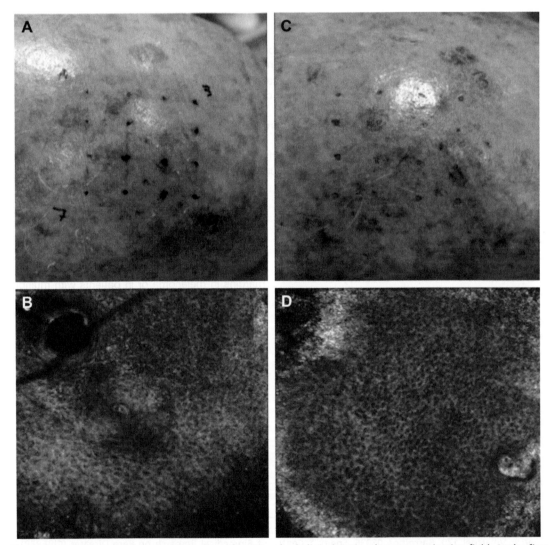

Fig. 1. Patient treated with topical imiquimod for AK and subclinical AK in a large cancerization field. At the first visit (A) the area to treat was assessed with clinical, RCM, and HD-OCT examination. At epidermal level, RCM reveals an atypical honeycomb pattern (B). At the end of the treatment in clinical evaluation (C) a little inflammation is shown. Evaluation with RCM (D) shows the improvement with a typical honeycomb in the same area compared with baseline (B).

or after treatment because the tissue is removed. The main limitation of RCM in AK is in thick tumors with marked hyperkeratosis because of the reduced depth penetration of 200 μm to 300 μm of the microscope. However, in thin AKs or in field cancerization RCM seems to be the best option for monitoring the response to topical treatment; photodynamic therapy (PDT); or ablative options, such as laser or cryotherapy.

There are several studies concerning the efficacy of RCM in monitoring treatments. In 2009 Ulrich and colleagues[3] demonstrated the applicability of RCM for noninvasive monitoring and detection of field cancerization and subclinical AK. The authors in this study described the clinical response of AKs and subclinical AKs to topical treatment in 11 volunteers with imiquimod 5% cream. In nine patients the clinical and RCM evaluation showed clearance of AKs. In one volunteer the clearance was clinical but on RCM examination showed persistence of AK features. The limitation in the evaluation with RCM was in skin areas with intense superficial inflammation or crusting because in these areas the penetration depth was limited, interfering with resolution, and impeding the visualization of cellular detail.[3]

In 2015 Malvehy and colleagues[4] published a study of monitoring treatment with 3% diclofenac sodium plus 2.5% hyaluronic acid and their correlation with histopathology. At RCM the degree of atypical honeycomb decreased and an elevated level of inflammation persisted during the entire period of study. Changes in parakeratosis, inflammation, and dermal collagen remodeling were also observed.

Ulrich and colleagues[5] in 2015 published a case series of eight patients with RCM monitoring for AKs and cancerization field. They suggested the

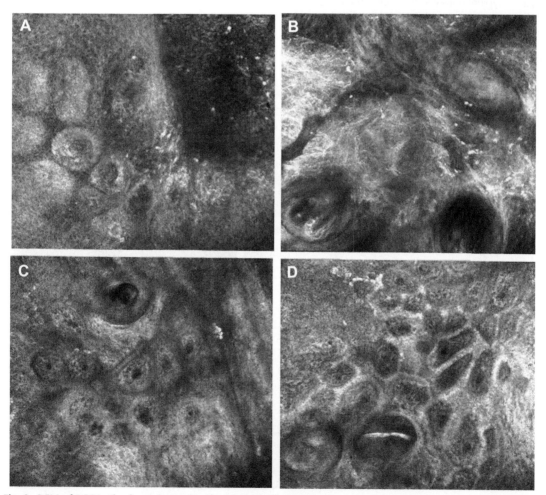

Fig. 2. RCM of BCC in the frontal area (*A, B*) with dark silhouettes of tumor islands and the typical palisade, dark clefting spaces, and reflective stroma. In the control posttreatment (*C, D*) all the structures described before indicate complete clinical response and small bright cells corresponding to macrophages are seen.

in vivo evaluation with RCM was a promising management approach for subclinical AKs.

A study by Maier and colleagues[6] to evaluate the response of AKs to topical ingenol mebutate using RCM and OCT showed that both tools are noninvasive methods that allow the monitoring of the clinical response to treatment. The combination of RCM and OCT was superior to the naked eye and may help the clinician to decide the therapeutic approach.

Malvehy and colleagues[7] used the combination of RCM and OCT in a clinical trial with 20 patients with diagnosis of AK and subclinical AK treated with a combination of 0.5% 5-FU plus 10% salicylic acid once daily for 6 weeks. The authors evaluated the lesions and field cancerization with RCM and OCT before the treatment and 2 weeks after the end of treatment. The study showed a significant improvement in the imaging scores used to evaluate this lesion (scaling, detached corneocytes, atypical honeycomb, round nucleated cells in the spinosum granulosum layer, round vessels, inflammatory cells).

Recently, Longo and colleagues[8] described the RCM findings of topical treatment response with ingenol mebutate in two patients. At baseline, RCM revealed typical findings seen in AKs, such as the presence of parakeratosis and irregular keratinocytes. Approximately a week after treatment vesicle formation with several inflammatory and necrotic cells was seen. With complete recovery, the RCM shows an epidermis with keratinocytes well-defined and a regular honeycomb pattern.

RCM has also been used in the monitoring of PDT therapy in this indication.[9] In a recent study by Jafari and colleagues efficacy of daylight PDT was assessed in 40 grade I and II AKs in 20 patients. Complete resolution and partial resolution was proved in 80% and 17.5% of lesions, respectively. This study confirmed that vivo RCM examination correlated with clinical findings and that this technology can be used to monitor the efficacy of this treatment modality. The authors in their study proposed a new RCM atypia scoring system based on atypia and cell sizes.

Basal Cell Carcinoma

In the case of superficial basal cell carcinoma (sBCC) topical treatment with imiquimod, PDT, or

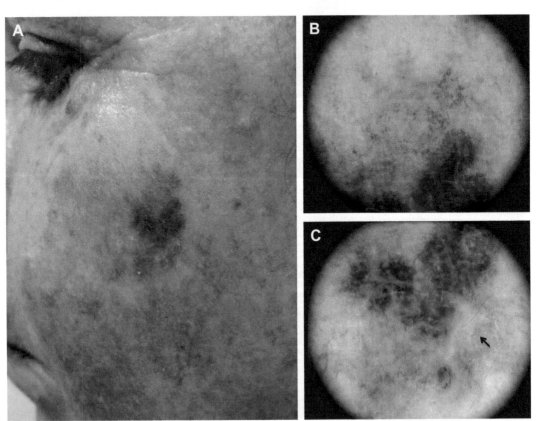

Fig. 3. A 63-year-old woman with a brown and grayish macule in her cheek corresponding to lentigo maligna (LM) (*A*). At dermoscopy irregular perifollicular pigmentation with peppering and milky-red areas around the scar of previous biopsy is shown (*arrow*) (*B, C*).

ablative treatments can be used with excellent results (Fig. 2). However, the precise diagnosis of this subtype needs to be confirmed. For this reason in addition to clinical judgment, dermoscopy, RCM, or OCT have been proposed for an accurate diagnosis.

In the case of patients with advanced BCC under treatment with hedgehog inhibitors, RCM has been used to study the changes in tissue.[10] RCM can be used in patients with special conditions, such as Gorlin syndrome with many BCCs.[11]

Ahlgrimm-Siess and colleagues[12] evaluated 10 histologically proven sBCCs located on the trunk and the response to cryotherapy treatment. RCM imaging was performed in each sBCC before cryotherapy and after 5 and 24 hours to monitor resulting tissue injury. Tumor clearance was assessed 3 months after therapy by RCM and histopathologic examination. Characteristic RCM features of BCC were present in all lesions before cryotherapy. Five hours after cryotherapy, all 10 sBCCs showed small bright round to polygonal structures at basal layer and black round to oval areas of varying size with bright structures floating therein, correlating to cell necrosis and incipient blistering. Eight sBCCs also showed cell necrosis in upper dermis. After 24 hours all sBCCs showed necrotic cells beneath collagen bundles. Tumor clearance on later histopathologic examination was only proven in those lesions showing damage to the upper dermis in RCM after 5 hours.

Segura and colleagues[11] evaluated the response to PDT in patients with Gorlin syndrome and xeroderma pigmentosum. RCM was performed before and 3 months after treatment. Tumor remissions and residual subclinical tumor persistence could be assessed by this technique. Complete clinical remission was obtained in 25% to 67% of the lesions. RCM could identify already described confocal features for BCC.

Authors from University of Modena and Reggio Emilia (Italy) valued 12 BCCs treated with PDT.[13] Dermoscopy and RCM imaging were performed at baseline and 7 days, 30 days, and 18 months

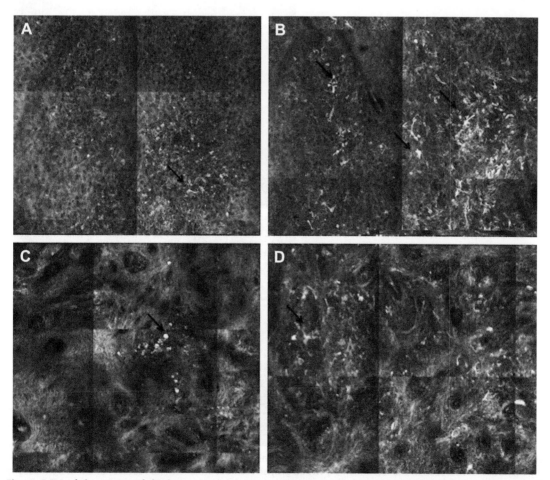

Fig. 4. RCM of the center of the lesion in Fig. 3. At the epidermis (*A*), dermal-epidermal (*B*), and dermis (*C, D*) exhibiting large and nucleated dendritic cells (*arrows*), in favor of LMM diagnosis (confirmed by histopathology).

after treatment. Biopsy was performed at baseline and in case of BCC persistence. RCM showed the persistence of two BCCs that escaped the clinical and dermoscopic diagnosis.

Maier and colleagues[10] described RCM findings in six BCCs in five patients receiving vismodegib or sonidegib, before and during treatment. Characteristic features were compared with histopathologic findings. The criteria of BCC decreased or disappeared during treatment. Half of the clinically complete responding tumors still featured tumor residue. They describe new findings, pseudocystic structures, and widespread fibrosis, and their correlation with response to oral hedgehog inhibitors.

Finally RCM can also be used in the assessment of margins of BCC during surgical excision.[14–16] In Mohs micrographic surgery in vivo RCM facilitated by aluminum chloride as a contrast enhancer has been used in patients with BCC.

Reflectance Confocal Microscopy in Trials in Melanoma

RCM allows the in vivo study of melanocytic tumors at the cellular level.[1,2] This method shows great accuracy with clinical diagnostic evidence in several studies. RCM in combination with dermoscopy is the most accurate method for the diagnosis in vivo of equivocal lesions. Otherwise RCM allows the study of hypo or amelanotic melanocytic lesions because of the reflectance of the immature melanosomes of these tumors.[17] In some particular situations, such as in flat pigmented lesions in sun-damaged skin, or in sensitive anatomic sites, such as the face or in mucosae, RCM has been proved to allow a precise diagnosis, avoid unnecessary biopsies, and orientate the clinician to biopsy site in the case that this procedure is needed.[2]

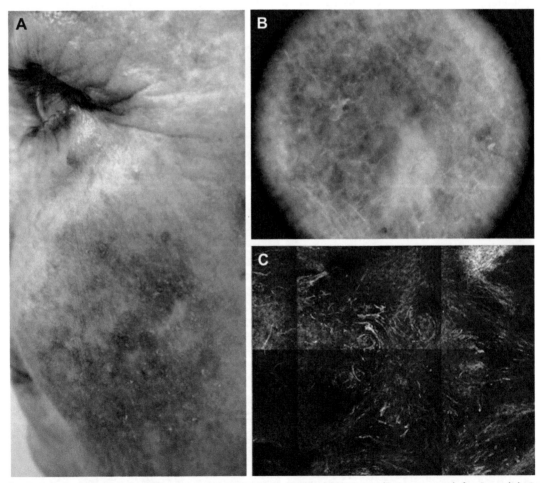

Fig. 5. Tumor of **Fig. 3** at 4 weeks after treatment with imiquimod 5% cream (3 times a week for 8 weeks). An inflammation area is seen in the left cheek (A) with a grayish residual area, with no features of LM at dermoscopy (B). RCM was performed, showing dendritic cells with criteria of persistence LM (C). A surgical approach was finally indicated of the area affected by tumor.

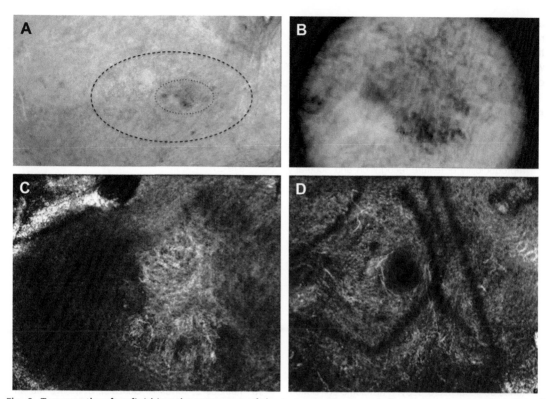

Fig. 6. Two months after finishing the treatment of the tumor in **Fig. 3**, no inflammation is seen. The affected area of LM by dermoscopy (*A*, *B*) in the minor circle and the affected area by RCM in the major circle. The RCM showed dendritic cells in the same place as the dermoscopy-positive area (*C*) and some atypical cells around the hair follicles (*D*). Surgical excision is performed in this area.

In LMM on the face the diagnosis and limits of the tumor cannot be determined well with clinical examination (**Figs. 3–6**).[18] Dermoscopy and Wood light may add information for the map of tumor limits before surgery.[19] However, RCM is clearly superior in this indication because of the cellular resolution of this method. In LMM the tumor can be detected in superficial layers of the skin in subclinical areas beyond the pigmented lesion. Guitera and coworkers[18] validated the diagnostic criteria for LMM in a series of 219 patients. They comprised two major criteria (non-edged papillae and round large pagetoid cells) and four minor features (three or more atypical cells at the dermal-epidermal junction in five of 0.5×0.5 mm^2 fields, follicular localization of atypical cells, nucleated cells within the dermal papillae, and a broadened honeycomb pattern). Only the last one has a negative punctuation in the diagnostic score proposed by these authors.

In different studies monitoring of treatment of LMM with imiquimod has been proposed. Alarcon and colleagues[20] used in vivo RCM in the evaluation and monitoring the response of LM to topical imiquimod in patients when surgery was contraindicated. They evaluated prospectively 20 patients with confirmed facial LM, when surgical treatment or radiation therapy was not indicated. In 75% of the patients in this study histologic tumor clearance was presented. In vivo RCM identified 70% of these responders with no false-negative results, and when compared with histopathology, there was no significant difference in evaluating the response to imiquimod.

Guitera and colleagues[18] showed the role of RCM combined with dermoscopy in the diagnosis of treatment failure. They describe a dust appearance with very fine brown dots highly correlated with treatment failure in LM (73% sensitivity and 88% specificity) and also the presence of pagetoid cells on RCM.

SUMMARY

RCM alone or in combination with dermoscopy or OCT has been shown to significantly improve accuracy in detection of tumor margins and recurrences in skin cancer. This tool is useful in clinical trials and in clinical practice with this indication in melanocytic and nonmelanocytic tumors using either a handheld device or the standard RCM device to produce vivablocks. The main advantage of the first technical option is the reduced time of examination to a few minutes. In the future faster scanners with higher resolution will be available in the market with the possibility of anatomic mapping of the tumor.

REFERENCES

1. Farnetani F, Scope A, Braun RP, et al. Skin cancer diagnosis with reflectance confocal microscopy: reproducibility of feature recognition and accuracy of diagnosis. JAMA Dermatol 2015;151(10): 1075–80.

2. González S, Swindells K, Rajadhyaksha M, et al. Changing paradigms in dermatology: confocal microscopy in clinical and surgical dermatology. Clin Dermatol 2003;21(5):359–69.

3. Ulrich M, Krueger-Corcoran D, Roewert-Huber J, et al. Reflectance confocal microscopy for noninvasive monitoring of therapy and detection of subclinical actinic keratoses. Dermatology 2010;220(1): 15–24.

4. Malvehy J, Roldán-Marín R, Iglesias-García P, et al. Monitoring treatment of field cancerisation with 3% diclofenac sodium 2.5% hyaluronic acid by reflectance confocal microscopy: a histologic correlation. Acta Derm Venereol 2015;95(1):45–50.

5. Ulrich M, Alarcon I, Malvehy J, et al. In vivo reflectance confocal microscopy characterization of field-directed 5-fluorouracil 0.5%/salicylic acid 10% in actinic keratosis. Dermatology 2015;230(3): 193–8.

6. Maier T, Cekovic D, Ruzicka T, et al. Treatment monitoring of topical ingenol mebutate in actinic keratoses with the combination of optical coherence tomography and reflectance confocal microscopy: a case series. Br J Dermatol 2015;172(3):816–8.

7. Malvehy J, Alarcon I, Montoya J, et al. Treatment monitoring of 0.5% 5-fluorouracil and 10% salicylic acid in clinical and subclinical actinic keratoses with the combination of optical coherence tomography and reflectance confocal microscopy. J Eur Acad Dermatol Venereol 2016;30(2):258–65.

8. Longo C, Borsari S, Benati E, et al. Dermoscopy and reflectance confocal microscopy for monitoring the treatment of actinic keratosis with Ingenol Mebutate Gel: report of two cases. Dermatol Ther (Heidelb) 2016;6(1):81–7.

9. Jafari SM, Timchik T, Hunger RE. In-vivo confocal microscopy efficacy assessment of daylight photodynamic therapy in actinic keratosis patients. Br J Dermatol 2016 Aug;175(2):375–81.

10. Maier T, Kulichova D, Ruzicka T, et al. Noninvasive monitoring of basal cell carcinomas treated with systemic hedgehog inhibitors: pseudocysts as a sign of tumor regression. J Am Acad Dermatol 2014;71(4): 725–30.

11. Segura S, Puig S, Carrera C, et al. Non-invasive management of non-melanoma skin cancer in patients with cancer predisposition genodermatosis: a role for confocal microscopy and photodynamic therapy. J Eur Acad Dermatol Venereol 2011;25(7): 819–27.

12. Ahlgrimm-Siess V, Horn M, Koller S, et al. Monitoring efficacy of cryotherapy for superficial basal cell carcinomas with in vivo reflectance confocal microscopy: a preliminary study. J Dermatol Sci 2009; 53(1):60–4.

13. Longo C, Casari A, Pepe P, et al. Confocal microscopy insights into the treatment and cellular immune response of Basal cell carcinoma to photodynamic therapy. Dermatology 2012;225(3): 264–70.

14. Marra DE, Torres A, Schanbacher CF, et al. Detection of residual basal cell carcinoma by in vivo confocal microscopy. Dermatol Surg 2005;31(5): 538–41.

15. Tannous Z, Torres A, González S. In vivo real-time confocal reflectance microscopy: a noninvasive guide for Mohs micrographic surgery facilitated by aluminum chloride, an excellent contrast enhancer. Dermatol Surg 2003;29(8):839–46.

16. Torres A, Niemeyer A, Berkes B, et al. 5% imiquimod cream and reflectance-mode confocal microscopy as adjunct modalities to Mohs micrographic surgery for treatment of basal cell carcinoma. Dermatol Surg 2004;30(12 Pt 1):1462–9.

17. Braga JC, Scope A, Klaz I, et al. The significance of reflectance confocal microscopy in the assessment of solitary pink skin lesions. J Am Acad Dermatol 2009;61(2):230–41.

18. Guitera P, Haydu LE, Menzies SW, et al. Surveillance for treatment failure of lentigo maligna with dermoscopy and in vivo confocal microscopy: new descriptors. Br J Dermatol 2014;170(6):1305–12.

19. Chen CS, Elias M, Busam K, et al. Multimodal in vivo optical imaging, including confocal microscopy, facilitates presurgical margin mapping for clinically complex lentigo maligna melanoma. Br J Dermatol 2005;153(5):1031–6.

20. Alarcon I, Carrera C, Alos L, et al. In vivo reflectance confocal microscopy to monitor the response of lentigo maligna to imiquimod. J Am Acad Dermatol 2014;71(1):49–55.

Fluorescence (Multiwave) Confocal Microscopy

J. Welzel, MD[a],*, Raphaela Kästle[a], Elke C. Sattler, MD[b]

KEYWORDS

- Fluorescence confocal microscopy • Staining • Fluorescent dyes • Fluorophores • Quenching
- Photobleaching • Selective featuring of target structures

KEY POINTS

- Fluorescence confocal microscopy (FCM) improves the contrast between the epithelium and the surrounding soft tissue and allows the depiction of certain structures, like epithelial tumors, nerves, and glands.
- Main indications include instant margin control in basal cell carcinoma (BCC) on the excised tissue and studies on barrier function and skin protection in vivo and ex vivo.
- Further optimizations on FCM parameters and fluorophores are needed to improve FCM, offering in addition to the reflection mode, valuable image information for the selective imaging of certain target structures in the human skin in vivo and ex vivo.

INTRODUCTION

In reflectance confocal microscopy contrasts are achieved due to different refractive indices of cell structures and organelles. Keratin and melanin serve as endogenous chromophores in the reflection mode due to a higher refractive index than water.

With the development of so-called multiwave devices, additional lasers with wavelengths of 445/488 nm, 658 nm, and 785 nm were added to an 830-nm laser. By using exogenous fluorescent dyes and different filters, they offer a fluorescence mode in addition to the reflectance mode. Corresponding to the different laser wavelengths, each fluorophore has a certain excitation and emission maximum. Because the emitted fluorescence spectrum has longer wavelengths with respect to the absorption spectrum, it is, therefore, usually red-shifted. The reflection light is much brighter than the fluorescence light, so filters are needed to keep out the reflection light and to gather only the fluorescent light. Fluorescence microscopy can be performed with a laser light source with correct wavelength and laser power, a filter system allowing for display of reflection, fluorescence, or both, and fluorophores matching these parameters.

The range of possible indications for FCM is growing rapidly. FCM is used in vivo for studies on skin barrier function, nanocarriers, and penetration.[1–4] For ex vivo FCM, the main indication is instant tumor margin control of BCCs during Mohs micrographic surgery by increasing the contrast between epithelial tumor and stroma.[5–9]

This article offers information on the staining modalities in FCM. Suitable fluorophores for the available laser wavelengths with corresponding excitation and emission maxima, their applicability in vivo and ex vivo in different concentrations (especially in terms of toxicity), and how to overcome problems, such as photobleaching, quenching, and pH sensitivity (specific and different for each particular dye), are reviewed.

[a] Department of Dermatology and Allergology, General Hospital Augsburg, Sauerbruchstrasse 6, 86179 Augsburg, Germany; [b] Department of Dermatology and Allergology, Ludwig-Maximilian University of Munich, Frauenlobstrasse 9-11, 80337 Munich, Germany
* Corresponding author. Department of Dermatology and Allergology, Klinikum Augsburg, Sauerbruchstraße 6, Augsburg D-86179, Germany.
E-mail address: julia.welzel@klinikum-augsburg.de

Dermatol Clin 34 (2016) 527–533
http://dx.doi.org/10.1016/j.det.2016.06.002
0733-8635/16/$ – see front matter © 2016 Elsevier Inc. All rights reserved.

CONTENT
Devices

The multilaser confocal microscopes suitable for FCM are the VivaScope 1500 Multilaser for in vivo and the VivaScope 2500 Multilaser for examination of freshly excised tissue (MAVIG, Munich, Germany). Both devices offer cellular resolution. In vivo, the penetration depth is limited to approximately 250 μm to 300 μm. For the ex vivo examination, there is no limitation to the depth as the tissue is placed on the cutting edge. Depending on the wavelength of the different lasers and dependent on the features of the devices (filters and so forth), reflection, fluorescence, or both are possible. Detailed technical data of both devices are as follows (new parameters of the latest device generation in parentheses).

VivaScope 1500 Multilaser for in vivo use

- Reflection mode wavelengths 445 (488) nm, 658 nm, and 830 (785) nm
- Fluorescence mode wavelengths 445 (488) nm, 658 nm, and 830 (785) nm
- Filter position only reflection, only fluorescence, both reflection and fluorescence
- Field of view 0.5 mm × 0.5 mm up to 8 mm × 8 mm
- Optical resolution horizontal less than 1.25 μm, vertical less than 5 μm

VivaScope 2500 Multilaser for ex vivo use

- Reflection mode wavelength 830 nm
- Fluorescence mode wavelengths 445 (488) nm and 658 nm
- Filter position fixed: 830-nm only reflection, 445 (488) nm, and 658-nm only fluorescence
- Field of view 0.75 mm × 0.75 mm (0.63 mm × 0.63 mm) up to 12 mm × 12 mm (20 mm × 20 mm)
- Optical resolution horizontal less than 1.25 μm, vertical less than 5 μm

Fluorophores

For the optimal dye, certain properties have to be fulfilled: excitation and emission wavelength have to correspond with the given lasers and filters. Tissue toxicity and patient safety have to be considered. Best concentrations for in vivo and ex vivo use and adequate staining procedures have to be established. Also, further biological and chemical properties, such as stability, specificity of binding, and membrane penetration, have to be taken into account. Last, but not least, important properties, such as availability and prize, should not result in major restrictions.

Fluorescein, acridine orange, methylene blue, patent blue, Nile blue, and indocyanine green (ICG) were identified as suitable candidate fluorophores according to their excitation maxima (supplier in parentheses):

445 (488) nm
- Fluorescein (Alcon Pharma, Freiburg, Germany), approved for angiography of the eye
- Acridine orange (Sigma-Aldrich Chemie, Munich, Germany), approved for ex vivo use

658 nm
- Methylene blue (Sigma-Aldrich Chemie), approved as a drug
- Patent blue (Guerbet, Sulzbach, Germany), approved for lymphatic mapping
- Nile blue (Sigma-Aldrich Chemie), approved for ex vivo use

758 nm
- ICG (Pulsion Medical Systems, Feldkirchen, Germany), approved for angiography of the eye

Depending on their tissue toxicity, the fluorophore can be used in vivo (topically or intracutaneously) and/or ex vivo in different concentrations.

In Vivo Fluorescence Confocal Microscopy

The issue of patient safety is the most important one for in vivo examinations. ICG is approved for in vivo use but is generally also toxic to tissue and can cause pain and necrosis; the authors have used it intradermally in low concentrations. Without restrictions in terms of toxicity and therefore appropriate for in vivo use are fluorescein, patent blue and methylene blue, although the latter bears the risk of permanent tattooing.

Due to the barrier function of the skin, different results can be expected, if the fluorophores are applied topically or intracutaneously in vivo.

Topical application

To mark the superficial layers of the stratum corneum, topical application of the dye is sufficient. The dye is dropped on the skin surface and wiped off with a paper cloth.

Fluorescein, methylene blue, patent blue V, and ICG are suitable for topical application.

Intradermal injection

To look at the lower epidermal layers and the upper dermis and to omit the barrier function of the stratum corneum, fluorescein or ICG can be injected intradermally after disinfection with a standard alcoholic disinfectant. ICG has to be used with caution because it is not approved for intradermal use, and tissue necrosis and pain at the injection site are possible. In the authors' studies, discoloration of the injection site for more than 24 hours and slight pain during injection were the only noticed side effects (**Fig. 1**).

Ex Vivo Fluorescence Confocal Microscopy

Due to tissue toxicity, Nile blue and acridine orange, possible carcinogenic agents, are restricted to ex vivo use. Fluorescein and methylene blue also can be used for tissue staining.

Tissue staining

Different staining protocols are used. In the authors' experience, best results were achieved as follows: freshly excised tissue was transferred in sodium chloride solution and slices of 2 mm to 3 mm thickness were prepared by the histopathologic technician. Using acetowhitening to get better contrast and to enlighten the nuclei, the tissue slices were put in citric acid 10% (pH 1.6) for 1 minute and afterwards buffered with Dulbecco's Phosphate Buffered Saline (100 mL, Sigma-Aldrich Chemie) at pH 7.5 (important to leave the cell structures unaltered) for 1 minute. Then the probe was placed in the staining solution for another minute and buffered again for 1 minute. After drying off (probe was not rinsed with distilled water to avoid alteration due to osmosis), measurements were performed immediately. Citric acid, as with acetowhitening, has also no influence on the following preparation and staining for histopathology.

Concentrations

According to suggested concentrations from the literature and from the authors' extensive experience in which many different dilution steps from the supplied concentrations were tested, optimal concentrations were derived: these were correlated with the image quality in addition to the visual impression quantified by measuring and comparing the intensities of light in different parts of the images, using the software ImageJ.

Advantages and Challenges of the dyes

All six fluorophores inherit different dye-specific challenges that have to be considered and overcome, such as tissue toxicity, light sensitivity, pH sensitivity, tendency for photobleaching, and quenching. These are briefly described for each dye and some exemplary images are shown.

The time window of fluorescence differs markedly between the fluorophores when injected into the skin. While fluorescein only shows a short window of up to 20 minutes when applied intracutaneously, ICG works up to 48 hours. For methylene blue, the time window is also restricted, due to photobleaching. Fading of the fluorescence was found within a few minutes (**Fig. 2**).

A way to cope with photobleaching is to lower the concentration or the laser power as much as tolerable. The effect of photobleaching, however, is not always a challenge, but can also be used on purpose for denoising.[10,11]

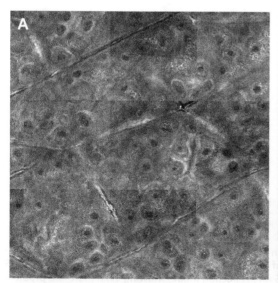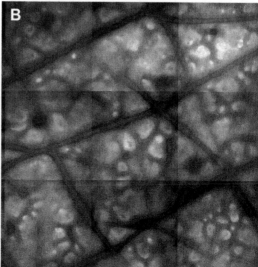

Fig. 1. Confocal mosaics after intradermal injection of fluorescein (0.2%) (*A*) in the reflection mode at 758 nm and (*B*) in the fluorescence mode at 445 nm; size of the mosaics (so-called VivaBlocks): 1.5 mm × 1.5 mm.

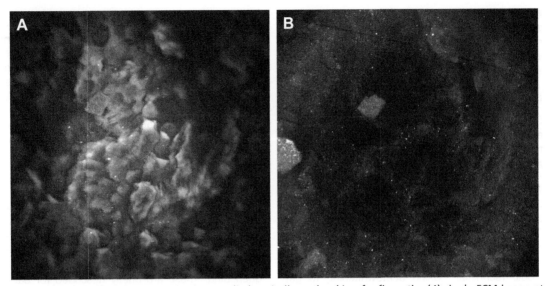

Fig. 2. Methylene blue, 20 mg/mL, in vivo, applied topically to the skin of a fingertip: (*A*) single FCM image at 658 nm right after application and (*B*) single FCM image of the same site taken only 1 minute later than in (*A*), also at 658 nm (size: 500 μm × 500 μm each), demonstrating the phenomenon of photobleaching encountered with methylene blue.

Another problem can be that the fluorophore itself can shade off the emitted light and cause artifacts. This should be omitted by using lower concentrations.

A further challenge the authors encountered with fluorescein is the topic of quenching. This process decreases the fluorescence intensity and can have several causes, such as complex-formation,

collisional quenching, or energy transfer to a so-called quencher (**Fig. 3**).

The Förster resonance energy transfer refers to a distinct mechanism by which energy is transferred from one dye to another, from the donor dye to the acceptor dye.[12] This process has to be taken into account, especially if trying to combine two dyes or examine

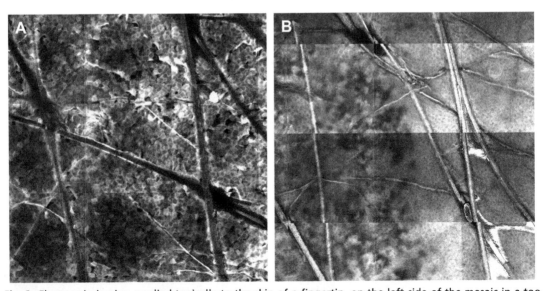

Fig. 3. Fluorescein in vivo, applied topically to the skin of a fingertip, on the left side of the mosaic in a too high concentration of 5% vs 0.2% on the right side of the mosaic. In comparison, (*A*) confocal image at 445 nm, fluorescence mode, and (*B*) confocal image at 445 nm, reflection mode, showing even more the problem of quenching due to a too high concentration (5%) of the fluorophore on the left side of the mosaic (size of the mosaics: 1.5 mm × 1.5 mm).

the same probe consecutively with different fluorophores.

The authors' tests revealed also that pH sensitivity can be a challenge. Fluorescein and Nile blue showed an especially strong pH dependency. Although the strong yellow fluorescence of fluorescein fades with lowering of the pH, in Nile blue the excitation and emission spectra differ significantly depending on the solvent used.

Considering these properties, the authors' recommendations for in vivo and ex vivo FCM are as follows:

Recommendations for In Vivo Fluorescence Confocal Microscopy

- Fluorescein ++, 0.2 %, well established for in vivo use and no tissue toxicity; challenges: quenching, short window of intradermal fluorescence (20 minutes after intracutaneous injection), and spectral absorption strongly pH dependent
- Methylene blue +, 2 mg/mL and no tissue toxicity; challenges: risk of permanent tattooing and photobleaching
- Patent blue +, less than 6 mg/mL (0.4 mg/mL) and no tissue toxicity; challenges: after subcutaneou injection, blue coloring up to 48 hours
- ICG +, 0.5% (intracutaneously), long window of fluorescence up to 48 hours; challenges: tissue toxicity and laser power too low in the authors' device

Recommendations for Ex Vivo Fluorescence Confocal Microscopy

- Acridine orange ++, 1.2 mg/mL, very good contrast epithelial versus stroma; challenges: possibly carcinogenic properties
- Fluorescein +, 0.4 %, strong fluorescence and no toxicity; challenges: quenching and spectral absorption strongly pH dependent
- Nile blue ++, 0.2 mg/mL in ethanol 70%, very good contrast epithelial versus stroma; challenges: pH value and solvent dependent
- Patent blue +, <6 mg/mL (0.4 mg/ml), no toxicity
- Methylene blue +, 2 mg/mL, no tissue toxicity; challenges: photobleaching

INDICATIONS FOR FLUORESCENCE CONFOCAL MICROSCOPY
In Vivo Fluorescence Confocal Microscopy

In vivo FCM is already used for different indications. In an in vivo study with fluorescein topically incorporated in a protective lotion, data could be collected on how long this protection lasted in an everyday setting, showing the value of FCM for pharmaceutical and cosmetic questions.[13] Also a study on the penetration of silver nanoparticles was conducted with FCM, opening up a wide field for future studies on nanocarriers and skin penetration properties.[14]

Ex Vivo Fluorescence Confocal Microscopy

For ex vivo FCM, recently a study on healthy skin specimens could underpin the excellent correlation to histopathology.[15] It enhances the contrast between epithelium and stroma, as shown in **Fig. 4**, depicting a sweat gland.

The main indication in dermatology for ex vivo FCM is the examination of BCC containing tissue and margin control similar to Mohs surgery right after excision on the fresh tissue.[5,16–20] Tumor nests can be detected very clearly with higher contrast (**Fig. 5**).

Recently, this method was also applied for cutaneous squamous cell carcinoma. Also the differentiation of 2 facial papules, the ex vivo identification of herpes viruses, the differentiation of oral potentially malignant lesions, and the intraoperative performance of FCM in the diagnosis of nonpigmented nail tumors have been described as new indications for FCM and suggest the value of this method for rapid bedside pathology.[21–24]

In addition, a spectral analysis for digital staining has been developed to mimic hematoxylin-eosin histology, offering images close to routine histologic slides. With these developments and

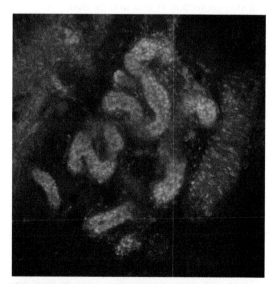

Fig. 4. Eccrine sweat gland in healthy tissue stained with acridine orange, 1.2 mg/mL, confocal single image at 445 nm, fluorescence mode; 0.75 mm × 0.75 mm.

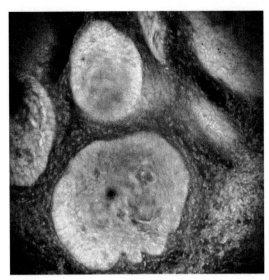

Fig. 5. BCC-containing tissue stained with Nile blue, 0.2 mg/mL, in ethanol 70%, confocal single image at 658 nm, fluorescence mode, showing prominently the tumor nests.

advancements, further studies on a wider range of indications for the use of FCM can be expected.[25]

SUMMARY

FCM improves contrast between the epithelium and the surrounding soft tissue and allows depiction of certain structures, such as epithelial tumors, nerves, and glands. Main indications include instant margin control in BCC on the excised tissue and studies on barrier function and skin protection in vivo and ex vivo.

Further optimizations on FCM parameters and fluorophores are needed to improve FCM offering, in addition to the reflection mode, valuable image information for the selective imaging of certain target structures in the human skin in vivo and ex vivo.

REFERENCES

1. Lademann J, Patzelt A, Richter H, et al. Comparison of two in vitro models for the analysis of follicular penetration and its prevention by barrier emulsions. Eur J Pharm Biopharm 2009;72:600–4.
2. Lademann J, Richter H, Golz K, et al. Influence of microparticles on the homogeneity of distribution of topically applied substances. Skin Pharmacol Physiol 2008;21:274–82.
3. Lademann J, Richter H, Schanzer S, et al. Penetration and storage of particles in human skin: perspectives and safety aspects. Eur J Pharm Biopharm 2011;77(3):465–8.
4. Lange-Asschenfeldt B, Alborova A, Kruger-Corcoran D, et al. Effects of a topically applied wound ointment on epidermal wound healing studied by in vivo fluorescence laser scanning microscopy analysis. J Biomed Opt 2009;14:054001.
5. Gareau DS, Karen JK, Dusza SW, et al. Sensitivity and specificity for detecting basal cell carcinomas in Mohs excisions with confocal fluorescence mosaicing microscopy. J Biomed Opt 2009;14:034012.
6. Gareau DS, Li Y, Huang B, et al. Confocal mosaicing microscopy in Mohs skin excisions: feasibility of rapid surgical pathology. J Biomed Opt 2008;13: 054001.
7. Gareau DS, Patel YG, Li Y, et al. Confocal mosaicing microscopy in skin excisions: a demonstration of rapid surgical pathology. J Microsc 2009;233: 149–59.
8. Gareau DS, Jeon H, Nehal KS, et al. Rapid screening of cancer margins in tissue with multimodal confocal microscopy. J Surg Res 2012;178: 533–8.
9. Rossi AM, Sierra H, Rajadhyaksha M, et al. Novel approaches to imaging basal cell carcinoma. Future oncology (London, England) 2015;11:3039–46.
10. Rodrigues I, Sanches J. Denoising of LSFCM images with compensation for the photoblinking/photobleaching effects. Conf Proc IEEE Eng Med Biol Soc 2010;2010:4292–5.
11. Rodrigues I, Xavier J, Sanches J. Fluorescence confocal microscopy imaging denoising with photobleaching. Conf Proc IEEE Eng Med Biol Soc 2008; 2008:2205–8.
12. Peng X, Chen H, Draney DR, et al. A nonfluorescent, broad-range quencher dye for Forster resonance energy transfer assays. Anal Biochem 2009;388: 220–8.
13. Sattler E, Kästle R, Arens-Corell M, et al. How long does protection last?–in vivo fluorescence confocal laser scanning imaging for the evaluation of the kinetics of a topically applied lotion in an everyday setting. Skin Res Technol 2012;18:370–7.
14. Zhu Y, Choe CS, Ahlberg S, et al. Penetration of silver nanoparticles into porcine skin ex vivo using fluorescence lifetime imaging microscopy, Raman microscopy, and surface-enhanced Raman scattering microscopy. J Biomed Opt 2015;20:051006.
15. Hartmann D, Ruini C, Mathemeier L, et al. Identification of ex-vivo confocal scanning microscopic features and their histological correlates in human skin. J Biophotonics 2016;9(4):376–87.
16. Bennassar A, Carrera C, Puig S, et al. Fast evaluation of 69 basal cell carcinomas with ex vivo fluorescence confocal microscopy: criteria description, histopathological correlation, and interobserver agreement. JAMA Dermatol 2013;149:839–47.
17. Bennassar A, Vilata A, Puig S, et al. Ex vivo fluorescence confocal microscopy for fast evaluation of tumour margins during Mohs surgery. Br J Dermatol 2014;170:360–5.

18. Karen JK, Gareau DS, Dusza SW, et al. Detection of basal cell carcinomas in Mohs excisions with fluorescence confocal mosaicing microscopy. Br J Dermatol 2009;160:1242–50.

19. Longo C, Ragazzi M, Gardini S, et al. Ex vivo fluorescence confocal microscopy in conjunction with Mohs micrographic surgery for cutaneous squamous cell carcinoma. J Am Acad Dermatol 2015;73:321–2.

20. Longo C, Rajadhyaksha M, Ragazzi M, et al. Evaluating ex vivo fluorescence confocal microscopy images of basal cell carcinomas in Mohs excised tissue. Br J Dermatol 2014;171:561–70.

21. Bennassar A, Vilalta A, Carrera C, et al. Rapid diagnosis of two facial papules using ex vivo fluorescence confocal microscopy: toward a rapid bedside pathology. Dermatol Surg 2012;38:1548–51.

22. Cinotti E, Perrot JL, Labeille B, et al. First identification of the herpes simplex virus by skin-dedicated ex vivo fluorescence confocal microscopy during herpetic skin infections. Clin Exp Dermatol 2015;40(4):421–5.

23. Debarbieux S, Gaspar R, Depaepe L, et al. Intraoperative diagnosis of non pigmented nail tumors with ex vivo fluorescence confocal microscopy: about 10 cases. Br J Dermatol 2014;172(4):1037–44.

24. El Hallani S, Poh CF, Macaulay CE, et al. Ex vivo confocal imaging with contrast agents for the detection of oral potentially malignant lesions. Oral Oncol 2013;49:582–90.

25. Bini J, Spain J, Nehal K, et al. Confocal mosaicing microscopy of human skin ex vivo: spectral analysis for digital staining to simulate histology-like appearance. J Biomed Opt 2011;16:076008.

Quick Evidence Synopsis
Minocycline for Acne Vulgaris

Date completed: July 14, 2015
Elsevier EBM Center contributors: Megan Sands-Lincoln, PhD, MPH and David R. Goldmann, MD

What is the clinical question? What are the benefits and harms of oral minocycline for moderate to severe acne vulgaris?

Intervention	Quality of Evidence	Balance Between Benefits and Harms
Minocycline vs placebo	Low	Trade-off between benefits and harms

Quality of evidence: quality of evidence scale (GRADE [Grading of Recommendations Assessment, Development, and Evaluation]): high, moderate, low, and very low. For more information on the GRADE rating system, see http://www.grade-workinggroup.org/index.htm.

Balance between benefits and harms: The Guideline Elements Model: beneficial, likely to be beneficial, unknown effectiveness, trade-off between benefits and harms, likely harmful, and harmful. For more information, see http://gem.med.yale.edu/default.htm.

What are the parameters of the evidence search?

Population: adults and adolescents ($\geq$12 years old) with moderate to severe acne vulgaris

Setting: outpatient

Intervention: minocycline (oral)

Comparator: placebo

Outcomes: change in lesion count, adverse events

What is the basis for the conclusions?

Population: adults and adolescents ($\geq$12 years old) with moderate to severe acne vulgaris
Intervention: minocycline (oral)
Comparator: placebo
Setting: outpatient (Table 1)

What do clinical guidelines say?

Guidelines of Care for the Management of Acne Vulgaris. American Academy of Dermatology, 2016[2] (AGREE II [Appraisal of Guidelines for Research and Evaluation II] score: unavailable).

- Tetracyclines, including minocycline, doxycycline, and tetracycline, are recommended as first-line therapy in the treatment of moderate to severe acne and forms of inflammatory acne that are difficult to treat (Strength of recommendation: A. level of evidence: I, II)
- Tetracyclines should not be used when contraindicated, such as in pregnant women or children less than or equal to 8 years of age, or allergy, in which case oral erythromycin and azithromycin can be administered.
- Doxycycline and minocycline are more effective than tetracycline, but neither is superior to the other.
- Erythromycin use should be restricted, because of its increased risk of bacterial resistance. Use of systemic antibiotics, other than the tetracyclines and macrolides, is discouraged, because there are limited data for their use in acne.

Dermatol Clin 34 (2016) 535–538
http://dx.doi.org/10.1016/j.det.2016.08.004
0733-8635/16

Table 1

Outcomes	Assumed Risk[a] Placebo	Corresponding Risk[a] Minocycline	Relative Effect (95% CI)	Number of Participants (Studies)	Confidence in the Effect Estimates (GRADE)	Comments
Mean % decrease in total lesion count (SD) at 12-wk follow-up	23.9 (41.9) N = 364	35.6 (41.9) N = 674	9.84 (4.84–14.84)	1038 (3 RCTs)[1]	Low	Favors minocycline
Adverse drug reactions[b]	28 out of 76	106 out of 186	1.25 (0.95–1.65)	262 (2 RCTs)[1]	Low	No difference

Abbreviations: CI, confidence interval; GRADE, Grading of Recommendations Assessment, Development and Evaluation; RCT, randomized controlled trial; SD, standard deviation.

  [a] Illustrative comparative risks.

  [b] Adverse drug reactions include gastrointestinal disorders, nausea, vertigo, drug-induced lupus, autoimmune hepatitis, autoimmune vasculitis, rheumatoid arthritis, hyperpigmentation, intracranial hypertension, liver damage, inflammatory bowel disease, and antineutrophil antibody and antineutrophil cytoplasmic antibody positivity.

Evidence-Based Recommendations for the Diagnosis and Treatment of Pediatric Acne. American Academy of Pediatrics, 2013[3] (AGREE II score: unavailable)

- Extended-release minocycline dosed at 1 mg/kg/d (administered as 1 tablet daily) is US Food and Drug Administration (FDA) approved for the treatment of moderate to severe inflammatory acne vulgaris that is not predominantly nodular in patients greater than or equal to 12 years of age.
- Both immediate-release doxycycline and immediate-release minocycline have the indication listed in their FDA-approved labeling of adjunctive use for severe acne, although this was not based on formal submission for FDA approval for either drug.
- For children more than 8 years old, the commonly used oral antibiotics are minocycline, tetracycline, and doxycycline.
- For children less than 8 years old or those with allergies, alternative antibiotics (azithromycin, erythromycin, trimethoprim/sulfamethoxazole) may be used judiciously.

European Evidence-based (S3) Guidelines for the Treatment of Acne. European Academy of Dermatology and Venereology, 2012.[4–6] (AGREE II score: 81.8%)

- The use of topical and systemic antibiotics should be optimized by using appropriate combinations for a predefined duration to reduce the development of antibiotic resistance.
- When choosing a treatment, different skin types, ethnic groups, and subtypes of acne must also be considered.
- The efficacies of doxycycline, lymecycline, minocycline, and tetracycline are comparable.
- Tetracycline has a lower practicability and patient preference compared with doxycycline, lymecycline, and minocycline.
- More severe drug reactions are experienced during treatment with minocycline compared with doxycycline, lymecycline, and tetracycline.

Antibiotic resistance:

- The first relevant changes in *Propionibacterium acnes* antibiotic sensitivity were found in the United States shortly after the introduction of the topical formulations of erythromycin and clindamycin.
- Combined resistance to clindamycin and erythromycin is much more common (the highest prevalence is 91% in Spain) than resistance to the tetracyclines, which includes minocycline (the highest prevalence is 26% in the United Kingdom).

- Use of topical antibiotics can lead to resistance largely confined to the skin of treated sites, whereas oral antibiotics can lead to resistance in commensal flora at all body sites.

AUTHOR COMMENTARY

Acne vulgaris is an inflammatory skin disease that can affect the face, back, and chest. It is characterized by open or closed comedones (blackheads and whiteheads) and inflammatory lesions, including papules, pustules, or nodules. It is generally characterized as mild, moderate, or severe, but according to the American Academy of Dermatology there is no consensus on a universal acne grading/classifying system.[2] Although topical agents constitute the usual first-line treatment of mild to moderate acne, in cases of moderate to severe acne, oral antibiotics are often included in the regimen.

The authors searched PubMed, EMBASE, and the Cochrane Database of Systematic Reviews for meta-analyses, randomized controlled trials, and guidelines for studies on the use of oral minocycline compared with placebo in the treatment of acne. Forty-three studies were retrieved, including 1 high-quality Cochrane Review on oral minocycline in the treatment of acne vulgaris from 2012, and relevant guidelines,[1–5] as well as descriptive studies and narrative reviews, which were excluded from our analysis. An older review comparing the use of different oral tetracyclines in patients with acne was found by hand searching.[7]

The data forming the basis of our analysis suggest that oral minocycline decreases lesion count in adults and adolescents with moderate to severe acne (Table 1). The overall quality of the evidence is low because of limited available data from placebo-controlled trials, significant variability in outcome measures, and use of multiple different scales and approaches to lesion count measurement. Studies comparing effectiveness of minocycline with other tetracyclines also showed comparable outcomes over 12 weeks of follow-up, but there was significant heterogeneity across studies.[1] These findings were further supported by a systematic review identified through hand searching that suggested similar efficacy across the drug class regardless of formulation or dosing regimen.[7]

Although minocycline is associated with a lower lesion count than placebo,[1] it has side effects, which may be more severe than those of other antibiotics in the tetracycline class of drugs. The most common side effect is gastrointestinal manifestations, and other reported but less frequent effects include skin discoloration, drug-induced lupus, hepatitis, dizziness, and vertigo.[8] It should also be noted that oral tetracyclines are generally not indicated in children younger than 8 years of age and are contraindicated in pregnant women.

The American Academy of Dermatology recommends minocycline along with tetracycline and doxycycline for treatment of moderate to severe acne.[2] The European Academy of Dermatology and Venereology notes the similar efficacy of minocycline compared with doxycycline, lymecycline, and tetracycline but also highlights the issue of antibiotic resistance to the systemic tetracycline class. It voices concerns regarding antimicrobial resistance, which is an important population health issue, but also concerns about resistance in commensal flora in all body sites with oral antibiotics, unlike topical antibiotics, which do not pose the same risks.[9]

Several questions remain about the use of oral minocycline and oral antibiotics in general in the treatment of acne. These questions include optimal dose, duration of treatment, role in combination treatment, and differences in side effect profiles. Additional research on the comparative effectiveness, safety, and tolerability of these drugs in trials using standardized outcome measures for lesion count, quality of life, and long-term treatment harms is needed.

ADDITIONAL INFORMATION ON MINOCYCLINE INDICATION AND DOSING

http://www.clinicalpharmacology-ip.com/Forms/Monograph/monograph.aspx?
cpnum=407&sec=mondesc&t=0
http://www.clinicalpharmacology-ip.com/Forms/Monograph/monograph.aspx?
cpnum=407&sec=monindi&t=0

GLOSSARY

AGREE II, Appraisal of Guidelines for Research and Evaluation; CI, confidence interval; FDA, US Food and Drug Administration; GRADE, Grading of Recommendations Assessment, Development and Evaluation; RCT, randomized controlled trial; SD, standard deviation.

RECOMMENDED CITATION

DISCLAIMER

REFERENCES

1. Garner SE, Eady A, Bennett C, et al. Minocycline for acne vulgaris: efficacy and safety. Cochrane Database Syst Rev 2012;(8):CD002086.
2. Zaenglein AL, Pathy AL, Schlosser BJ, et al. Guidelines of care for the management of acne vulgaris. J Am Acad Dermatol 2016;74(5):945–73.e33.
3. Eichenfield LF, Krakowski AC, Piggott C, et al. Evidence-based recommendations for the diagnosis and treatment of pediatric acne. Pediatrics 2013;131(Suppl 3):S163–86.
4. Nast A, Dreno B, Bettoli V, et al. European evidence-based (S3) guidelines for the treatment of acne. J Eur Acad Dermatol Venereol 2012;26(Suppl 1):1–29.
5. Nast A, Rosumeck S, Sammain A, et al. Methods report on the development of the European S3 guidelines for the treatment of acne. J Eur Acad Dermatol Venereol 2012;26(Suppl 1):e1–39.
6. Kawala C, Fernando D, Tan JK. Quality appraisal of acne clinical practice guidelines, 2008-2013. J Cutan Med Surg 2014;18(6):385–91.
7. Simonart T, Dramaix M, De Maertelaer V. Efficacy of tetracyclines in the treatment of acne vulgaris: a review. Br J Dermatol 2008;158(2):208–16.
8. Tripathi SV, Gustafson CJ, Huang KE, et al. Side effects of common acne treatments. Expert Opin Drug Saf 2013; 12(1):39–51.
9. US Centers for Disease Control and Prevention. Antibiotic Resistance Threats in the United States, 2013. Available at: http://www.cdc.gov/drugresistance/pdf/ar-threats-2013-508.pdf.

Quick Evidence Synopsis
Oral Contraceptives for Acne Vulgaris in Women

Date completed: July 21, 2015
Elsevier EBM Center contributors: Megan Sands-Lincoln PhD, MPH and David R. Goldmann, MD

What is the clinical question? What are the benefits and harms of oral contraceptives for acne vulgaris in women?

Intervention	Quality of Evidence[a]	Balance Between Benefits and Harms[b]
Oral contraceptives vs placebo	Low	Likely to be beneficial

[a] Quality of evidence scale (GRADE [Grading of Recommendations Assessment, Development, and Evaluation]): high, moderate, low, and very low. For more information on the GRADE rating system, see http://www.gradeworkinggroup.org/index.htm.
[b] The Guideline Elements Model: http://gem.med.yale.edu/default.htm.

What are the parameters of our evidence search?

Population: menstruating women with acne

Sociodemographic status, including age, ethnicity, and geographic location; diet; weight; physical activity level; menstrual history; use of helmets and sports gear; cosmetic use; medication use (eg, lithium, isoniazid, phenytoin, steroids, anabolic steroids); presence or absence of hyperandrogenism; acne lesion count and grade (various systems); comorbidities.

Setting: outpatient

Intervention: oral contraceptives containing an estrogen and a progestin

Dose, frequency, duration.

Comparator: placebo

Outcomes: change in lesion count, participant self-assessment of improvement, adverse events (outcomes assessed at 24 weeks or 6 cycles)

What is the basis for our conclusions?

Population: menstruating women with acne
Settings: outpatient
Intervention: combined oral contraceptives(various types and doses), combinations among and with topical and nondrug treatments
Comparator: placebo

See data in **Table 1**

What do clinical guidelines say?
Although our initial search did not retrieve any relevant guidelines, the following was retrieved through hand searching:

Diagnosis and Treatment of Acne. American Academy of Family Physicians, 2012.[12] (AGREE II score: unavailable)

Dermatol Clin 34 (2016) 539–543
http://dx.doi.org/10.1016/j.det.2016.08.005
0733-8635/16

Table 1
Intervention for OCP containing dienogest

Outcomes	Assumed Risk[a] Placebo	Corresponding Risk[a] COC	Relative Effect (95% CI)	Number of Participants (Studies)	Confidence in the Effect Estimates (GRADE)	Comments
Intervention: Oral Contraceptives Containing Levonorgestrel 100 µg/EE 20 µg						
Change in (mean decreased) lesion count ≤168 d	−9.8 N = 291	−19.95 N = 281	−9.98 (−16.51, −3.93)	572 (2 RCTs)[1-3]	Moderate	Favors treatment
Lesion improvement (based on participant self-assessment) ≤168 d	193 out of 291	228 out of 281	2.13 (1.47, 3.09)	572 (2 RCTs)[1-3]	Low	Favors treatment
Adverse event (discontinuation) ≤168 d	6 out of 176	9 out of 174	1.54 (0.55, 4.31)	350 (1 RCT)[1,3]	Low	No difference
Intervention: Oral Contraceptives Containing Norethindrone Acetate 1 mg/EE 20/30/35 µg						
Adverse event (discontinuation) 168 d	7 out of 296	20 out of 297	2.73 (1.26, 5.90)	593 (1 RCT)[1,4]	Low	Favors control
Intervention: Oral Contraceptives Containing Norgestimate 180/215/250 µg/EE 35 µg						
Change in total lesion count (mean) 168 d	−16.7 N = 194	−26.5 N = 193	−9.32 (−14.19, −4.45)	387 (2 RCTs)[1,5,6]	Low	Favors treatment
Lesion improvement (based on participant self-assessment) 168 d	38 out of 80	68 out of 83	4.50 (2.37–8.56)	163 (1 RCT)[1,6]	Low	Favors treatment
Adverse event (discontinuation) 168 d	9 out of 242	18 out of 246	1.98 (0.91–4.30)	488 (2 RCTs)[1,5,6]	Low	No difference
Intervention: Oral Contraceptives Containing Dienogest 2 mg/EE 30 µg						
Total lesion count; mean reduction (%)	−39.4% (SD=33.6) N = 259	−54.7% (SD=26.3) N = 515	−15.30 (−19.98, −10.62)	774 (1 RCT)[1,7]	Low	Favors treatment
Adverse event (discontinuation) 168 d	3 out of 264	8 out of 525	1.33 (0.38–4.67)	789 (1 RCT)[1,7]	Low	No difference
Intervention: Oral Contraceptives Containing Drospirenone 3 mg/EE 20 µg						
Change in total lesion count; mean(%) 168 d	37.7 (118.7) N = 86	66.8 (31.5) N = 87	29.08 (3.13, 55.03)	173 (1 RCT)[1,8]	Low	Favors treatment
Lesion improvement (based on participant self-assessment) 168 d	62 out of 73	75 out of 79	3.06 (1.06, 8.85)	152 (1 RCT)[1,8]	Low	Favors treatment
Adverse event (discontinuation) 168 d	24 out of 626	37 out of 625	1.57 (0.94, 2.62)	1251 (3 RCTs)[1,8-11]	Moderate	No difference

Note: 6 × 28-day cycles = 168 days.
Abbreviations: CI, confidence interval; COC, combined oral contraception; EE, ethinyl estradiol; GRADE, Grading of Recommendations Assessment, Development and Evaluation; RCT, randomized controlled trial.
[a] Illustrative comparative risks.

- Combined oral contraceptives can be used to treat inflammatory and noninflammatory acne (evidence rating: A).
- Several estrogen-containing oral contraceptives are US Food and Drug Administration (FDA)–approved for the treatment of acne.
- Oral contraceptives are considered second-line therapies.
- In certain cases, oral contraceptives may be considered first-line treatments in women with adult-onset acne or perimenstrual flare-ups.

AUTHOR COMMENTARY

The authors searched PubMed, EMBASE, and the Cochrane Database of Systematic Reviews for studies on the treatment of acne vulgaris with oral contraceptives. The search retrieved 1 systematic review[1] and 1 additional recent randomized trial.[9] One relevant guideline was found through hand searching.[12]

The Cochrane Review included 6 trials comparing various contraceptives with placebo and an additional 18 comparative effectiveness trials of different specific oral contraceptives.[1] The quality of the studies was compromised by high risk of bias, because most of the included studies were industry sponsored and had inconsistency and variation in the measurement of outcomes.

The systematic review suggested that oral contraceptives are effective in significantly reducing lesion count (measured after six 28-day cycles) compared with placebo (see **Table 1**) and are an effective treatment option for acne vulgaris. Data from comparative effectiveness trials included in the review were conflicting, making it difficult to determine which specific combinations of oral contraceptives are better than others. Contraceptive composition (estrogen/progesterone) and phasing (monophasic, biphasic, triphasic) have also been considered in recent trials, which have shown that there are no differences in acne outcomes between multiphasic and biphasic oral contraceptives.[13]

The review reported some adverse events, including headache, loss of appetite, moodiness, and breakthrough bleeding, but no serious side effects.[9] The duration of the component trials was not long enough to provide comprehensive data on adverse events, and longer-term observational studies to explicitly evaluate harms were not included. However, it should be noted that oral contraceptives are not indicated in all patients and are specifically contraindicated in those with cardiovascular risk factors, including arterial thrombosis, pulmonary embolism, and deep vein thrombosis, as well as in women with liver or biliary disease or breast neoplasm, and in those who are lactating.[14] The increased estrogenic effect may promote increased risk of venous thromboembolism and myocardial infarction and affect estrogen-dependent tissues, including the liver and breast.[14] Female smokers more than 35 years of age should not take oral contraceptives, and patients with renal dysfunction should not use drospirenone, a synthetic hormone (see **Table 1**).

Current acne guidelines support the use of topical therapy combinations, including retinoids and topical antimicrobial agents (benzoyl peroxide); however, a recent meta-analysis showed that oral contraceptives are similar to antibiotics in treating acne.[15] The American Academy of Family Physicians recommends combined oral contraceptives as second-line treatment of inflammatory and noninflammatory acne in women, except in cases of adult-onset or perimenstrual acne, in which case it can be considered first-line treatment.[12] This evidence supporting these guideline recommendations was derived from a 2009 Cochrane Review,[16] an older version of the systematic review included here.[1]

The FDA has approved 3 combination oral contraceptives for treatment of acne: norgestimate, norethindrone acetate, and drospirenone.

FOOD AND DRUG ADMINISTRATION BLACK BOX WARNING

Tobacco smoking and hormonal contraceptive use

Hormonal contraceptive agents are contraindicated in patients with a current or past history of stroke, cerebrovascular disease, coronary artery disease, coronary thrombosis, myocardial infarction, thrombophlebitis, and thromboembolic disease. Hormonal contraceptive agents have been associated with thromboembolic disease such as deep venous thrombosis (DVT). A positive relationship between estrogen dosage and thromboembolic disease has been shown. Oral products containing 50 μg of ethinyl estradiol should not be used unless medically indicated. Certain progestins (eg, desogestrel) may also increase thromboembolic risk (see Adverse Reactions at https://www.clinicalpharmacology-ip.com/Forms/Monograph/monograph.aspx?cpnum=2388&sec=monadve&t=0).

Because tobacco smoking increases the risk of DVT, myocardial infarction, stroke, and other thromboembolic disease, estrogen-progestin contraceptives should be used cautiously, if at all, in smokers. Risk is especially high for female smokers 35 years of age or older or in those women who smoke 15 cigarettes or more per day. Women receiving combination hormonal contraceptives should be advised not to smoke. Desogestrel has minimal androgenic activity; there is some evidence that the risk of myocardial infarction associated with hormonal contraceptives is lower when the progestogen has minimal androgenic activity than when the activity is greater. Preexisting high blood pressure, renal disease, hypercholesterolemia, hyperlipidemia, morbid obesity, or diabetes may increase the potential for embolism.

GLOSSARY

CI, confidence interval; COC, combined oral contraceptives; FDA, US Food and Drug Administration; GRADE, Grading of Recommendations Assessment, Development and Evaluation; RCT, randomized controlled trial.

RECOMMENDED CITATION

Sands-Lincoln M, Goldmann DR; Elsevier Evidence-Based Medicine Center. Evidence Review: Oral Contraceptives for Acne Vulgaris in Women. Dermatol Clin 2016;34(4).

DISCLAIMER

Knowledge and best practice in this field are constantly changing. As new research and experience broaden clinicians' understanding, changes in research methods, professional practices, or medical treatment may become necessary.

Practitioners and researchers must always rely on their own experience and knowledge in evaluating and using any information, methods, compounds, or experiments described herein. In using such information or methods they should be mindful of their own safety and the safety of others, including parties for whom they have a professional responsibility.

To the fullest extent of the law, neither the publisher nor the authors, contributors, or editors assume any liability for any injury and/or damage to persons or property as a matter of product liability, negligence or otherwise, or from any use or operation of any methods, products, instructions, or ideas contained in the material herein.

REFERENCES

1. Arowojolu AO, Gallo MF, Lopez LM, et al. Combined oral contraceptive pills for treatment of acne. Cochrane Database Syst Rev 2012;(7):CD004425.
2. Leyden J, Shalita A, Hordinsky M, et al. Efficacy of a low-dose oral contraceptive containing 20 microg of ethinyl estradiol and 100 microg of levonorgestrel for the treatment of moderate acne: A randomized, placebo-controlled trial. J Am Acad Dermatol 2002;47(3):399–409.
3. Thiboutot D, Archer DF, Lemay A, et al. A randomized, controlled trial of a low-dose contraceptive containing 20 microg of ethinyl estradiol and 100 microg of levonorgestrel for acne treatment. Fertil Steril 2001;76(3):461–8.
4. Maloney J, Arbit D, Flack M, et al. Use of a low-dose oral contraceptive containing norethindrone acetate and ethinyl estradiol in the treatment of moderate acne vulgaris. Womens Health 2001;1(3):123–31. Available at: https://www.researchgate.net/publication/244871891_Use_of_low-dose_oral_contraceptive_containing_norethindrone_acetate_and_ethinyl_estradiol_in_the_treatment_of_moderate_acne_vulgaris.
5. Lucky AW, Henderson TA, Olson WH, et al. Effectiveness of norgestimate and ethinyl estradiol in treating moderate acne vulgaris. J Am Acad Dermatol 1997;37(5 Pt 1):746–54.
6. Redmond GP, Olson WH, Lippman JS, et al. Norgestimate and ethinyl estradiol in the treatment of acne vulgaris: a randomized, placebo-controlled trial. Obstet Gynecol 1997;89(4):615–22.
7. Palombo-Kinne E, Schellschmidt I, Schumacher U, et al. Efficacy of a combined oral contraceptive containing 0.030 mg ethinylestradiol/2 mg dienogest for the treatment of papulopustular acne in comparison with placebo and 0.035 mg ethinylestradiol/2 mg cyproterone acetate. Contraception. 2009;79(4):282–9.
8. Bayer. GA YAZ ACNE in China Phase III. In: ClinicalTrials.gov [Internet]. Bethesda (MD): National Library of Medicine (US); 2015. Available at: https://clinicaltrials.gov/show/NCT00818519. NLM Identifier: NCT00818519.

9. Palli MB, Reyes-Habito CM, Lima XT, et al. A single-center, randomized double-blind, parallel-group study to examine the safety and efficacy of 3mg drospirenone/0.02 mg ethinyl estradiol compared with placebo in the treatment of moderate truncal acne vulgaris. J Drugs Dermatol 2013;12(6):633–7.

10. Maloney JM, Dietze P Jr, Watson D, et al. Treatment of acne using a 3-milligram drospirenone/20-microgram ethinyl estradiol oral contraceptive administered in a 24/4 regimen: a randomized controlled trial. Obstet Gynecol 2008; 112(4):773–81. Available at: https://www.researchgate.net/publication/23291812_Treatment_of_Acne_Using_a_3-Milligram_Drospirenone20-Microgram_Ethinyl_Estradiol_Oral_Contraceptive_Administered_in_a_244_Regimen.

11. Koltun W, Lucky AW, Thiboutot D, et al. Efficacy and safety of 3 mg drospirenone/20 mcg ethinylestradiol oral contraceptive administered in 24/4 regimen in the treatment of acne vulgaris: a randomized, double-blind, placebo-controlled trial. Contraception. 2008;77(4):249–56.

12. Titus S, Hodge J. Diagnosis and treatment of acne. Am Fam Physician 2012;86(8):734–40.

13. Jaisamrarn U, Chaovisitsaree S, Angsuwathana S, et al. A comparison of multiphasic oral contraceptives containing norgestimate or desogestrel in acne treatment: A randomized trial. Contraception. 2014;90(5):535–41.

14. Evans G, Sutton EL. Oral contraception. Med Clin North Am 2015;99(3):479–503.

15. Koo EB, Petersen TD, Kimball AB. Meta-analysis comparing efficacy of antibiotics versus oral contraceptives in acne vulgaris. J Am Acad Dermatol 2014;71(3):450–9.

16. Arowojolu AO, Gallo MF, Lopez LM, et al. Combined oral contraceptive pills for treatment of acne. Cochrane Database Syst Rev 2009;(3):CD004425.

Quick Evidence Synopsis
Selected Nonpharmacologic Therapies for Acne Vulgaris

Date completed: June 12, 2015

Elsevier EBM Center contributors: Megan Sands-Lincoln, PhD, MPH, and David R. Goldmann, MD

What is the clinical question? What are the benefits and harms of selected nonpharmacologic dietary and topical therapies for acne vulgaris?

What does the evidence conclude?

Intervention	Quality of Evidence[a]	Balance Between Benefits and Harms[b]
Low glycemic load or ginger	Low	Unknown effectiveness
Topical aloe vera as a supplement to tretinoin	Low	Unknown effectiveness

[a] Quality of evidence scale (GRADE [Grading of Recommendations Assessment, Development, and Evaluation]): high, moderate, low, and very low. For more information on the GRADE rating system, see http://www.gradeworkinggroup.org/index.htm.
[b] The Guideline Elements Model: http://gem.med.yale.edu/default.htm.

What are the parameters of our search?

Population: adults with acne vulgaris

Setting: outpatient

Intervention: nonpharmacologic treatments, including low-glycemic-load diet and topical aloe vera

Comparator: placebo, higher glycemic load diet

Outcomes: lesion count, quality of life (QOL), harms

What is the basis for our conclusions?

Population: adults with acne vulgaris
Setting: outpatient
Intervention: low-glycemic-load diet
Comparator: high-glycemic-load diet (Table 1)

Dermatol Clin 34 (2016) 545–548
http://dx.doi.org/10.1016/j.det.2016.08.006
0733-8635/16

Table 1
Diets with high or low glycemic loads in adults with acne vulgaris

Outcomes	Assumed Risk[a] High Glycemic Load (95% CI)	Corresponding Risk[a] Low Glycemic Load (95% CI)	Relative Effect (95% CI) NNT	Number of Participants (Studies)	Confidence in the Effect Estimates (GRADE)	Comments
Change in noninflammatory lesion count at 12 weeks	1.15 lesions	−3.89 lesions (−10.07, 2.29)	—	75 (2 RCTs)[1–3]	Low	No difference

Abbreviations: CI, confidence interval; GRADE, Grading of Recommendations Assessment, Development, and Evaluation; NNT, number needed to treat; RCT, randomized controlled trial.
[a] Illustrative comparative risks.

Population: adults with acne vulgaris
Setting: outpatient
Intervention: *Zingiber officinale* (ginger capsule)
Comparator: placebo, active comparator (**Table 2**)

Population: adults with acne vulgaris
Setting: outpatient
Intervention: aloe vera (topical)
Comparator: placebo, active comparator (**Table 3**)

WHAT DO CLINICAL GUIDELINES SAY?

Malaysian Ministry of Health. Clinical Practice Guidelines on Management of Acne, 2012[6] (AGREE II [Appraisal of Guidelines for Research and Evaluation II] score: 84%).

- A low-glycemic-load diet and high-fiber diet should be encouraged for patients with acne (grade B).
  - Low-glycemic-load diet significantly reduces total acne lesion count compared with high-glycemic-load diet in individuals aged 15 to 25 years (evidence level I).
  - Risk of acne increased significantly with increasing dietary glycemic load (evidence level II).
  - There is no good evidence for oily foods, chocolate, or nuts in the pathogenesis of acne (evidence level II).

Table 2
Ginger capsules to treat acne vulgaris in adults

Outcomes	Assumed Risk[a] Baseline	Corresponding Risk[a] Intervention at 6-mo Follow-up	Relative Effect (95% CI)	Number of Participants (Studies)	Confidence in the Effect Estimates (GRADE)	Comments
Mean Acne -QOL[4] Total Score (95% CI)	60.4 (54.1–66.7)	88.2 (84.2–92.2)	QOL increased by 27.8 units (33.4–22.1)	31 (1 open-label trial)[4]	Very low	Favors intervention
Mean Lesion Count (95% CI)	120 (95.1–144.9)	57.7 (39.9–75.5)	Mean lesion reduction 48%	31 (1 open-label trial)[4]	Very low	Favors intervention

[a] Illustrative comparative risks.

Table 3
Aloe vera to treat acne vulgaris in adults

Outcomes	Baseline Lesion Count (Trentinoin)	Follow-up Lesion Count at 2-mo (Aloe Vera/Trentinoin)	Risk Difference (RD)	Number of Participants (Studies)	Confidence in the Effect Estimates (GRADE)	Comments
Change in total lesion count	6.20	8.63	RD = 23.3% greater reduction in total lesion score	75 (1 RCT)[5]	Very low	Favors intervention

Abbreviation: RD, risk difference.

- ○ A weak association exists between all types of milk with worsening of acne among adolescent girls (evidence level III).
- There is insufficient evidence to recommend any specific complementary and alternative medicine (CAM) therapies for the treatment of acne.

AUTHOR COMMENTARY

This evidence synopsis on treatment of acne vulgaris with specific complementary therapies is supported only by low-quality evidence because of inconsistency (heterogeneity between trials), indirectness, risk of bias (lack of blinding and allocation concealment), and incomplete reporting of appropriate data. There were also several concerns regarding measurement and quantifying the dose of various interventions.

The major results are supported by 1 systematic review[3] and 2 single studies.[4,5] The systematic review focused on complementary treatments of diet and herbal treatment approaches and less on mind-body interventions, bioelectromagnetics, and other folk remedies. The included meta-analysis on dietary interventions indicated no difference in lesion count between participants on a low-glycemic index diet compared with a high-glycemic-index diet at 12-week follow-up (see **Table 1**). Essentially none of the additional meta-analyses from the 33 studies in this systematic review on a variety of complementary-alternative therapies supported a significant impact on lesion count.[3] One nonrandomized study on Zingiber officinale (ginger) indicated a reduced lesion count and increased QOL among the intervention group (see **Table 2**), and an additional study supported the use of aloe vera with tretinoin, which also reduced total lesion count (see **Table 3**). Both studies were of very low quality, and additional evidence on these treatments is needed.

In a systematic review addressing the quality of guidelines on acne vulgaris, which itself was critically appraised for quality using the AGREE II tool, significant variability in the quality and methodological rigor of the guidelines[7] was observed. Only 2 of the 6 guidelines were recommended.[7] Several of the guidelines were limited in quality because of stakeholder involvement, rigor of guideline development, and applicability. Only 2 guidelines clearly reported on patient-important outcomes such as efficacy and QOL.[6,8] The current clinical practice guidelines vary in their consideration of complementary-alternative therapy and do not make any recommendations regarding specific CAM treatments for acne because of insufficient evidence. This lack of recommendations is consistent with the findings in this evidence synopsis.

Acne treatment is intended to reduce inflammation while minimizing the adverse effects of the treatment. No major adverse effects were reported in the studies reviewed; however, minor skin irritation (scaling, erythema),[5] gastrointestinal effects, and nausea were reported as minor adverse symptoms of these treatments.[3]

A more recent systematic review on botanic therapies, which supported each individual herb and plant extract studied in single low-quality studies, suggested that they may be helpful in treatment mild to moderate, but not severe, acne.[9]

This synopsis focuses primarily on diet and herbal CAM therapies; however, the literature contains studies on other alternative therapies for acne that are beyond the scope of this synopsis, including bee venom, moxibustion, cupping, tea tree, and acupuncture. In addition, it has been suggested in the past that specific foods such as chocolate, dairy, and oil may be associated with increased risk of acne. However, as noted in the Cochrane Review, there are limited systematic reviews and randomized controlled trials specific to these interventions, and additional evidence is needed.

GLOSSARY

AGREE II, Appraisal of Guidelines for Research and Evaluation; CAM, complementary and alternative medicine; CI, confidence interval; GRADE, Grading of Recommendations Assessment, Development and Evaluation; NNT, number needed to treat; QOL, quality of life; RCT, randomized controlled trial; RD, risk difference.

RECOMMENDED CITATION

Sands-Lincoln M, Goldmann DR. Elsevier Evidence-Based Medicine Center. Evidence Review: Selected Nonpharmacologic Therapies for Acne Vulgaris. Dermatol Clin 2016;34(4).

DISCLAIMER

Knowledge and best practice in this field are constantly changing. As new research and experience broaden clinicians' understanding, changes in research methods, professional practices, or medical treatment may become necessary.

Practitioners and researchers must always rely on their own experience and knowledge in evaluating and using any information, methods, compounds, or experiments described herein. In using such information or methods they should be mindful of their own safety and the safety of others, including parties for whom they have a professional responsibility.

To the fullest extent of the law, neither the publisher nor the investigators, contributors, or editors assume any liability for any injury and/or damage to persons or property as a matter of product liability, negligence or otherwise, or from any use or operation of any methods, products, instructions, or ideas contained in the material herein.

REFERENCES

1. Kwon HH, Yoon JY, Hong JS, et al. Clinical and histological effect of a low glycaemic load diet in treatment of acne vulgaris in Korean patients: a randomized, controlled trial. Acta Derm Venereol 2012;92(3):241–6.
2. Smith RN, Mann NJ, Braue A, et al. The effect of a high-protein, low glycemic-load diet versus a conventional, high glycemic-load diet on biochemical parameters associated with acne vulgaris: a randomized, investigator-masked, controlled trial. J Am Acad Dermatol 2007;57(2):247–56.
3. Cao H, Yang G, Wang Y, et al. Complementary therapies for acne vulgaris. Cochrane Database Syst Rev 2015;(1):CD009436.
4. Miglani A, Manchanda RK (2014). Prospective, non-randomised, open-label study of homeopathic *Zingiber officinale* (ginger) in the treatment of acne vulgaris. Focus on Alternative and Complementary Therapies, 19:191–7. http://dx.doi.org/10.1111/fct.12140.
5. Hajheydari Z, Saeedi M, Morteza-Semnani K, et al. Effect of *Aloe vera* topical gel combined with tretinoin in treatment of mild and moderate acne vulgaris: a randomized, double-blind, prospective trial. J Dermatolog Treat 2014; 25(2):123–9.
6. MOH. Clinical practice guidelines: Management of acne. Malaysia Ministry of Health, Dermatological Society of Malaysia, Academy of Medicine Malaysia; 2012. p. 1–82. Available at: http://www.acadmed.org.my/index.cfm?&menuid=67.
7. Sanclemente G, Acosta JL, Tamayo ME, et al. Clinical practice guidelines for treatment of acne vulgaris: a critical appraisal using the AGREE II instrument. Arch Dermatol Res 2014;306(3):269–77.
8. Nast A, Bayerl C, Borelli C, et al. S2k-guideline for therapy of acne. J Dtsch Dermatol Ges 2010;(8 Suppl 2):s1–59.
9. Fisk WA, Lev-Tov HA, Sivamani RK. Botanical and phytochemical therapy of acne: a systematic review. Phytother Res 2014;28(8):1137–52.

Index

Note: Page numbers of article titles are in **boldface** type.

Dermatol Clin 34 (2016) 549–554
http://dx.doi.org/10.1016/S0733-8635(16)30094-8
0733-8635/16/$ – see front matter

UNITED STATES POSTAL SERVICE ®
Statement of Ownership, Management, and Circulation
(All Periodicals Publications Except Requester Publications)

1. Publication Title	2. Publication Number		3. Filing Date
DERMATOLOGIC CLINICS	000 – 705		3/18/2016

4. Issue Frequency	5. Number of Issues Published Annually	6. Annual Subscription Price
JAN, APR, JUL, OCT	4	$346.00

7. Complete Mailing Address of Known Office of Publication (Not printer) (Street, city, county, state, and ZIP+4®)

ELSEVIER INC.
360 PARK AVENUE SOUTH
NEW YORK, NY 10010-1710

Contact Person
STEPHEN R. BUSHING

Telephone (Include area code)
215-239-3688

8. Complete Mailing Address of Headquarters or General Business Office of Publisher (Not printer)

ELSEVIER INC.
360 PARK AVENUE SOUTH
NEW YORK, NY 10010-1710

9. Full Names and Complete Mailing Addresses of Publisher, Editor, and Managing Editor (Do not leave blank)

Publisher (Name and complete mailing address)

ADRIANNE BRIGIDO, ELSEVIER INC.
1600 JOHN F KENNEDY BLVD. SUITE 1800
PHILADELPHIA, PA 19103-2899

Editor (Name and complete mailing address)

JESSICA MCCOOL, ELSEVIER INC.
1600 JOHN F KENNEDY BLVD. SUITE 1800
PHILADELPHIA, PA 19103-2899

Managing Editor (Name and complete mailing address)

PATRICK MANLEY, ELSEVIER INC.
1600 JOHN F KENNEDY BLVD. SUITE 1800
PHILADELPHIA, PA 19103-2899

10. Owner (Do not leave blank. If the publication is owned by a corporation, give the name and address of the corporation immediately followed by the names and addresses of all stockholders owning or holding 1 percent or more of the total amount of stock. If not owned by a corporation, give the names and addresses of the individual owners. If owned by a partnership or other unincorporated firm, give its name and address as well as those of each individual owner. If the publication is published by a nonprofit organization, give its name and address.)

Full Name	Complete Mailing Address
WHOLLY OWNED SUBSIDIARY OF REED/ELSEVIER US HOLDINGS	1600 JOHN F KENNEDY BLVD. SUITE 1800 PHILADELPHIA, PA 19103-2899

11. Known Bondholders, Mortgagees, and Other Security Holders Owning or Holding 1 Percent or More of Total Amount of Bonds, Mortgages, or Other Securities. If none, check box. ▶ ☐ None

Full Name	Complete Mailing Address
N/A	

12. Tax Status (For completion by nonprofit organizations authorized to mail at nonprofit rates) (Check one)
The purpose, function, and nonprofit status of this organization and the exempt status for federal income tax purposes:
☐ Has Not Changed During Preceding 12 Months
☐ Has Changed During Preceding 12 Months (Publisher must submit explanation of change with this statement)

13. Publication Title

DERMATOLOGIC CLINICS

14. Issue Date for Circulation Data Below

JULY 2016

15. Extent and Nature of Circulation		Average No. Copies Each Issue During Preceding 12 Months	No. Copies of Single Issue Published Nearest to Filing Date
a. Total Number of Copies (Net press run)		395	593
b. Paid Circulation (By Mail and Outside the Mail)	(1) Mailed Outside-County Paid Subscriptions Stated on PS Form 3541 (Include paid distribution above nominal rate, advertiser's proof copies, and exchange copies)	84	105
	(2) Mailed In-County Paid Subscriptions Stated on PS Form 3541 (Include paid distribution above nominal rate, advertiser's proof copies, and exchange copies)	0	0
	(3) Paid Distribution Outside the Mails Including Sales Through Dealers and Carriers, Street Vendors, Counter Sales, and Other Paid Distribution Outside USPS®	61	93
	(4) Paid Distribution by Other Classes of Mail Through the USPS (e.g. First-Class Mail®)	0	0
c. Total Paid Distribution (Sum of 15b (1), (2), (3), and (4))	▶	145	198
d. Free or Nominal Rate Distribution (By Mail and Outside the Mail)	(1) Free or Nominal Rate Outside-County Copies included on PS Form 3541	54	70
	(2) Free or Nominal Rate In-County Copies Included on PS Form 3541	0	0
	(3) Free or Nominal Rate Copies Mailed at Other Classes Through the USPS (e.g. First-Class Mail)	0	0
	(4) Free or Nominal Rate Distribution Outside the Mail (Carriers or other means)	0	0
e. Total Free or Nominal Rate Distribution (Sum of 15d (1), (2), (3) and (4))	▶	54	70
f. Total Distribution (Sum of 15c and 15e)	▶	199	268
g. Copies not Distributed (See Instructions to Publishers #4 (page #3))	▶	196	325
h. Total (Sum of 15f and g)	▶	395	593
i. Percent Paid (15c divided by 15f times 100)		73%	74%

* If you are claiming electronic copies, go to line 16 on page 3. If you are not claiming electronic copies, skip to line 17 on page 3.

16. Electronic Copy Circulation		Average No. Copies Each Issue During Preceding 12 Months	No. Copies of Single Issue Published Nearest to Filing Date
a. Paid Electronic Copies	▶	0	0
b. Total Paid Print Copies (Line 15c) + Paid Electronic Copies (Line 16a)	▶	145	198
c. Total Print Distribution (Line 15f) + Paid Electronic Copies (Line 16a)	▶	199	268
d. Percent Paid (Both Print & Electronic Copies) (16b divided by 16c × 100)	▶	73%	74%

☒ I certify that 50% of all my distributed copies (electronic and print) are paid above a nominal price.

17. Publication of Statement of Ownership

☒ If the publication is a general publication, publication of this statement is required. Will be printed in the OCTOBER 2016 issue of this publication.

☐ Publication not required.

18. Signature and Title of Editor, Publisher, Business Manager, or Owner

[signature]

STEPHEN R. BUSHING - INVENTORY DISTRIBUTION CONTROL MANAGER

Date 3/18/2016

I certify that all information furnished on this form is true and complete. I understand that anyone who furnishes false or misleading information on this form or who omits material or information requested on the form may be subject to criminal sanctions (including fines and imprisonment) and/or civil sanctions (including civil penalties).

PS Form 3526, July 2014 (Page 3 of 4) PSN: 7530-01-000-9931   PRIVACY NOTICE: See our privacy policy on www.usps.com.

Moving?

Make sure your subscription moves with you!

To notify us of your new address, find your **Clinics Account Number** (located on your mailing label above your name), and contact customer service at:

Email: journalscustomerservice-usa@elsevier.com

800-654-2452 (subscribers in the U.S. & Canada)
314-447-8871 (subscribers outside of the U.S. & Canada)

Fax number: 314-447-8029

Elsevier Health Sciences Division
Subscription Customer Service
3251 Riverport Lane
Maryland Heights, MO 63043

*To ensure uninterrupted delivery of your subscription, please notify us at least 4 weeks in advance of move.

Printed and bound by CPI Group (UK) Ltd, Croydon, CR0 4YY

03/10/2024

01040306-0002